Infant Vision

The European Brain and Behaviour Society Publications Series

Series editor
TERJE SAGVOLDEN

Institute of Basic Medical Sciences, Department of Neurophysiology, University of Oslo, Norway

Infant Vision

Edited by

FRANÇOIS VITAL-DURAND

INSERM U. 371,
Cerveau et Vision,
Bron, France

JANETTE ATKINSON

Visual Development Unit, Department of Psychology,
University College London

and

OLIVER J. BRADDICK

Department of Psychology,
University College London

Oxford   New York   Tokyo

OXFORD UNIVERSITY PRESS

1996

Oxford University Press, Walton Street, Oxford OX2 6DP

Oxford New York
Athens Auckland Bangkok Bombay
Calcutta Cape Town Dar es Salaam Delhi
Florence Hong Kong Istanbul Karachi
Kuala Lumpur Madras Madrid Melbourne
Mexico City Nairobi Paris Singapore
Taipei Tokyo Toronto
and associated companies in
Berlin Ibadan

Oxford is a trade mark of Oxford University Press

Published in the United States
by Oxford University Press Inc., New York

A catalogue record for this book is available from the British Library

Library of Congress Cataloging in Publication Data
Infant vision / edited by François Vital-Durand, Janette Atkinson, and
Oliver J. Braddick.
(European brain and behaviour society ; 2)
Includes bibliographical references and index.
1. *Vision in infants.*   2. *Vision disorders in infants.*   I. *Vital-Durand, François.*
II. *Atkinson, Janette.*   III. *Braddick, O. J. (Oliver John), 1944-*
IV. *European Brain and Behaviour Society.*
V. *Series: Ebbs publications series ; 2.*
[*DNLM: 1. Vision Disorders–in infancy & childhood.*   2. *Vision–physiology.*
3. *Vision Perception–in infancy & childhood.*
4. *Vision Disorders–in infancy & childhood.*   W1 EB888 v.2 1996 /
WW 103 I43 1996]
RE48.2.C5I53   1996   612.8'4'0832–dc20   95-30844
ISBN 0 19 852316 5 (Hbk)

Typeset by Advance Typesetting Ltd, Oxford
Printed in Great Britain by
Biddles Ltd
Guildford & King's Lynn

Preface

Twenty years ago, 'infant vision' barely existed as a scientific field. Some fragments of the field could be found in developmental psychology, paediatrics, and clinical ophthalmology, but they were isolated from each other and had a very limited base of experimental findings. This book demonstrates the range and vigour of the science that has developed from those fragments.

This rapid development came about for several reasons. Several scientists in North America and Europe, with expertise in vision or in behavioural and cognitive development, realized that there was a potential to fuse the methods of these two domains; the precisely controlled stimuli that had been designed to probe visual function psychophysically and electrophysiologically in adults and in animals could be combined with behavioural measures of discrimination that were well adapted to human infants. A second, very powerful, influence was the excitement coming from discoveries in the electrophysiology and anatomy laboratories, especially that of Wiesel and Hubel (1963). Their experiments and those of others showed that the immature visual function could be analysed at a detailed level, and gave a very direct view of how the developing visual system could be modified by the pattern of stimulation. To many of us, these results cried out for a comparative approach with normal and abnormal human development, and this approach needed exactly the same information that could be provided by uniting up-to-date visual science with the analysis of infant behaviour. We regard it as particularly important that this book includes examples of such comparative approaches. These include both comparisons between parallel behavioural measures from human and other species, and comparisons of functional measures of vision with sophisticated explorations of the development of neural structure.

Researchers soon recognized the potential relevance of their work to clinical problems in the assessment, diagnosis, and therapy of childhood vision disorders, and some clinicians became aware at an early stage that they could contribute to, and their practice could gain from, this growing enterprise. However, the contributions from psychology, physiology, anatomy, ophthalmology, and optometry have led to a literature that has been scattered across different journals. It has taken a while for the people involved to form a community, an evolution nicely chronicled by Teller and Movshon (1986). The widespread community of infant vision devotees—a mosaic of scientists and clinicians—now recognizes its common interests and is organized enough to come together regularly in large and small meetings in North America and Europe, and hopefully soon elsewhere. However, it is valuable for the health of this enterprise that the community recognizes itself as part of several wider communities in neuroscience, psychology, and the clinical sciences, and the occasions when it meets often reflect this. This book grew out of a meeting in Lyon in July 1993 which was organized jointly by the Child Vision Research Society—an association whose existence speaks to the fact of a coherent infant vision community—and the European Brain and Behaviour Society, representing a wider unity of neuroscience with the function of the whole organism.

Despite the development of this community, there has not been, until very recently, any single book where students and specialists could find the most prominent contributions brought together in a single convenient source. The recent publication of a magnificent volume edited by Kurt Simons (1993) has changed this. However, in a field as active and diverse as infant vision, no one single book can be comprehensive and we believe that the present book has its own distinctive range and balance that valuably complements that of Simons.

The 27 original contributions come from many of the leading teams world-wide working in the realm of infant vision, most of whom participated in the Lyon meeting. Each chapter gives an overview of its topic as well as presenting, in some cases for the first time, the latest findings from the author's work. The range is from receptor function at the cellular level to the cognitive and social abilities that depend on visual development. It also presents side by side the findings of pure scientific enquiry into development, the analysis of abnormal function, and the application of this research in diagnosis, therapy, and rehabilitation.

At the start of the 20-year period in which the study of infant vision has matured, the general view of the newborn was already beginning to change. For most people, the newborn infant was a being whose sensory, motor, and neural immaturity implied total dependence and incompetence in all domains. However, some developmental psychologists were arguing the case for the 'competent infant' (Stone *et al.* 1973) who possessed an intrinsic organization that was well adapted to the needs of that stage of life, in particular the need to take in and structure a prodigious amount of information about the physical and social world. The growth of knowledge about infant vision, reflected in this book, has contributed to a much richer and more detailed understanding of infant competence. The result is a dramatic change in attitudes towards the beginning of life. We now know a great deal about what sensory information, and what sensory–motor capabilities, are available to the infant at different ages. In some respects this reinforces the picture of the competent infant, who within the first few months can analyse contrast, pattern, colour, motion, and depth; in other respects it reveals specific, subtle, and unsuspected limitations that can be very revealing about the immaturity of some underlying mechanisms. We do not need to take up simplistic positions of treating the infant as a blank slate, or as having fully adapted competences. We are beginning to understand the biological constraints that determine how, and to what degree, the infant's competence is less than that of the mature individual.

In the face of this new-found depth of knowledge, a better understanding of the nature of development comes within our grasp. Any simply polarized debate on nature *versus* nurture is now of historical interest only. We are appreciating how to consider the combinations of internal and external requisites for development of a function, rather than to assign particular functions to the command of the genes or the formative power of the environment. The quest is rather for how early we can track the course of development, what we can do to correct deviations from the best course, and what damaging interactions we can avoid between the developing functions and external pressures. The benefit is that infant vision is not only a field of research for scholars, but is also applicable to the needs of clinical practice and health care managers.

We hope that this book contributes to the idea that a better knowledge of developmental mechanisms will make those who care for the world's infants, more able to help those children to achieve the best of their potential.

F. V.-D.
J. A.
O. J. B.

REFERENCES

Simons, K. (ed.) (1993). *Early visual development: normal and abnormal*. Oxford University Press, New York.

Stone, L. J., Smith, H. T. and Murphy, L. B. (1973). *The competent infant*. Basic Books, New York.

Teller, D. Y. and Movshon, J. A. (1986). Visual development. *Vision Research*, **26**, 1483–506.

Wiesel, T. N. and Hubel, D. H. (1963). Single-cell responses in striate cortex of kittens deprived of vision in one eye. *Journal of Neurophysiology*, **26**, 1003–17.

Contents

Contributors

M. Abrahamsson Department of Ophthalmology, University of Goteborg, Sweden

M. R. Angi Department of Ophthalmology, University of Padua, Italy

Patricia Apkarian Department of Physiology I, Medical Faculty, Erasmus University, Rotterdam, The Netherlands

Janette Atkinson Visual Development Unit, Department of Psychology, University College, London, UK

Louis Ayzac Unité d'Hygiène, Epidémiologie et Information Médicale, (Pr J. Fabry), CHLS Pierre-Bénite, France

Joseph Bauer Department of Brain and Cognitive Sciences, Massachusetts Institute of Technology, Cambridge, Massachusetts, USA

Michelle Bieber Department of Psychology, University of Colorado, Boulder, Colorado, USA

H. Bloch Laboratoire de Psychobiologie du Développement, EPHE-CNRS, Paris, France

Ronald G. Boothe Departments of Psychology and Ophthalmology, and Yerkes Regional Primate Research Center, Emory University, Atlanta, Georgia, USA

Oliver Braddick Visual Development Unit, Department of Psychology, University College London, UK

David C. Burr Istituto di Neurofisiologia del CNR, Pisa, and Dipartimento di Psicologia, Università di Roma 'la Sapienza', Rome, Italy

Cathy Buquet U279 INSERM, Lille, France

E. Byhr Department of Ophthalmology, University of Goteborg, Sweden

R. Canapicchi Department of Neuroradiology, S. Chiara Hospital, Pisa, Italy

I. Carchon Laboratoire de Psychobiologie du Développement, EPHE-CNRS, Paris, France

Jacques R. Charlier U279 INSERM, Lille, France

G. Cioni Institute of Developmental Neurology, Psychiatry and Educational Psychology, University of Pisa and Stella Maris Foundation, Pisa, Italy

Helen Davis Department of Ophthalmology and Orthoptics, University of Sheffield, S10 2JF, UK

C. Deruelle Developmental Neurocognition Group, Laboratory of Cognitive Neurosciences (LNC), and Group of Research in Neuropsychology (GDR), CNRS, Marseille, France

S. de Schonen Developmental Neurocognition Group, Laboratory of Cognitive Neurosciences (LNC), and Group of Research in Neuropsychology (GDR), CNRS, Marseille, France

Elizabeth Dorn Departments of Ophthalmology and Biological Structure, University of Washington, Seattle, Washington, USA

E. Fazzi Institute of Developmental Neurology, Psychiatry and Educational Psychology, University of Pisa and Stella Maris Foundation, Pisa, Italy

Alistair R. Fielder Department of Ophthalmology, University of Birmingham, UK

Adriana Fiorentini Istituto di Neurofisiologia del CNR, Pisa, Italy

Anne Fulton Department of Ophthalmology, Children's Hospital and Harvard Medical School, Boston, Massachusetts, USA

Jane Gwiazda Department of Brain and Cognitive Sciences, Massachusetts Institute of Technology, Cambridge, Massachusetts, USA

Louise Hainline Infant Study Center, Brooklyn College, Brooklyn, New York, USA

Ronald Hansen Department of Ophthalmology, Children's Hospital and Harvard Medical School, Boston, Massachusetts, USA

Richard Held Department of Brain and Cognitive Sciences, Massachusetts Institute of Technology, Cambridge, Massachusetts, USA

Anita Hendrickson Departments of Ophthalmology and Biological Structure, University of Washington, Seattle, Washington, USA

Bruce Hood Visual Development Unit, Department of Psychology, University College, London, UK

A. E. Ipata Institute of Developmental Neurology, Psychiatry and Educational Psychology, University of Pisa and Stella Maris Foundation, Pisa, Italy

Kenneth Knoblauch Vision Research Laboratory, The Lighthouse Research Institute, New York, USA

Lynne Kiorpes Center for Neural Science and Department of Psychology, New York University, USA

Sarah Lewin Department of Orthoptics, University of Liverpool, L7 8XP, UK

J. Mancini Service de Neuropédiatrie, and Groupement de Recherche en Neuropsychologie, CHU La Timone, Marseille, France

M. Concetta Morrone Istituto di Neurofisiologia del CNR, Pisa and Scuola Normale Superiore, Pisa, Italy

Merrick J. Moseley Department of Ophthalmology, University of Birmingham, UK

O. Pascalis Developmental Neurocognition Group, Laboratory of Cognitive Neurosciences (LNC), and Group of Research in Neuropsychology (GDR), CNRS, Marseille, France

E. Pilotto Department of Ophthalmology, University of Padua, Italy

Gabriel Pinzaru Unité d'Hygiène, Epidémiologie et Information Médicale, (Pr J. Fabry), CHLS Pierre-Bénite, France

J. W. R. Pott Department of Physiology I, Erasmus University, Rotterdam, The Netherlands

Patricia M. Riddell Department of Psychology, University of Reading, UK

Paulette P. Schmidt Exceptional Child and Infant Vision Testing Laboratory, College of Optometry, The Ohio State University, Columbus, Ohio, USA

Ruxandra Sireteanu Max-Planck-Institute for Brain Research, Frankfurt, Germany

J. Sjöstrand Department of Ophthalmology, University of Goteborg, Sweden

A. Sjöström Department of Ophthalmology, University of Goteborg, Sweden

Alan Slater Department of Psychology, Washington Singer Laboratories, Exeter, UK

Frank Thorn New England College of Optometry and Department of Brain and Cognitive Sciences, Massachusetts Institute of Technology, Cambridge, Massachusetts, USA

J. van Hof-van Duin Department of Physiology I, Erasmus University, Rotterdam, The Netherlands

François Vital-Durand Cerveau et Vision, INSERM Unité 371, Bron et Service d'Ophtalmologie (Dr A. Hullo) CHLS, Pierre-Bénite, France

John R. B. Wattam-Bell Visual Development Unit, University College London, UK

John S. Werner Department of Psychology, University of Colorado, Boulder, Colorado, USA

Ivan C. J. Wood Department of Optometry and Vision Science, University of Manchester Institute of Science and Technology, Manchester M60 1QD, UK

Part I
Basic coding of spatial and chromatic vision

This first section brings together contributions devoted to the initial coding and processing of spatial, temporal, and chromatic signals. It was in these areas that the modern study of infant vision was initiated; the chapters demonstrate the depth and detail in which it is now possible to analyse human visual development. These are also the areas in which our understanding of the underlying neural mechanisms is most advanced. This understanding has necessarily depended heavily on a comparative approach, linking human work to anatomical, physiological, and behavioural studies with animals. Consequently, the first three contributions in this section include a genuinely comparative perspective, in which the development of visual mechanisms in monkeys, rats, and cats is used to throw light on the processes of visual development in human infants.

This section does not include directly the physiological and anatomical study of how the visual pathways become organized and how visual properties are represented in patterns of neural activity. This has been another key contribution of comparative work; however, we had to set some limit to the scope and size of this book. Single-unit electrophysiology, beginning with the classic work of Hubel and Wiesel, has had a period of truly ground-breaking achievements whose mark will be found in almost every chapter of this section and throughout the book. However, the pace of the advance does not now appear so fast as it was a few years ago. Visual neuroscientists are now exploring a diverse range of techniques: in physiology, measuring oscillation, synchronization, and cross-correlation; in neuroanatomy, exploiting the possibilities of a wealth of new tracing and labelling techniques. In the future these new approaches will, no doubt, have an increasing impact on our understanding of the functional development of human vision.

The first approaches to basic visual capacities in infancy were intended to chart the course of normal development; however, the motivation to understand abnormal development was never far away both in human and comparative studies. In particular, amblyopia, since it is a pathology that arises as a result of developmental plasticity, has been of special interest to developmental visual scientists, and questions related to its cause, nature, and therapy recur in all four sections of this book. In this part, Kiorpes describes, in Chapter 1, work with a well controlled animal model, investigating how sensitivity to spatial contrast develops in normal and amblyopic eyes. As this work shows, the loss of sensitivity in amblyopia, and its increase in normal development, are not necessarily uniform across the field of view. Chapter 2, by Sireteanu, shows what can be learned from the limits of the visual field, in particular the asymmetries between the temporal and nasal field, which appear both in development and in pathology.

It is clear that normal visual development is not limited by any single level of the visual pathways but that constraints at every level may play a part, depending on the age and the specific function that is being considered. A first requirement is that the receptors should be sufficiently mature to transduce light energy into visual signals. Fulton and her colleagues bring together, in Chapter 3, immuno-chemistry, electroretinography, and behaviour, showing that the developing structure of the rod outer segments is a significant constraint that can largely account for differences in dark-adapted sensitivity between infants and adults. Like the studies of spatial sensitivity in Chapters 1 and 2, this is a clinically significant area because receptor dystrophies are an important cause of visual disability in children and adults.

It is still controversial how far the development of colour sensitivity is also limited by photoreceptor structure, and also how far it reflects the maturation of the neural systems required to extract chromatic information from receptor output. In Chapter 4, Knoblauch, Bieber, and Werner and Burr, Morrone, and Fiorentini in Chapter 5, illustrate and explain the sophisticated methods that are now being applied to isolate in infants the responses of the chromatic system and the contributions to discrimination of individual cone classes.

Colour sensitivity is a scattered ability among species and its evolution in primates is quite a recent phylogenetic process. In contrast, sensitivity to motion is one of the most ancient and universal properties of vision among both invertebrates and vertebrates. None the less, perhaps because it has come to depend on central brain mechanisms in higher mammals, it is not a particularly early function to develop in infants, as shown by the evidence Wattam-Bell presents in Chapter 6. It is, of course, closely associated with the refinement of ocular movements—an issue to which we shall return in Part III. While specific pathologies of visual motion processing are rare, motion is still of importance to those involved with clinical issues. As will appear in the final section of this book, motion can aid rehabilitation as a function that may be spared in children when other aspects of vision are seriously impaired.

The findings of this first part, therefore, as well as having intrinsic importance for the developmental neurobiology of vision, provide a basis for the understanding of higher function, of assessment and therapy in ways that will be reflected in the remaining parts of this book.

1
Development of contrast sensitivity in normal and amblyopic monkeys

Lynne Kiorpes

INTRODUCTION

The aim of this chapter is to discuss the development of spatial vision in primates and explore the possible underlying neural limitations on visual performance in infants. The basic measure of spatial vision for the purposes of this chapter is the spatial contrast sensitivity function. The development of contrast sensitivity is described, both in the central and peripheral visual field, in non-human primates, and parallels are drawn between development in animals and in humans. To explore the neural basis for behaviourally assessed development, parallels between anatomical and physiological development of the retina and lateral geniculate nucleus (LGN) are discussed, together with measured performance in infant monkeys. Finally, the effects of abnormal visual experience on the development of contrast sensitivity and on development of the visual nervous system are described.

Several conclusions are drawn from the data presented. First, the basic form of contrast sensitivity development is quite consistent across individuals and primate species. Second, development follows an essentially normal sequence in animals whose visual experience is abnormal, such as results from strabismus and anisometropia; the primary effect of the abnormal visual experience is to slow development. Finally, behavioural development seems to reflect anatomical and physiological changes in the retina and LGN under normal conditions. However, in amblyopes, performance seems to reflect compromised development at the level of the striate cortex.

NORMAL DEVELOPMENT OF CONTRAST SENSITIVITY

The spatial contrast sensitivity function describes the performance of the visual system in terms of the range of resolvable spatial frequencies and the minimum detectable contrast for patterns within that range. The contrast sensitivity function therefore provides information about the spatial scale and overall sensitivity of the visual system under study. There has been much interest in describing the development of contrast sensitivity. It is well known that spatial resolution in newborn primates is a factor of 30–50 times poorer than in adults

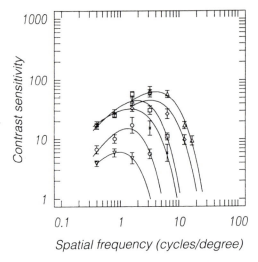

Fig. 1.1 The development of contrast sensitivity in an infant monkey. Different functions show contrast sensitivity at different ages: ∇ = 10 weeks, $\bigcirc$ = 11 weeks, × = 14 weeks, $\square$ = 15 weeks, $\lozenge$ = 26 weeks, $\triangle$ = 38 weeks (data from Boothe *et al.* 1988).

and approaches adult levels with a characteristic time course (Boothe *et al.* 1985). Sensitivity to contrast is also immature in newborns, approximately a factor of 10 poorer than in adults. Changes in the form of the contrast sensitivity function during development provide a window into the anatomical and physiological processes that limit performance in infants.

A series of contrast sensitivity functions measured in an individual infant monkey at several ages during development (Boothe *et al.* 1988) is shown in Fig. 1.1. The youngest data set was collected at the age of 10 weeks (inverted triangles, lower left function); the oldest data set was collected at 38 weeks (triangles, upper right function). Between the youngest and oldest test ages, the function shifted systematically to both higher spatial frequencies and higher contrast sensitivity. These changes can be characterized as changes in *spatial scale* and *sensitivity*. Spatial scale is the horizontal position of the curve that captures the spatial frequency range of the system; sensitivity is the vertical position of the curve which captures the range of contrasts to which the system is sensitive. As the function shifts with age toward higher spatial frequency and sensitivity it is shifting from coarse to fine spatial scale and from low to high sensitivity to contrast.

Some models of contrast sensitivity development suggest that different spatial frequency components develop at different rates (Wilson 1988). If this were the case, the function would change shape over the course of development. An analysis by Movshon and Kiorpes (1988) confirmed the observation, apparent from inspection of the functions in Fig. 1.1, that the contrast sensitivity function does not change shape during development. Therefore, it is not

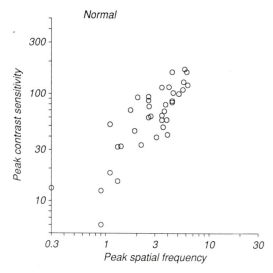

Fig. 1.2 The relationship between peak spatial frequency and peak contrast sensitivity for 13 infant monkeys ranging in age from 5–57 weeks. Data derived from the analysis presented in Movshon and Kiorpes (1988).

likely to be the case that the underlying frequency components of the function develop independently. Given that the function does not change shape but instead shifts rigidly horizontally and vertically, the developmental relationship between shifts in spatial scale and sensitivity can be determined. This relationship is illustrated in Fig. 1.2, where peak contrast sensitivity is plotted as a function of peak spatial frequency; the data are derived from contrast sensitivity functions of monkeys ranging in age from 5–57 weeks (Movshon and Kiorpes 1988). Fig. 1.2 shows that the changes in spatial scale and sensitivity occur simultaneously.

The pattern of development found for the monkeys, a concurrent shift to finer spatial scale and higher contrast sensitivity, is also apparent in contrast sensitivity data from human infants, when measured using behavioural techniques (Banks and Dannemiller 1987). It is worth noting, though, that contrast sensitivity development charted using electrophysiological techniques (sweep VEP measurement) shows an early predominant increase in sensitivity followed by a later increase in spatial scale (Norcia *et al.* 1990).

The primary difference between spatial vision development in monkeys and humans is that macaque monkeys develop about four times faster than humans (Teller and Boothe 1979). Direct comparison of the time courses for the development of spatial resolution in monkeys and humans reveals that the functions roughly compare if human age is plotted in months and monkey age is plotted in weeks. In both cases, newborn resolution is near 1 cycle/degree and adult resolution is between 30 and 50 cycles/degree. The many similarities in visual function between monkeys and humans support the study of the macaque monkey as a model system for humans. More direct questions can

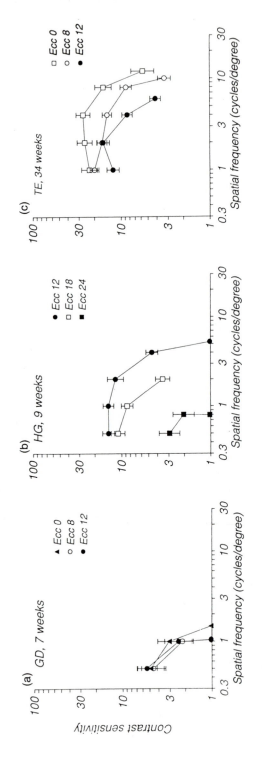

Fig. 1.3 Contrast sensitivity in the peripheral visual field is shown for three monkeys at 3 ages: (a) contrast sensitivity at 0, 8, and 12° eccentric for a 7-week-old; (b) contrast sensitivity at 12, 18, and 24° eccentric for a 9-week-old; (c) contrast sensitivity at 0, 8, and 12° eccentric for a 34-week-old.

then be asked, in the monkey, about the limitations placed on visual performance by the developing visual system.

To understand the limitations on vision in infants it is important to establish what locus (or loci) in the visual system is setting important limits on the measured performance. In adults the fovea is the area of highest sensitivity. Thus contrast sensitivity measurements typically reflect the capability of the central visual field. It is natural to assume that contrast sensitivity data collected from infants also reflect the function of the central visual field. However, recent data from humans and macaque monkeys show that the infant primate fovea is under-developed (Abramov *et al.* 1982; Yuodelis and Hendrickson 1986; Hendrickson and Kupfer 1976; Packer *et al.* 1990). The density of cones in the central retina is low in newborns and increases dramatically during the early post-natal months. Yuodelis and Hendrickson (1986) also reported morphological immaturities in the foveal cones that are likely to reduce the efficiency of light capture (Banks and Bennett 1988; Brown *et al.* 1987). It was suspected, based on these data, that the contrast sensitivity of the central visual field in young monkeys might not be superior to that of the near periphery.

The development of contrast sensitivity across the visual field was then investigated in monkeys to confirm the suspicion that, initially, central field sensitivity is similar to that of the near periphery (Kiorpes and Kiper 1995). In Fig. 1.3(a) contrast sensitivity data from a young infant monkey are shown. The sensitivity under free-viewing conditions (eccentricity of 0) was similar to that measured at locations in the peripheral visual field (eccentricities of 8 and 12°). At more peripheral locations, there was a progressive decrease in contrast sensitivity with increasing eccentricity. This result is illustrated in Fig. 1.3(b) where data from a second slightly older infant monkey are shown. Over the next 4–6 post-natal months, there was differential development of contrast sensitivity as a function of location in the visual field. In Fig. 1.3(c) contrast sensitivity data from an 8-month-old monkey are shown for eccentricities between 0 and 12°. There was a shift to lower sensitivity and reduced spatial scale with increasing eccentricity for this older animal; this pattern is consistent with that found in fully mature animals and adult humans tested under the same conditions.

It is clear that the post-natal development of contrast sensitivity reflects predominantly the development of the central visual field. An analysis of the pattern of development across the visual field showed that the central field undergoes substantially greater improvement in spatial scale and sensitivity than is seen at more peripheral locations. However, the same developmental pattern shown in Fig. 1.1 was also apparent at peripheral locations. At each location within at least the central 12°, there was a concurrent improvement in both spatial scale and sensitivity with increasing age. At 24° eccentricity there was little change in either spatial scale or sensitivity over the age ranges tested. The improvements in foveal sensitivity and spatial scale were greater and continued over a longer period of time than at more peripheral locations; moreover, the extent of post-natal development declined with increasing eccentricity.

The pattern found for contrast sensitivity development across the visual field is consistent with that expected based on concurrent changes in cone density already mentioned. In accord with the anatomical immaturity of the fovea in newborns, contrast sensitivity is similar for the central visual field and near periphery. Superiority of foveal contrast sensitivity becomes significant between about 12 and 24 weeks, which is the time during which foveal cone density increases dramatically in monkeys (Packer *et al.* 1990). Given that visual performance in the monkey develops about four times faster than in the human, one might expect to find superiority of foveal contrast sensitivity in the second post-natal year in humans.

The apparent concordance between retinal development and the pattern of behavioural changes in contrast sensitivity suggests that the retina may be providing a crucial limit on visual function in infants. Banks and Bennett (1988) modelled quantitatively the extent to which the immaturities in photoreceptor density and cone morphology could account for measured post-natal changes in contrast sensitivity in human infants. They concluded that, while these factors may contribute to the relatively poor acuity and contrast sensitivity of the infant, a significant proportion of the developmental changes cannot be accounted for at the level of the photoreceptors. A similar conclusion was reached by Brown (1990). Therefore, it is likely that neural factors central to the photoreceptors impose a second important limitation on visual behaviour.

The earliest post-receptoral level at which the development of neural processing has been studied is the lateral geniculate nucleus. Blakemore and Vital-Durand (1986a) studied the development of spatial resolving power and overall responsiveness in macaque monkey LGN neurones. They reported three features of LGN development that are of interest for the analysis of behavioural development. First, there is an overall increase in responsiveness and spatial resolution during the first post-natal year that is reminiscent of the improvement in contrast sensitivity and spatial scale seen behaviourally. Second, the progressive improvement in spatial resolving power is similar in time course and extent to that measured behaviourally in macaques (Jacobs and Blakemore 1988; Kiorpes 1992a; Movshon and Kiorpes 1993). The time course for development of grating acuity measured behaviourally is shown in Fig. 1.4 (open circles; from Kiorpes 1992a) along with spatial resolution for the LGN cell with the highest resolution at each age (filled triangles; from Blakemore and Vital-Durand 1986a). The performance of the best LGN cells is slightly better than the monkey behaviour at each age and parallels the behavioural data well. It is important to note that, particularly at the youngest ages, neither behaviour nor geniculate physiological measures achieve the resolution permitted by the photoreceptor mosaic (Movshon and Kiorpes 1993).

Finally, Blakemore and Vital-Durand (1986a) reported differential development of resolution depending on receptive field position. Neurones with receptive field positions within the central 10° showed a considerably greater post-natal increase in spatial resolution than those at more peripheral locations. This result is consistent with behavioural data described above on the

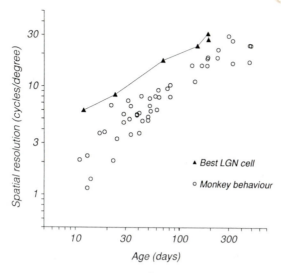

Fig. 1.4 The development of spatial resolution in monkeys as measured behaviourally is compared with the development of spatial resolving power of neurones in the LGN. The behavioural data (circles) are from Kiorpes (1992*a*). The physiological data (triangles) represent the highest resolution shown by an LGN neurone at each age; the data are from Blakemore and Vital-Durand (1986*a*).

development of contrast sensitivity across the visual field. Taken together, the remarkable consistency between the development of spatial contrast sensitivity and the development of receptive field properties of LGN neurones suggests that neural processing between the photoreceptors and the LGN may provide a crucial limit for visual development.

Additional data on the development of LGN cell contrast sensitivity lend further weight to the suggestion that a critical limitation on the development of visual performance is set at or before this level of the system. Blakemore and Hawken (1985; and unpublished observations) measured contrast sensitivity over a range of spatial frequencies for individual LGN neurones. Composite contrast sensitivity 'functions' for newborn, 2-month-old, and 8-month-old macaque LGN show the same bandpass character that behavioural functions show. Importantly, the shift in the composite contrast sensitivity functions with age is consistent with the pattern measured behaviourally. That is, the composite neural functions show a simultaneous shift to both higher contrast sensitivity and spatial frequency as do the behavioural functions for individual monkeys (see Figure 1.1).

The preceding discussion documented the post-natal changes in macaque monkey spatial vision that are consistent with what is known about spatial vision development in humans. These changes seem to unfold according to a prescribed maturational plan, since there is considerable consistency across individual monkeys, across locations in the visual field, and across primate species. Comparisons of quantitative behavioural and physiological data from the macaque reveal remarkable similarities in the pattern of development reflected at the level of the LGN and that measured behaviourally, suggesting that maturation of neural processing at or before the LGN may be underlying behavioural contrast sensitivity in infants. While under normal conditions the development of spatial vision appears to proceed according to a prescribed maturational plan, it is clear that this plan can be disrupted.

DEVELOPMENT OF CONTRAST SENSITIVITY IN AMBLYOPIA

Numerous visual disorders in infancy and early childhood are associated with a condition called amblyopia. Amblyopia is generally defined as a deficit in visual function that cannot be corrected optically and appears in the absence of obvious ocular pathology. Conditions such as cataracts, strabismus (misalignment of the visual axes), and anisometropia (unequal refractive errors for the two eyes) are associated with the development of amblyopia when they occur during the early childhood years; the same conditions are not associated with amblyopia when they occur in adults. Thus abnormal visual imput during an early *sensitive period*, when the visual system is susceptible to influence by the visual environment, leads to relatively permanent deficits in visual performance (Harwerth *et al.* 1986; Movshon and Kiorpes 1990; Kiorpes 1992*b*).

While amblyopia is typically measured as a deficit in acuity, the character of the amblyopic deficit can be specified by examination of the contrast sensitivity function. Human amblyopes typically show deficits in contrast sensitivity throughout the middle-to-high spatial frequency range (Hess *et al.* 1980). Monkeys raised with visual conditions that simulate those associated with amblyopia in humans also show deficits in contrast sensitivity (Harwerth *et al.* 1983; Smith *et al.* 1985; Kiorpes 1989; Kiorpes *et al.* 1993). Contrast sensitivity functions for each eye of four amblyopic monkeys are shown in Fig. 1.5; two monkeys were raised with esotropic strabismus (Fig. 1.5(a,b)) and two were raised with anisometropia induced by an extended-wear contact lens (Fig. 1.5(c,d)). Two of the amblyopic animals show modest deficits with the amblyopic eye (filled circles; Fig. 1.5(a,c)); while two show severe deficits (Fig. 1.5(b,d)). In all cases, the animals show the same pattern of contrast sensitivity loss in the amblyopic eye as typically shown by human amblyopes; the largest deficits are in the mid-to-high spatial frequency range.

Given that amblyopia is a disorder of visual development, it is important to understand how it arises. Our studies have followed the development of spatial resolution and contrast sensitivity, as well as other visual functions such as vernier acuity, in monkeys raised with either esotropic strabismus oranisometropia. The development of vision in these amblyopic animals appears to be slowed compared with development in normal animals (Kiorpes *et al.* 1989;

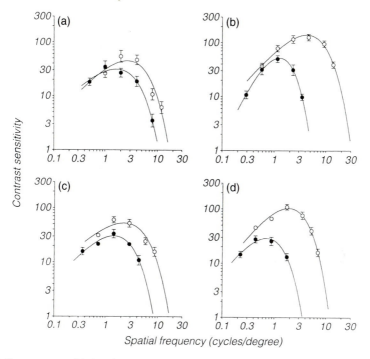

Fig. 1.5 Contrast sensitivity functions are shown for each eye of four monkeys with experimentally produced amblyopia. Filled and open symbols represent data from the amblyopic and fellow eyes, respectively. Panels (a) and (b) show data from two strabismic amblyopes; panels (c) and (d) show data from two lens-reared anisometropic amblyopes (induced with a −10 dioptre extended-wear contact lens). See Kiorpes *et al.* (1993) for details.

Kiorpes 1989; Kiorpes 1992*b*). In Fig. 1.6 the development of grating acuity for normally-raised monkeys (open circles) and amblyopic eyes of monkeys raised with esotropic strabismus (filled circles) is shown. The amblyopic eyes lag behind normal eyes during development. Kiorpes (1992*b*) found this pattern of development for vernier acuity in amblyopes as well as for grating acuity.

This slowed progress of visual development is also apparent in the contrast sensitivity data. As shown in Fig. 1.5, the contrast sensitivity functions for the amblyopic eyes are shifted to lower spatial frequencies and contrast sensitivities compared with the non-amblyopic eyes. This pattern is consistent with that of younger normal animals. Recall that the progress of contrast sensitivity development in normal animals, already described, is one of progressive shifting up toward both higher sensitivity and spatial scale so that functions from younger animals show both lower contrast sensitivity and a lower range of spatial frequencies than older animals. It is important to note that the amblyopic contrast sensitivity function does not differ in shape from non-amblyopic

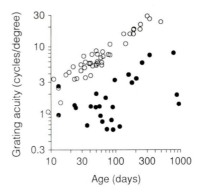

Fig. 1.6 The developmental time course for amblyopic eyes is compared with that for normal monkeys. The open circles represent development for normal eyes; the filled symbols represent development for the amblyopic eyes of strabismic amblyopes. Data from Kiorpes (1992*b*).

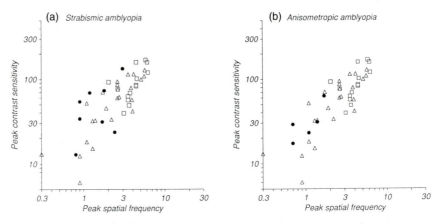

Fig. 1.7 The relationship between peak spatial frequency and peak contrast sensitivity is shown for amblyopic eyes. The filled circles in (a) and (b) show data from strabismic and anisometropic amblyopes, respectively. The open symbols reproduce subsets of the normal data in Fig. 1.2: triangles show the relationship for monkeys younger than 20 weeks; squares show the relationship for monkeys older than 26 weeks. The relationship for the amblyopic eyes is similar to that of the young normal animals.

functions (Kiorpes 1989; Kiorpes and Movshon 1989). Consistent with this result, the relationship between overall contrast sensitivity and spatial scale for amblyopic eyes is similar to that of normal contrast sensitivity development. This point is illustrated in Fig. 1.7 where the relationship between peak contrast sensitivity and peak spatial frequency is shown for strabismic amblyopic (Fig. 1.7(a)) and anisometropic amblyopic (Fig. 1.7(b)) eyes. The relationship for normal animals (see Fig. 1.2) is reproduced in Fig. 1.7 but here data from animals younger than 20 weeks are shown as open triangles and data from more mature animals are shown as open squares. It is clear that the amblyopic eyes (represented with filled circles in each panel) perform similarly to young normal animals rather than visually mature animals.

As the studies described above show, under normal visual conditions development proceeds according to a particular maturational plan. However, when visual imput is abnormal during the early sensitive period, the maturational plan is disrupted. In amblyopia, the disruption appears to be a slowing of development. Slowed development will have the effect of leaving the visual system in an immature state at the end of the sensitive period. Therefore, the performance of amblyopes is like that of young normals. It is worth noting that this process describes well the development of amblyopia as results from strabismus and anisometropia. However, given more severe forms of deprivation, for example, lid suture, the developmental process can be halted or even reversed. In such cases, the performance of the visual system can be compromised to levels poorer than would be expected in a newborn (Harwerth *et al.* 1983; Blakemore 1990; Movshon and Kiorpes 1993).

While there is good evidence for placing the critical limitations on visual development in normal individuals at or before the level of the LGN, there is no evidence to suggest that the same limitations apply in the case of amblyopes. Monkeys raised with monocular deprivation show extremely severe deficits in visual performance (Harwerth *et al.* 1983); however, spatial resolution of LGN cells in monocularly deprived monkeys is normal (Blakemore and Vital-Durand 1986*b*; Levitt *et al.* 1989). Similarly, there is no evident abnormality of retinal anatomy in amblyopic animals (Hendrickson *et al.* 1987). The effects of abnormal visual experience must therefore appear more centrally in the visual pathways than the LGN. Indeed, several studies have reported deficits in spatial resolution and/or contrast sensitivity of striate cortical neurones from amblyopic monkeys (Movshon *et al.* 1987; Eggers *et al.* 1984).

To conclude, it appears that, in normal development, limitations set early in the visual pathways are relayed faithfully through the striate cortex and subsequent processing regions. However, when visual experience is abnormal, the striate cortex appears to develop abnormally and loses information available at the LGN. Additional studies comparing behavioural, physiological, and anatomical development in monkeys will be needed to determine precisely how it is that experience exerts its effects on visual processing.

REFERENCES

Abramov, I., Gordon, J., Hendrickson, A., Dobson, V., and LaBossiere, E. (1982). The retina of the newborn human infant. *Science*, **217**, 265–7.

Banks, M. S. and Bennett, P. J. (1988). Optical and photoreceptor immaturities limit the spatial and chromatic vision of human neonates. *Journal of the Optical Society of America*, **A5**, 2059–79.

Banks, M. S. and Dannemiller, J. L. (1987). Infant visual psychophysics. In *Handbook of infant perception, Vol. 1, From sensation to perception*, (ed. P. Salapatek and L. Cohen), Academic Press, Orlando.

Blakemore, C. (1990). Maturation of mechanisms for efficient spatial vision. In *Vision: coding and efficiency*, (ed. C. Blakemore), Cambridge University Press, Cambridge.

Blakemore, C. and Hawken, M. (1985). Contrast sensitivity of neurones in the lateral geniculate nucleus of the neonatal monkey. *Journal of Physiology*, **369**, 37P.

Blakemore, C. and Vital-Durand, F. (1986a). Organization and post-natal development of the monkey's lateral geniculate nucleus. *Journal of Physiology*, **380**, 453–91.

Blakemore, C. and Vital-Durand, F. (1986b). Effects of visual deprivation on the development of the monkey's lateral geniculate nucleus. *Journal of Physiology*, **380**, 493–511.

Boothe, R. G., Dobson, M. V., and Teller, D. Y. (1985). Post-natal development of vision in human and nonhuman primates. *Annual Review of Neuroscience*, **8**, 495–545.

Boothe, R. G., Kiorpes, L., Williams, R. A., and Teller, D. Y. (1988). Operant measurements of contrast sensitivity in infant macaque monkeys during normal development. *Vision Research*, **28**, 387–96.

Brown, A. M. (1990). Development of visual sensitivity to light and color vision in human infants: a critical review. *Vision Research*, **30**, 1159–88.

Brown, A. M., Dobson, M. V., and Maier, J. (1987). Visual acuity of human infants at scotopic, mesopic and photopic luminances. *Vision Research*, **27**, 1845–58.

Eggers, H. M., Gizzi, M. S., and Movshon, J. A. (1984). Spatial properties of striate cortical neurons in esotropic macaques. *Investigative Ophthalmology and Visual Science*, **25** (suppl.), 278.

Harwerth, R. S., Smith III, E. L., Boltz, R. L., Crawford, M. L. J., and von Noorden, G. K. (1983). Behavioral studies on the effect of abnormal early visual experience in monkeys: spatial modulation sensitivity. *Vision Research*, **23**, 1501–10.

Harwerth, R. S., Smith III, E. L., Duncan, G. C., Crawford, M. L. J., and von Noorden, G. K. (1986). Multiple sensitive periods in the development of the primate visual system. *Science*, **232**, 235–8.

Hendrickson, A. and Kupfer, C. (1976). The histogenesis of the fovea in the macaque monkey. *Investigative Ophthalmology and Visual Science*, **15**, 746–56.

Hendrickson, A., Movshon, J. A., Boothe, R. G., Eggers, H. M., Gizzi, M. S., and Kiorpes, L. (1987). Effects of early unilateral blur on the macaque's visual system: II. Anatomical observations. *Journal of Neuroscience*, **7**, 1327–39.

Hess, R. F., Campbell, F. W., and Zimmern, R. (1980). Differences in the neural basis of human amblyopia: the effect of mean luminance. *Vision Research*, **80**, 295–305.

Jacobs, D. S. and Blakemore, C. (1988). Factors limiting the postnatal development of visual acuity in the monkey. *Vision Research*, **28**, 947–58.

Kiorpes, L. (1989). The development of spatial resolution and contrast sensitivity in naturally strabismic monkeys. *Clinical Vision Sciences*, **4**, 279–93.

Kiorpes, L. (1992a). The development of vernier acuity and grating acuity in normally-reared monkeys. *Visual Neuroscience*, **9**, 243–51.

Kiorpes, L. (1992b). The effect of strabismus on the development of vernier acuity and grating acuity in monkeys. *Visual Neuroscience*, **9**, 253–9.

Kiorpes, L. and Kiper, D. C. (1995). Development of contrast sensitivity across the visual field in macaque monkeys (*Macaca nemestrina*). *Vision Research*, in press.

Kiorpes, L. and Movshon, J. A. (1989). Vernier acuity and contrast sensitivity in monkeys and humans. *Optical Society of America Technical Digest Services*, **18**, 142.

Kiorpes, L., Carlson, M. R., and Alfi, D. (1989). Development of visual acuity in experimentally strabismic monkeys. *Clinical Vision Sciences*, **4**, 95–106.

Kiorpes, L., Kiper, D. C., and Movshon, J. A. (1993). Contrast sensitivity and vernier acuity in amblyopic monkeys. *Vision Research*, **33**, 2301–11.

Levitt, J. B., Movshon, J. A., Sherman, S. M., and Spear, P. D. (1989). Effects of monocular deprivation on macaque LGN. *Investigative Ophthalmology and Visual Science*, **30** (suppl.), 296.

Movshon, J. A. and Kiorpes, L. (1988). Analysis of the development of spatial contrast sensitivity in monkey and human infants. *Journal of the Optical Society of America*, **A5**, 2166–72.

Movshon, J. A. and Kiorpes, L. (1990). The role of experience in visual development. In *The development of sensory systems in mammals*, (ed. J. R. Coleman), John Wiley and Sons, New York.

Movshon, J. A. and Kiorpes, L. (1993). Biological limits on visual development in primates. In *Early visual development, normal and abnormal*, (ed. K. Simons), Oxford University Press, New York.

Movshon, J. A., Eggers, H. M., Gizzi, M. S., Hendrickson, A. E., Kiorpes, L., and Boothe, R. G. (1987). Effects of early unilateral blur on the macaque's visual system: III. Physiological observations. *Journal of Neuroscience*, **7**, 1340–51.

Norcia, A. M., Tyler, C. W., and Hamer, R. D. (1990). Development of contrast sensitivity in the human infant. *Vision Research*, **30**, 1475–86.

Packer, O., Hendrickson, A. E., and Curcio, C. A. (1990). Developmental redistribution of photoreceptors across the *Macaca nemestrina* (pigtail macaque) retina. *Journal of Comparative Neurology*, **298**, 472–93.

Smith, E. L. III, Harwerth, R. S., and Crawford, M. L. J. (1985). Spatial contrast sensitivity deficits in monkeys produced by optically induced anisometropia. *Investigative Ophthalmology and Visual Science*, **26**, 330–42.

Teller, D. Y. and Boothe, R. G. (1979). The development of vision in infant primates. *Transactions of the Ophthalmological Society of the UK*, **99**, 333–7.

Wilson, H. R. (1988). Development of spatiotemporal mechanisms in infant vision. *Vision Research*, **28**, 611–28.

Yuodelis, C. and Hendrickson, A. E. (1986). A qualitative and quantitative analysis of the human fovea during development. *Vision Research*, **26**, 847–55.

2

Development of the visual field: results from human and animal studies

Ruxandra Sireteanu

INTRODUCTION

The extent of the adult visual field gives important clues on brain functioning. Visual field deficits often accompany, and sometimes predict, the onset of neurological problems. It is therefore of utmost importance to have reliable methods of early assessment of the visual field, in addition to the assessment of visual resolution.

In recent years a rapid progress in the means of assessing visual acuity in infants and children has been seen. The method of forced-choice preferential looking, originally developed for purposes of basic research (Teller *et al.* 1974), has gained wide popularity. Its derivative, the Teller Acuity Card method (McDonald *et al.* 1985), is now used extensively in clinical settings as a complement to clinical observation. This method has proven useful when testing infants with a variety of ophthalmological and neurological disorders (Preston *et al.* 1987; Mohn *et al.* 1988; Vital-Durand and Hullo 1989; Katz and Sireteanu 1990).

The behavioural function that is used for visual acuity assessment is the spontaneous orienting towards a salient visual stimulus in preference to a homogeneous field. Recently, the same behavioural function was introduced in visual field testing. Several perimetry methods have been developed, and then refined, to give rapid and reliable information on the extent of the visual fields in infants and children from clinical populations.

In this chapter, an overview on the achievements and limitations of the methods of visual perimetry used with infants and children is given, including correlative data from cats and monkeys.

BEHAVIOURAL PERIMETRY IN KITTENS AND CATS

During the 1970s, Sherman (1973) and van Hof-van Duin (1977) independently developed methods of food perimetry to be used with adult cats. Visually deprived cats were trained to fixate a small visual target presented in front of them. On presentation of a peripheral stimulus (a food pellet), the cats were trained to produce an orienting response, which was rewarded by food. Consistent field losses (e.g. monocular and binocular deprivation, strabismus, eye rotation, callosal split, asymmetric alternating occlusion) were described in cats with a variety of early induced experimental manipulations. Almost invariably, the cats showed deficits in the extent of the nasal visual field (van Hof-van Duin 1977; Ikeda and Jacobson 1977; Heitländer and Hoffmann 1978; Kalil 1977; Gordon *et al.* 1979; Elberger 1979; Tumosa *et al.* 1980; Elberger *et al.* 1983; see also Berman and Murphy 1981), sometimes accompanied by restrictions of the temporal visual field (Kalil 1977; see Fig. 2.1).

The nasal field losses might be caused by a delay in the maturation of the visual field. Indeed, the ipsilateral retinocortical projection (on which orienting toward the nasal visual field is based) is phylogenetically more recent than the contralateral projection (Currie and Cowan 1974; So *et al.* 1978; Anker 1977). Responses to stimuli presented in the nasal visual field appear later in ontogenetic development (Albus and Wolf 1984). In addition, the pathway that goes through the visual cortex to the superior colliculus and which, in the cat, is necessary for orienting toward the nasal visual field, also develops relatively late (Stein *et al.* 1973; Norton 1974).

To test this hypothesis, Sireteanu and Maurer (1982) measured the development of the visual field in very young kittens. Since the methods of food perimetry developed for adult cats cannot be used for young kittens, they capitalized on the tendency of the kittens to orient toward salient stimuli, without reinforcement or training. They developed a method of static perimetry, based on the unreinforced orienting to a novel, salient visual stimulus, presented at different positions in the peripheral visual field.

With this method, kittens could be tested from eye opening. It was found that the visual field is incomplete at 13–14 days of age (with responses to objects presented in the nasal visual field being virtually absent and the temporal visual field also showing a substantial limitation). Both the nasal and the temporal fields expand progressively, and the adult extent is reached at about 8–10 weeks of age (Sireteanu and Maurer 1982; see Fig. 2.2).

Strabismic kittens tested with the same method show similar limitations; interestingly, a nasal field loss and a reduction in overall visual responsiveness was also seen in the non-operated eye (albeit less pronounced than in the operated eye; Sireteanu and Singer 1984; Sireteanu 1991).

VISUAL PERIMETRY IN NORMAL INFANTS

There are indications that the effective visual field of humans also expands with age. At first, babies orient only toward peripheral stimuli near the midline, and orient better toward objects in the temporal than in the nasal field. With age, the visual field expands (Tronick 1972; Harris and MacFarlane 1974; MacFarlane *et al.* 1976), and orienting toward the nasal field improves (Lewis *et al.* 1979; Lewis *et al.* 1985).

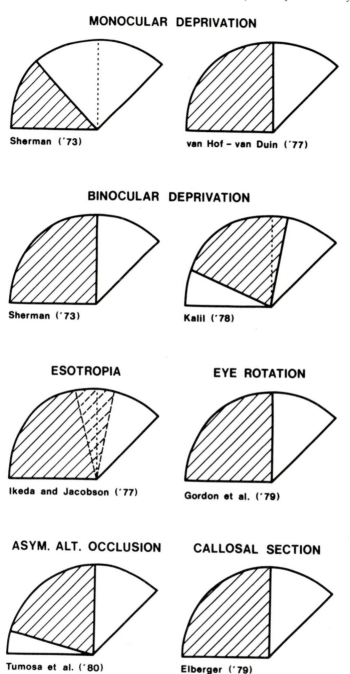

Fig. 2.1 Summary of visual-field testing in cats with different early induced experimental manipulations. Dashed area, remaining visual field; white area, visual field loss. Asym. alt. occlusion: asymmetric alternate occlusion

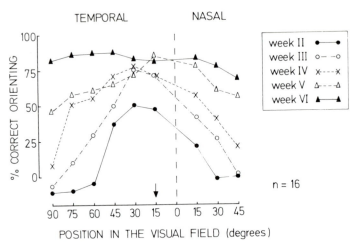

Fig. 2.2 Percentage correct orienting toward visual targets presented at different positions in the visual field of normal kittens. Data from Sireteanu and Maurer (1982). For each age group, chance orienting was subtracted, and the data were renormalized.

The success in the application of unreinforced perimetry in young kittens raised the question whether similar methods were applicable in infants and toddlers, in whom the classical perimetry methods based on verbal instructions cannot be applied.

In 1986, Mohn and van Hof-van Duin developed a method of kinetic perimetry for human infants. Visual stimuli were moved slowly from the periphery into the visual field, while the infants fixated a central visual stimulus. In agreement with the results obtained in very young kittens, 2-month-old infants show a very restricted visual field, both nasally and temporally. Both fields expand with age, with the nasal field lagging behind the temporal field; at about 1 year of age, the adult extent of the visual field is reached.

Schwartz and co-workers (1987) applied this method to study the visual fields of infants younger than 2 months of age and found that the binocular visual fields are similar in shape to those of adults but significantly smaller in size.

The advantages of the method of kinetic perimetry developed by Mohn and van Hof-van Duin are the relative speed with which field size measurements can be made (5–6 min, on average) and the portability of the testing equipment. The disadvantages are the variability in the speed and extent of movement of the hand-held peripheral stimuli, the relatively large size of the test stimuli, and the need for three or four adults to participate in testing.

To overcome these problems, Mayer, Fulton and Cummings (1988) developed a new perimetric technique (a modified Goldmann static perimetry), using a perimeter with LED stimuli and a forced-choice observation procedure.

Central fixation was elicited by four central, pulsing LEDs and maintained with the aid of auditory stimuli. Field extent was derived from the four alternative, forced-choice judgements of an adult who observed the infant's eye movements to peripherally illuminated LEDs. The binocular visual field of infants aged 6–7 months was similar (93%) to that of adults tested with the same apparatus. However, the infants' monocular fields were smaller than those of adults (74%), probably because of the discomfort of the monocular patch.

Lewis and Maurer (1992; see also Maurer and Lewis 1991, for an excellent review) independently developed a method of static perimetry to measure the development of the infants' monocular visual fields. The method was very similar to the method designed by Sireteanu and Maurer (1982) for kittens' field testing. Infants from birth to 6 months of age were shown a 3 or 6° flashing light at various locations along the horizontal meridian, between 15 and 120° in the temporal and the nasal visual fields.

The results are also reminiscent of the results obtained with kittens: with increasing age, the babies oriented toward increasingly peripheral targets, and also more frequently toward less peripheral targets. Thus, not only does the visual field expand but babies become more likely to orient toward any peripheral stimulus (increased visual responsiveness). At 6 months of age, the visual field of the infants was identical to that of adult observers.

Taken together, these results indicate that the effective visual field expands gradually during early infancy; with increasing age, infants become more responsive to peripheral targets and are more likely to produce an orienting response toward targets at increasing eccentricities. Orienting toward targets presented in the nasal visual field lags behind orienting toward the temporal field.

The exact age of maturation of the visual field depends on the testing procedure. With static perimetry, the adult extent is reached at about 6 months of age (Mayer *et al.* 1988; Lewis and Maurer 1992), while with kinetic perimetry, the field is adult-like at about 1 year of age (Mohn and van Hof-van Duin 1986). The pace of maturation is slower for smaller stimuli (Lewis and Maurer 1992).

It has to be kept in mind that, with all methods, the extent of the purely sensory visual field remains unknown and is likely to be underestimated. This is because all methods capitalize on an overt orienting behaviour, positive responses will be recorded only if the infants detect the stimulus as well as produce an adequate motor response (eye and head movement). However, these abilities are themselves immature in infancy. Although the motor immaturity of the infants cannot be the sole factor for their small visual field size (infants produce spontaneous eye and head movements to locations where visual targets are not effective—Lewis and Maurer 1992), it certainly plays a role. Evidence for this limitation comes from studies in which visual orienting and cardiac responses were recorded simultaneously; indeed, heart rate deceleration was seen for peripheral stimuli that did not elicit an overt orienting response (Finlay *et al.* 1982; Finlay and Ivinskis 1984).

VISUAL PERIMETRY IN INFANTS FROM CLINICAL POPULATIONS

In spite of the technological limitations of the perimetry methods based on un-reinforced visual orienting, these methods hold promise for the assessment of the visual field in neuropaediatric patients. Children with perinatal hypoxia/ ischaemia show clear visual field deficits, sometimes manifested as tunnel vision (van Hof-van Duin and Mohn 1984). Pre-term infants at high risk for neurological abnormalities often show severely restricted visual fields (van Hof-van Duin and Mohn 1986). Delayed maturation of the visual field is seen in infants with very low birthweight (VLBW) and in infants with perinatal hypoxia (van Hof-van Duin *et al.* 1989; Groenendaal *et al.* 1989). In infants with perinatal hypoxia, the visual field shows partial recovery when tested 2 years later (Groenendaal and van Hof-van Duin 1990).

Infants with stage 3 retinopathy of prematurity (ROP) or periventricular leucomalacia (PVL) also show a significant delay in the maturation of the visual field (Luna *et al.* 1989; Scher *et al.* 1989).

The clinical studies reported above were performed with kinetic perimetry; thus, the field limitation might be caused by a sensory loss or a slowing of the reaction time of the infants. In children with neurological abnormalities, motor retardation is very likely to occur, in addition to the sensory handicap. There-fore, whenever kinetic perimetry is used with neuropaediatric patients, an independent measure of reaction time would be useful.

This problem is avoided in static perimetry. Indeed, Mayer *et al.* (1988) tested one patient with a severe left hydrocephalus and noted a right homonymous hemianopsia at 14 months, which was confirmed at 22 months. Thus, although static perimetry is more time-consuming, it might give a more reliable measure of visual field deficits in children from clinical populations.

PERIPHERAL VISUAL ACUITY IN NORMAL INFANTS

The clear limitation and the nasotemporal asymmetry of the visual field in early infancy raise the question whether these immaturities might be reflected in the development of peripheral visual acuity. On one hand, the peripheral visual field is incomplete (Mohn and van Hof-van Duin 1986; Lewis and Maurer 1992); while, on the other, the peripheral retina is anatomically more mature than the foveal region (Hendrickson and Yuodelis 1986; Hendrickson

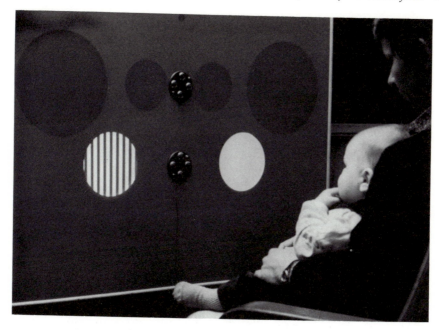

Fig. 2.3 Experimental set-up for testing peripheral grating acuity in human infants. From Sireteanu *et al.* (1988; 1994).

and Drucker 1992). If the development of acuity is the consequence of retinal maturation, much less development of spatial vision in the peripheral than in the central visual field might be expected. In addition, the nasotemporal asymmetry in the development of the visual field might be accompanied by an asymmetrical development of visual acuity.

To test these possibilities, Sireteanu and co-workers (Sireteanu *et al.* 1984; Sireteanu and Fronius 1987; Sireteanu *et al.* 1988; Sireteanu *et al.* 1990; Sireteanu *et al.* 1994) measured binocular and monocular grating acuity in the peripheral visual field. Their measure of peripheral acuity was the baby's first fixation away from a central stimulus. They found that both binocular and monocular acuity developed clearly during the first year but that adult acuity was not yet reached at 1 year of age. At all ages tested, monocular acuity was lower than binocular acuity; acuity in the nasal visual field was always lower than in the temporal field (Figs. 2.3 and 2.4). Similar findings were reported by Maurer *et al.* (1986; see also Jobson unpublished doctoral dissertation) and by Courage and Adams (1990).

Thus, a development of acuity is seen in the peripheral visual field, in spite of the relative maturity of the peripheral retina. The late development of the nasal visual field is accompanied by a delay of maturation of grating acuity in this field. Whether the development of these two functions is the result of a common neural mechanism, is still an open question.

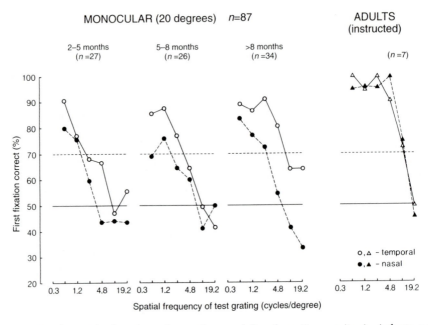

Fig. 2.4 Psychometric functions for testing peripheral grating acuity in infants and adults. Open symbols, stimuli were presented in the temporal visual field; closed symbols, stimuli were presented in the nasal visual field. Data from Sireteanu *et al.* (1988; 1994).

PERIPHERAL VISION IN HUMANS WITH ABNORMAL EARLY VISUAL EXPERIENCE

The clear limitation seen in the peripheral vision of young infants and the maturational delay in neuropaediatric patients lead to the question whether abnormal early visual experience might cause lasting deficits in the extent of the visual field, similar to the deficits seen in cats with early experimental manipulations. Of special interest in this respect are subjects with a congenital esotropia (convergent strabismus) or a monocular deprivation caused by a congenital cataract or ptosis. If the effect of deprivation is similar in the two species, a consistent nasal field loss must be expected in these subjects.

Sireteanu and Fronius (1981) measured monocular grating acuity at different eccentricities along the horizontal meridian in esotropic amblyopes and found a consistent reduction of acuity in the near temporal field (an asymmetry opposite to the expected one) but no deficit in the far periphery (Fig. 2.5). This asymmetry could be explained in terms of the long-term suppression of the deviated eye (Sireteanu 1982) but not in terms of a delayed maturation of the visual field.

A direct approach to test the visual field of strabismic amblyopes has led to conflicting results: while Mehdorn (1986), and later Herzau *et al.* (1992) report

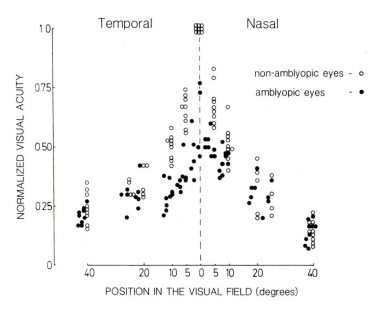

Fig. 2.5 Grating acuity at different positions in the visual field of adult esotropic amblyopes. Note the consistent loss of acuity in the near temporal visual field (5 and 10°), and the normality of acuity in the far periphery. Data from Sireteanu and Fronius (1981).

nasal field deficits in some strabismic amblyopes with very deep amblyopia, such deficits were not seen in any of 22 subjects with moderate-to-deep strabismic amblyopia tested by Sireteanu and Fronius (1990).

A nasal field loss was reported in one subject with a congenital monocular cataract removed at 19 years of age (Moran and Gordon 1982) and in 5–6-year-old children treated for congenital monocular cataracts (Bowering *et al.* 1989; Bowering *et al.* 1993) but not in five adults with congenital monocular deprivation or ptosis (Abdolvahab-Emminger and Sireteanu 1993).

An overall reduction of visual responsiveness throughout the visual field and a concentric shrinkage, affecting both the nasal and the temporal visual fields, were always seen in subjects with deep amblyopia (Sireteanu and Fronius 1990; Abdolvahab-Emminger and Sireteanu 1993).

In general, the nasal visual field losses in humans with abnormal visual experience are quite elusive; deep strabismic amblyopia might generate such losses but only in a few cases; congenital monocular cataract might also lead to nasal field losses but probably only if the cataract was complete. There are no reports of a nasal field loss after congenital monocular ptosis. Thus, humans appear to be different from kittens, in which nasal field losses were invariably found after an early surgical esotropia or monocular deprivation.

There are two ways to solve this apparent controversy. The first, and more direct one, is to perform prospective testing of the visual fields in infants and children in whom a congenital esotropia, cataract or ptosis has been confirmed; the second way is to resort to a species whose visual system is more similar to the human visual system.

BEHAVIOURAL PERIMETRY IN MONKEYS

The similarities between the monkey and the human visual system make the monkey appear more suitable than the cat for visual field studies. Indeed, in recent years, several studies were devoted to the measurement of the visual field in monkeys with different kinds of abnormal early visual experience.

Sparks and co-workers (1986) found no effect of monocular deprivation in rhesus monkeys with short periods of lid suture (1–2 weeks) and a complete lack of visual responsiveness at all visual field positions in monkeys lid sutured from 8–14 days to 18–26 months of age.

Using a method of static perimetry similar to the one used by Sireteanu and Maurer (1982) in young kittens, Wilson *et al.* (1989) confirmed that response levels and visual field extent are normal if the deprivation is initiated at approximately 3 weeks post-natally and lasts for about 1 year. They also found that the responses elicited through the deprived eye are slightly reduced but that the size of the visual field is unaffected in late lid-sutured monkeys deprived for 18 months. Monkeys having continuous monocular occlusion from near birth to 19 months of age showed either no responses or responses restricted to the temporal visual field. In the latter case, the responses in the monocular segment were better than those in the binocular segment. It therefore seems that, in monkeys, both age of onset and length of deprivation are important factors in altering visual field responses. Some of these results are compatible with a model of binocular competition in which the magnitude of competition declines along a naso-temporal gradient of visual field eccentricity.

Using the same method, Wilson and Nevins (1991) studied the visual field of squirrel monkeys monocularly deprived from birth for 3 years. The monkeys did not show any visual responses at any position in the visual field of the deprived eye, thus showing that binocular competition cannot be the only mechanism underlying this loss. Lack of patterned visual input obviously interferes with the development of neuronal connections in all segments of the visual cortex, resulting in complete loss of form vision.

Joosse and co-workers (1990) performed static perimetry in monkeys with a naturally occurring estropia of accommodative origin. The monkeys with alternating strabismus and no obvious eye preference had normal visual field extents and normal response levels across all segments of the visual field. From the animals with a clearly preferred eye for fixation, most had normal visual fields while, in some, a small field loss was seen in the far temporal periphery of the visual field of their non-preferred eye.

Thus, none of the strabismic monkeys exhibited the large, consistent field losses reported in the nasal fields of cats with experimentally induced strabismus (Ikeda and Jacobson 1977; Kalil 1977; Elberger *et al.* 1983; Sireteanu 1991), but are rather in agreement with the modest field losses in humans with mild-to-medium strabismic amblyopia (Sireteanu and Fronius 1990).

The discrepancies between the results obtained in primates (humans and monkeys), on the one hand, and in cats, on the other, might be caused by the fact that naturally occurring accommodative strabismus differs in several characteristics from surgically or optically induced strabismus: surgery produces a transient, paralytic strabismus (Sireteanu *et al.* 1993); an optical strabismus interferes with accommodation. Alternatively, the discrepancy might be the result of a genuine species difference. To resolve this issue, visual field testing in monkeys with a surgically induced strabismus might be helpful.

Recently, Harwerth and co-workers (1993) developed a method of computerized perimetry to be used with adult, extensively trained monkeys. Data from monkey and human observers were collected using the standard threshold programs of the Humphrey Field Analyzer. Fixation was controlled with a Maxwellian view system and an infrared-sensitive video camera connected to a microprocessor-based eye position monitor. The visual fields obtained for monkeys and humans were similar, thus showing that the techniques of computerized perimetry may be applied to monkey subjects without modification. These methods could be employed to study monkey models of ocular disorders (e.g. experimental glaucoma).

The results obtained with perimetry testing in macaque monkeys reinforce the idea that monkeys, with their high resolution, excellent stereopsis and good photopic vision, might be more suitable than cats for correlative developmental studies.

Unfortunately, data on normal visual field development are not yet available in monkeys. However, testing of peripheral contrast sensitivity proved feasible. As in human infants, peripheral visual acuity (this time evaluated by extrapolation of contrast sensitivity) showed a clear post-natal development. In the youngest monkeys tested at 7–10 weeks, contrast sensitivity of the fovea was similar to that of the near periphery, at least out to 8° in the periphery. For more peripheral eccentricities, contrast sensitivity declined systematically at all ages tested. The results show that, unlike adults, the sensitivity of the infant fovea is similar to that of the near periphery. The foveal region undergoes substantial post-natal development relative to the periphery (Kiorpes and Kiper 1992; see also Chapter 1).

CONCLUSIONS

Taken together, the studies mentioned in this chapter show that the effective visual field is incomplete at birth. In humans and kittens (and possibly also in monkeys), a substantial limitation is found, both nasally and temporally. Both fields expand with age, with the nasal field lagging behind the temporal one. Cats raised with an abnormal early visual experience almost invariably show deficits in the extent of their nasal visual field. Surprisingly, these deficits are erratic, and often absent, in primates (humans and monkeys) raised under comparable conditions.

The reasons for these discrepancies are still unclear. Nevertheless, the methods developed for visual field assessment, and especially the methods of static perimetry and their computerized versions, promise to be extremely useful as a complement of visual acuity assessment in neuropaediatric patients.

REFERENCES

Abdolvahab-Emminger, H. and Sireteanu, R. (1993). Residual visual properties in human amblyopia after monocular deprivation in early life. *Clinical Vision Sciences*, **8**, 263–79.

Albus, K. and Wolf, W. (1984). Early postnatal development of neuronal function in the kitten's visual cortex; a laminar analysis. *Journal of Physiology (London)*, **348**, 153–85.

Anker, R. L. (1977). The prenatal development of some of the visual pathways in the cat. *Journal of Comparative Neurology*, **173**, 185–204.

Berman, N. and Murphy, E. (1981). The critical period for alteration in cortical binocularity resulting from divergent and convergent strabismus. *Developmental Brain Research*, **2**, 181–202.

Bowering, E., Maurer, D., Lewis, T. L., Brent, P., and Brent, H. (1989). Development of the visual field in normal and binocularly deprived children. *Investigative Ophthalmology and Visual Science*, **30** (suppl.), 377.

Bowering, E. R., Maurer, D., Lewis, T. L., and Brent, H. P. (1993). Sensitivity in the nasal and temporal hemifields in children treated for cataract. *Investigative Ophthalmology and Visual Science*, **34**, 3501–9.

Courage, M. L. and Adams, R. J. (1990). The early development of visual acuity in the binocular and monocular peripheral fields. *Infant Behaviour and Development*, **13**, 123–8.

Currie, J. and Cowan, W. M. (1974). Evidence for the late development of the uncrossed retinothalamic projections in the frog, *Rana pipiens*. *Brain Research*, **71**, 133–9.

Elberger, A. J. (1979). The role of the corpus callosum in the development of interocular eye alignment and the organization of the visual field in the cat. *Experimental Brain Research*, **36**, 71–85.

Elberger, A. J., Smith, E. L. III, and White, J. M. (1983). Optically induced strabismus results in visual field losses in cats. *Brain Research*, **268**, 147–52.

Finlay, D. and Ivinskis, A. (1984). Cardiac and visual responses to moving stimuli presented either successively or simultaneously to the central and peripheral visual fields in 4-month-old infants. *Developmental Psychology*, **20**, 29–36.

Finlay, D., Quinn, K., and Ivinskis, A. (1982). Detection of moving stimuli in the binocular and nasal visual fields by infants three and four months old. *Perception*, **11**, 685–90.

Gordon, B., Moran, J., and Presson, J. (1979). Visual fields in cats with one eye rotated. *Brain Research*, **174**, 167–71.

Groenendaal, F. and van Hof-van Duin, J. (1990). Partial visual recovery in two full-term infants after perinatal hypoxia. *Neuropediatrics*, **21**, 76–8.

Groenendaal, F., van Hof-van Duin, J., Baerts, W., and Fetter, W. P. F. (1989). Effects of perinatal hypoxia on visual development during the first year of (corrected) age. *Early Human Development*, **20**, 267–79.

Harris, P. and MacFarlane, A. (1974). The growth of the effective visual field from birth to seven weeks. *Journal of Experimental Child Psychology*, **18**, 340–8.

Harwerth, R. S., Smith, E. L., and DeSantis, L. (1993). Behavioural perimetry in monkeys. *Investigative Ophthalmology and Visual Science*, **34**, 31–40.

Heitländer, H. and Hoffmann, K.-P. (1978). The visual field of monocularly deprived cats after late closure or enucleation of the non-deprived eye. *Brain Research*, **145**, 153–60.

Hendrickson, A. and Drucker, D. (1992). The development of parafoveal and mid-peripheral human retina. *Behavioural Brain Research*, **49**, 21–33.

Hendrickson, A. and Yuodelis, C. (1984). The morphological development of the human fovea. *Ophthalmology*, **91**, 603–12.

Herzau, V., Girrback, C., and Roth, A. (1992). Nasal-temporal asymmetry of the differential light threshold in strabismic amblyopia. In *Transactions of the 20th meeting of the European Strabismological Assocation*, (ed. H. Kaufmann), pp. 107–12.

Ikeda, H. and Jacobson, S. G. (1977). Nasal field loss in cats reared with convergent squint: behavioural studies. *Journal of Physiology (London)*, **270**, 367–81.

Jobson, S. A. (1985). Development of peripheral acuity in infants. Unpublished doctoral dissertation, McMaster University.

Joosse, M. V., Wilson, J. R., and Boothe, R. G. (1990). Monocular visual fields of macaque monkeys with naturally occurring strabismus. *Clinical Vision Sciences* **5**, 101–11.

Kalil, R. E. (1977). Visual field defects in strabismic cats. *Investigative Ophthalmology and Visual Science*, **16** (suppl.), 163.

Katz, B. and Sireteanu, R. (1990). The Teller Acuity Card Test: a useful method for the clinical routine? *Clinical Vision Sciences*, **5**, 307–23.

Kiorpes, L. and Kiper, D. C. (1992). Development of contrast sensitivity in the peripheral visual field of monkeys. *Perception*, **21** (suppl.), 3.

Lewis, T. L. and Maurer, D. (1992). The development of the temporal and nasal visual fields during infancy. *Vision Research*, **32**, 903–11.

Lewis, T. L., Maurer, D., and Milewski, A. (1979). The development of nasal detection in young infants. *Investigative Ophthalmology and Visual Science*, **19** (suppl.), 271.

Lewis, T. L., Maurer, D., and Blackburn, K. (1985). The development of young infants' ability to detect stimuli in the nasal field. *Vision Research*, **25**, 943–50.

Luna, B., Dobson, V., Carpenter, N., and Biglan, A. W. (1989). Visual field development in infants with Stage 3 retinopathy of prematurity. *Investigative Ophthalmology and Visual Science*, **30**, 580–2.

McDonald, M. A., Dobson, V., Sebris, S. L., Baitch, L., Varner, D., and Teller, D. Y. (1985). The acuity card procedure: A rapid test of infant acuity. *Investigative Ophthalmology and Visual Science*, **26**, 1158–62.

MacFarlane, A., Harris, P., and Barnes, I. (1976). Central and peripheral vision in early infancy. *Journal of Experimental Child Psychology*, **21**, 532–8.

Maurer, D. and Lewis, T. L. (1991). The development of peripheral vision and its physiological underpinnings. In *Newborn attention: biological constraints and the influence of experience*, (ed. M. J. Weiss and P. R. Zelazo), pp. 218–55. Norwood, New Jersey, Ablex.

Maurer, D., Jobson, S., and Lewis, T. L. (1986). The development of peripheral acuity. *Infant Behaviour and Development*, (suppl.), 245.

Mayer, D. L., Fulton, A. B., and Cummings, M. F. (1988). Visual fields of infants assessed with a new perimetric technique. *Investigative Ophthalmology and Visual Science*, **29**, 452–9.

Mehdorn, E. (1986). Nasal field defects in strabismic amblyopia. *Documenta Ophthalmologica Proceedings Series*, **45**, 318–29.

Mohn, G. and van Hof-van Duin, J. (1986). Development of the binocular and monocular visual fields during the first year of life. *Clinical Vision Sciences*, **1**, 51–64.

Mohn, G., van Hof-van Duin, J., Fetter, W. P. F., de Groot, L., and Hage, M. (1988). Acuity assessment of non-verbal infants and children: clinical experience with the acuity card procedure. *Developmental Medicine and Child Neurology*, **30**, 232–44.

Moran, J. and Gordon, B. (1982). Long-term visual deprivation in a human. *Vision Research*, **22**, 27–36.

Norton, T. T. (1974). Receptive-field properties of superior colliculus cells and development of visual behaviour in kittens. *Journal of Neurophysiology*, **37**, 674–90.

Preston, K. L., McDonald, M., Sebris, S. L., Dobson, V., and Teller, D. Y. (1987). Validation of the acuity card procedure for assessment of infants with ocular disorders. *Ophthalmology*, **94**, 644–53.

Scher, M. S., Dobson, V., Carpenter, N. A., and Guthrie, R. D. (1989). Visual and neurological outcome of infants with periventricular leukomalacia. *Developmental Medicine and Child Neurology*, **31**, 353–65.

Schwartz, T. L., Dobson, V., Sandstrom, D. J., and van Hof-van Duin, J. (1987). Kinetic perimetry assessment of binocular visual field shape and size in young infants. *Vision Research*, **27**, 2163–75.

Sherman, S. M. (1973). Visual field defects in monocularly and binocularly deprived cats. *Brain Research*, **49**, 25–45.

Sireteanu, R. (1982). Human amblyopia: consequence of long-term interocular suppression. *Human Neurobiology*, **1**, 31–3.

Sireteanu, R. (1991). Restricted visual fields in both eyes of kittens with a unilateral, surgically induced strabismus: relationship to extrastriate cortical binocularity. *Clinical Vision Sciences*, **6**, 277–87.

Sireteanu, R. and Fronius, M. (1981). Naso-temporal asymmetries in human amblyopia: consequence of long-term interocular suppression. *Vision Research*, **21**, 1055–63.

Sireteanu, R. and Fronius, M. (1987). The development of the peripheral visual acuity in human infants. In *Transactions of the 16th meeting of the European Strabismological Association*, (ed. H. Kaufmann), pp. 221–9. Giessen.

Sireteanu, R. and Fronius, M. (1990). Human amblyopia: structure of the visual field. *Experimental Brain Research*, **79**, 603–14.

Sireteanu, R. and Maurer, D. (1982). The development of the kitten's visual field. *Vision Research*, **22**, 1101–11.

Sireteanu, R. and Singer, W. (1984). Impaired visual responsiveness in both eyes of kittens with unilateral surgically induced strabismus. *Investigative Ophthalmology and Visual Science*, **25** (suppl.), 216.

Sireteanu, R., Kellerer, R., and Boergen, K.-P. (1984). The development of peripheral acuity in human infants: a preliminary study. *Human Neurobiology*, **3**, 81–5.

Sireteanu, R., Fronius, M., and Constantinescu, D.-H. (1988). The development of peripheral visual acuity in human infants: binocular summation and naso-temporal asymmetry. *Investigative Ophthalmology and Visual Science*, **29** (suppl.), 26.

Sireteanu, R., Fronius, M., and Katz, B. (1990). A perspective on psychophysical testing in children. *Eye*, **4**, 794–801.

Sireteanu, R., Singer, W., Fronius, M., Greuel, J., Best, J., Fiorentini, A., Bisti, S., Schiavi, C., and Campos, E. (1993). Eye alignment and cortical binocularity in strabismic kittens: a comparison between tenotomy and recession. *Visual Neuroscience*, **10**, 541–9.

Sireteanu, R., Fronius, M., and Constantinescu, D. H. (1994). The development of visual acuity in the peripheral visual field of human infants: binocular and monocular measurements. *Vision Research*, **34**, 1659–71.

So, K.-F., Schneider, G. E., and Frost, D. O. (1978). Postnatal development of retinal projections to the lateral geniculate body in Syrian hamsters. *Brain Research*, **142**, 343–52.

Sparks, D. L., Mays, L. E., Gurski, M., and Hickey, T. L. (1986). Long- and short-term monocular deprivation in the rhesus monkey: effects on visual fields and optokinetic nystagmus. *Journal of Neuroscience*, **6**, 1771–80.

Stein, B. E., Labos, E., and Kruger, L. (1973). Sequence of changes in properties of neurons of superior colliculus of the kitten during maturation. *Journal of Neurophysiology*, **36**, 667–79.

Teller, D. Y., Morse, R., Borton, R., and Regal, D. (1974). Visual acuity for vertical and diagonal gratings in human infants. *Vision Research*, **14**, 1433–9.

Tronick, E. (1972). Stimulus control and the development of infants' effective visual field. *Perception and Psychophysics*, **11**, 373–6.

Tumosa, N., Bliss-Tiemann, S., and Hirsch, V. B. (1980). Unequal alternating monocular deprivation causes asymmetric visual fields in cats. *Science*, **208**, 421–3.

van Hof-van Duin, J. (1977). Visual field measurements in monocularly deprived and normal cats. *Experimental Brain Research*, **30**, 353–68.

van Hof-van Duin, J. and Mohn, G. (1984). Visual defects in children after cerebral hypoxia. *Behavioural Brain Research*, **14**, 147–55.

van Hof-van Duin, J. and Mohn, G. (1986). Visual field measurements, optokinetic nystagmus and the visual threatening response: normal and abnormal development. *Documenta Ophthalmologica Proceedings Series*, **45**, 305–15.

van Hof-van Duin, J., Evenhuis-van Leunen, A., Mohn, G., Baerts, W., and Fetter, W. P. F. (1989). Effects of very low birthweight (VLBW) on visual development during the first year after term. *Early Human Development*, **20**, 255–66.

Vital-Durand, F. and Hullo, A. (1989). La mesure d'acuité visuelle du nourrisson en six minutes: Les Cartes d'Acuité de Teller. *Journal Français d'Ophtalmologie*, **3**, 221–5.

Wilson, J. R. and Nevins, C. L. (1991). Effects of monocular deprivation on the visual fields of squirrel monkeys. *Behavioural Brain Research*, **44**, 129–31.

Wilson, J. R., Lavallee, K. A., Joosse, M. V., Hendrickson, A. E., Boothe, R. G., and Harwerth, R. S. (1989). Visual fields of monocularly deprived macaque monkeys. *Behavioural Brain Research*, **33**, 13–22.

3

Development of primate rod structure and function

Anne Fulton, Ronald M. Hansen, Elizabeth Dorn, and Anita Hendrickson

INTRODUCTION

The rod-mediated sensitivity of infants is lower than that of adults while the scotopic sensitivity for full-field stimuli of infants approaches adult values earlier than those psychophysical sensitivities that are mediated by rods at the posterior pole (Hansen and Fulton 1993). For example, in 10-week-old infants, dark adapted scotopic sensitivity for full-field stimuli, whether assayed using an electroretinographic (ERG) or visually evoked potential procedures (Fulton and Hansen 1993; Hansen and Fulton 1995a), is only about 0.5 log unit less than that of adults, while psychophysical sensitivities for test spots falling only on more central retina are at least a log unit below those of adults (Brown 1986; Powers *et al.* 1981; Hansen *et al.* 1986). As a consequence, we have decided to examine the rod photoreceptors themselves for explanations of infants' low scotopic sensitivity.

Primate rod photoreceptor cells are immature at term (Hendrickson and Drucker 1992; Packer *et al.* 1990). All across the retina, the structure of the rods of infants and adults differs. Moreover, developmental increases in rod outer segment (ROS) length and in content of the photosensitive compound, rhodopsin, have been documented (Hendrickson and Drucker 1992; Fulton *et al.* 1991a). In addition, there appear to be regional variations in the rate of ROS maturation with both ROS and thresholds near the fovea relatively slow to mature (Hendrickson and Drucker 1992; Hansen and Fulton 1995b). Thus it is timely to examine the physical and functional characteristics of infants' rods for possible relationships.

Rod photoreceptors have their peak density at the eccentricity of the optic disc in a ring that encircles the fovea (Curcio *et al.* 1990; reviewed by Curcio and Hendrickson 1991). The near-central parafoveal rods are born and differentiate earlier than those in the rod ring (LaVail *et al.* 1991; Hendrickson and Kupfer 1976). This might suggest that the morphological development of rods in the ring should lag that of near-central rods. However, the only study comparing development of the parafovea and rod ring (Hendrickson and Drucker

1992) reports that human ROS in the ring develop before those in the parafovea and remain longer until well after term. This pattern suggests that primate ROS do not follow a central-to-peripheral developmental pattern.

This issue has been examined by using immunocytochemistry in a closely spaced series of macaque monkey eyes in which the sections contained the entire horizontal meridian. The expression of rod opsin was followed using monoclonal antibody rho-4D2 to the N-terminal region of opsin (Molday and MacKenzie 1983) which is situated on the extracellular surface of the ROS disc. Opsin is the protein part of rhodopsin and accounts for 90% of the protein in ROS discs (Hargrave and McDowell 1992). When rho-4D2 is visualized by a fluorescent marker such as Texas Red, it provides a very sensitive detector of ROS development at the light microscopic level, particularly since it is not compromised by adhering pigment epithelium. The development of rho-4D2 labelling was followed at five points across the horizontal meridian, beginning in early gestation and extending to 2 years post-natally, to determine: (i) where in the retina ROS first appeared; and (ii) the relationship of eccentricity to ROS length over development. The development of the sensitivity of the rod photoreceptors themselves was also examined. Besides short outer segments, the developing rods are known to have low rhodopsin content (Fulton *et al.* 1991). A model of the biochemical processes involved in the activation of the phototransduction cascade (Lamb and Pugh 1992; Pugh and Lamb 1993; Breton *et al.* 1993) has been fitted to a-waves of the ERG (Hood and Birch 1990*a,b,c*). The ERG a-wave voltage originates in the rods, and is proportional to the photocurrent of the rod (Pugh and Lamb 1993; Breton *et al.* 1993).

Control of the photoreceptor sensitivity of infants could be affected by steps in the phototransduction cascade occurring after photoisomerization of rhodopsin (Fulton *et al.* 1991*a,b*; Fulton *et al.* 1992). Opsin together with the vitamin-A-related chromophore, 11-*cis* retinal, forms rhodopsin. In the ROS, light activates rhodopsin and so initiates the cascade of processes involved in phototransduction (Pugh and Lamb 1993). Activated rhodopsin diffuses in the disc membrane to the G-protein on the membrane; G-protein then diffuses to phosphodiesterase. This leads to closure of the ionic channels in the outer segment membrane. The ROS channels are open in the dark and a 'dark current' circulates. In response to light, these channels close, and the dark current is lowered. The reduction in dark current is called the photocurrent. In the mature rod, channel density is constant along the ROS. The magnitude of the maximum photocurrent that the rod can generate is proportional to ROS length (Baylor *et al.* 1979).

METHODS

Immunocytochemistry

Retinas (n = 15) were obtained from fetal day (F) 55 (birth = F170) to post-natal (P) 9 months and compared with normal adult *Macaca nemestrina* retina. All eyes were immersion-fixed in 4% paraformaldehyde for 2–3 hours, cryo-protected and the entire horizontal meridian frozen in cryostat embedding compound. Coulottes were sectioned serially at 10 µm and every tenth slide stained with cresyl violet for morphological analysis. Sections were incubated sequentially as follows:

(1) in 10% goat serum in phosphate-buffered saline pH 7.4 (PBS) containing 0.25% Triton X-100 detergent for 30 min;
(2) overnight in mouse monoclonal antiserum rho-4D2 diluted 1/10 000 in PBS containing 1% goat serum (diluent);
(3) in PBS for 6 hours;
(4) biotinylated horse antimouse IgG (1/100 in diluent) at 37°C for 45 min;
(5) PBS for 45 min; and
(6) avidin/Texas Red (1/1000 in diluent) for 45 min at 37°C.

Slides were rinsed twice in phosphate buffer and then coverslipped with 80% glycerol in phosphate buffer and examined in a Nikon UFX microscope equipped with fluorescent filters specific for the wavelengths of rhodamine and Texas Red. Slides were photographed at ×180 magnification and the resulting colour transparencies projected onto a screen for measurements. Five different points were compared:

(1) fovea;
(2) parafovea, defined as 1.5 mm from the foveal edge;
(3) nasal rod ring just outside of the optic disc;
(4) temporal rod ring 4 mm peripheral to the fovea; and
(5) far peripheral temporal retina 2 mm from the ora serrata.

Morphology

A collection of pre-natal and post-natal human and monkey retinas embedded in glycol methacrylate and sectioned serially at 2 µm were analysed as reported by Hendrickson and Drucker (1992).

Rhodopsin assays

Rhodopsin was extracted from human eyes from patients aged from 32 weeks gestation to adulthood, using procedures for quantitative recovery of this photosensitive substance from the ocular tissues (Fulton *et al.* 1990; 1991*a*). Samples were assayed spectroscopically and the total quantity of rhodopsin per eye was determined from the difference spectrum (Fulton *et al.* 1990). A logistic growth curve (Hoglund *et al.* 1982) was fitted to the data ($n = 99$ eyes; 99 donors; 14 donors ≤ 10 years of age) using an iterative procedure that minimized the root-mean-square deviation from the function:

$$Y = Y_{max} \left[Age^n / (Age^n + \sigma^n) \right]$$

where Y is rhodopsin in nanomoles, Y_{max} the estimated adult value of rhodopsin and σ the age at which $Y = Y_{max}/2$.

Electroretinography

Responses to full-field stimuli were recorded from dark-adapted subjects using Burian Allen electrodes and signal averaging procedures (Fulton and Hansen 1992). A mathematical model of the a-wave (Hood and Birch 1994) based on the Lamb and Pugh (1992) model of the biochemical processes in the activation of phototransduction was fitted to the a-waves using an iterative procedure.

Dark-adapted psychophysical threshold

Modified preferential looking procedures (Hansen and Fulton 1981; Hansen *et al.* 1986; Brown 1986; Powers *et al.* 1981; Fulton *et al.* 1991) were used to obtain thresholds from dark-adapted subjects at eccentricities of 10° (within the rod ring) and 30° (peripheral to the rod ring) along the horizontal meridian. Test spots, 50 ms duration, 2° diam, were presented at 10° and 30°. A two-alternative forced-choice psychophysical method (Teller 1979) with a staircase procedure (Wetherill and Levitt 1966) was used (Fulton *et al.* 1991*b*) to estimate thresholds at the two retinal sites in each subject (Hansen and Fulton 1995*a*). The thresholds previously reported for normal 10-week olds and adults at 10° and 30° (Hansen *et al.* 1993) were compared with those of children with retinal disorders of early onset (Bardet-Biedl syndrome, $n = 5$; achromatopsia, $n = 4$).

RESULTS

Morphologically (Fig. 3.1), the first human ROS are found at the rod ring in the F24–26 week eye (Hendrickson and Drucker 1992). It is possible that the first ROS appear earlier but cannot be recognized in these sections. By F36 week ROS are also present in the parafovea; those in the rod ring are clearly longer. Rod ring ROS remain longer at P1 week but by P13 months the ROS in the ring

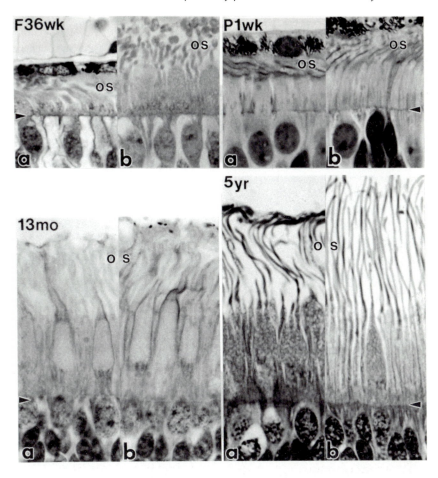

Fig. 3.1 Photomicrographs of human retina at late fetal and post-term ages (modified from Hendrickson and Drucker 1992). All photographs are aligned on the outer limiting membrane (arrowhead). In each pair of photographs the development of inner and outer segments (os) at the parafovea (a) and rod ring (b) is shown. All sections 2 μm glycol methacrylate stained with azure II-methylene blue; × 750.

and parafovea are more equal in length. By early childhood the ROS in the ring are only slightly longer than in the parafovea, and this relationship will remain into adulthood.

The pattern of monkey rod labelling for rho-4D2 is shown in Fig. 3.2. The earliest staining for opsin is seen at F66–70 in the parafovea when the entire cell membrane of scattered rods labels lightly but no ROS can be seen. By F83 the number of stained rods has increased and the staining is more intense. 'Stubs', 1–2 μm long, are present at the tip of the inner segment. Whether these are the first membranous discs in the newly formed ROS or the cilium that will form

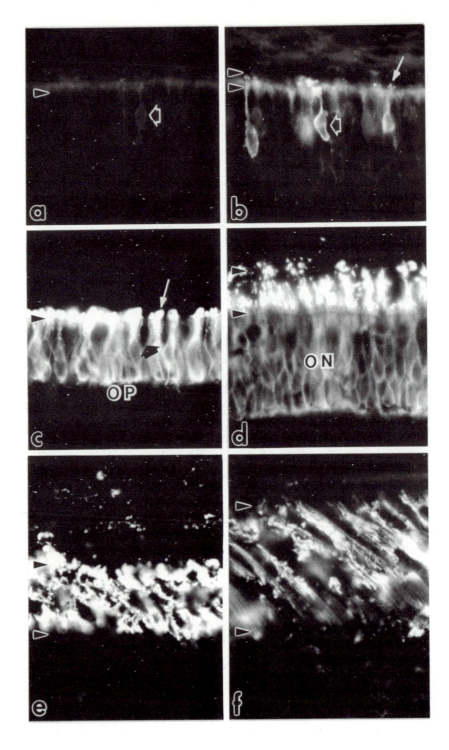

Fig. 3.2 Frozen sections of Macaca monkey retina immunocytochemically stained for rod opsin with rho-4D2 monoclonal antiserum and visualized by fluorescence using Texas Red. All photographs are from the temporal rod ring except (b), which is from the nasal rod ring. (a,b) F89; (c) F104; (d) F115; (e) F150; (f) P9mos. All photographs are aligned on the outer limiting membrane, which is marked by the inner arrowhead; the inner edge of the pigment epithelium is marked by the outer arrowhead in (b,d,e,f). The nasal rod ring (b) has clear cell body labelling for opsin at F89 (open arrow) and at least some rods have a tiny, intensely labelled 'stub' at the apical inner segment (white arrow), which may be either the cilium or forming the outer segment. In the temporal rod ring (a) at the same age only a very few rods stain faintly for opsin (open arrow). Cell-membrane staining increases with age so that by F105–115 (c,d) all of the rod cell bodies in the outer nuclear layer (ON) are stained to their synaptic spherules in the outer plexiform layer (OP). Cones (black arrow) are unstained. After late gestation (e) cell body membrane staining disappears, and only outer segments are labelled. Outer segment length increases markedly with age, demonstrated by the increasing distance between arrowheads in (b,d,f). All × 600.

the ROS at a later stage must be resolved by electron microscopic studies. By F80 both cell body and 'stubs' are rho-4D2$^+$ in the nasal rod ring (Fig. 3.2(b)). The temporal rod ring only shows faint cell membrane labelling in the same eye (Fig. 3.2(a)). Thus rho-4D2 immunocytochemical staining shows that parafoveal rods express rhodopsin 10–14 days before rods in the rod ring. By F105–108, distinct ROS can be identified across the central 4 mm of retina, including parafovea and rod ring (Fig. 3.2(c)), although the temporal rod ring is still less heavily labelled than the nasal one. Cell membrane staining is intense over the entire cell, including the synaptic spherule. Cell body labelling declines with age so that by F150 (Fig. 3.2(d)) the ROS are much longer and stain much more heavily than the cell body. By F140, rod cell membrane labelling reaches the ora and ROS can be detected in the far periphery just before birth. In late gestation (Fig. 3.2(d)) cell body labelling disappears centrally but stained cell bodies are present in the far periphery until several months after birth. In most of the retina after birth, only ROS are rho-4D2$^+$ (Fig. 3.2(e–f)).

   It can be seen in Fig. 3.2 that ROS growth is rapid in monkey retina but that it also continues over a long developmental period. ROS lengths at the five chosen retinal sites are shown for several ages in Fig. 3.3. The most central sites have the first detectable ROS but, after F90–110, ROS in both the nasal and temporal rod ring grow much faster, so that they are the longest in the retina in late gestation and just after term. Rod ring ROS are twice as long as ROS in the parafovea during this neonatal period. By P16 week ROS are of equal length across most of the retina, indicating that a late growth spurt takes place in central retina. There is a slight increase in both central and rod ring ROS length up to 9 months. Both the immunocytochemical staining and ROS length measurements show that, although rods in the rod ring may form ROS slightly later, once they are present they grow more rapidly than central rods. Rod ring ROS

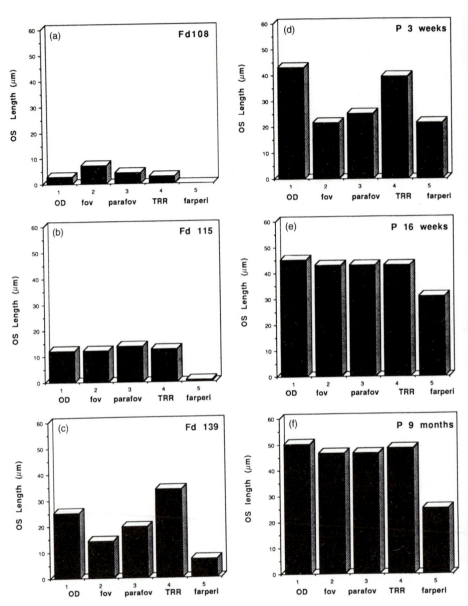

Fig. 3.3 Graphs of the growth of rod outer segments (os) over six stages of Macaca monkey retina development at the nasal rod ring (OD); in or near the fovea (fov); 1.5 mm from the fovea (parafov); 4 mm from the fovea in the temporal rod ring (TRR); and 2 mm from the ora serrata (farperi). Measurements were made from projected colour transparencies of frozen sections stained immunocytochemically for rod opsin (see Fig. 3.2). Rods near the fovea initially show the longest outer segments but, by late gestation, outer segments in both nasal and temporal rod ring have become longer. By 4 months after birth, outer segment length is uniform over most of the retina and is close to that of juveniles and adults.

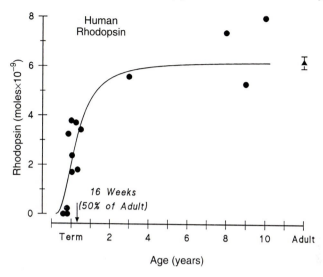

Fig. 3.4 The rhodopsin content of human eyes as a function of age. The circles plot data from the right eyes of 14 donors ≤10 years. The triangle (±1 SEM) plots the mean rhodopsin content for donors more than 10 years of age ($n = 85$). The smooth curve represents a logistic growth function fitted to the data.

dominate the retina at birth, suggesting that this region could be more sensitive in the newborn eye.

The rhodopsin content of human eyes also increases with age (Fulton *et al.* 1991*a*). The growth curve (Fig. 3.4) predicts that the rhodopsin content of human infants' eyes at term is 2.1 nmoles, or about 30% that of adult eyes. This is close to the values observed (Fig. 3.4). Near term, the human peripheral ROS lengths are at least 60% of adult length (Hendrickson and Drucker 1992). Thus the rhodopsin content per unit ROS length, that is rhodopsin per disc, of young human infants may be low as it is in 13–18 day infant rats (Fulton *et al.* 1995). Additional data at young ages are needed to define more completely the developmental increase in human rhodopsin and ROS length.

Electroretinographic records from a 10-week-old neonate and an adult show that at both ages a- and b-wave amplitudes increase and then saturate at high stimulus intensities (Fig. 3.5(a)).

Low rhodopsin content predicts low sensitivity because fewer photons can be captured. Further a-wave analysis (Fig. 3.5) indicates rod photoreceptor sensitivity in 10-week olds is about 50% of that of adults. At 10 weeks of age the rhodopsin growth curve (see Fig. 3.4) predicts rhodopsin content to be 45% of that of adults, meaning that the infants' sensitivity could be explained by low quantum catch.

The relationship of human rhodopsin to b-wave sensitivity over development (rather than only at age 10 weeks) shows that simple proportionality is

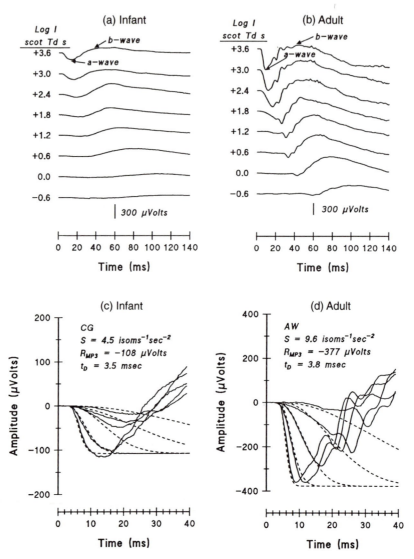

Fig. 3.5 Sample ERG records of human subjects, age 10 weeks and adult: (a,b) the numbers to the left of each trace specify stimuli in log Td s. These subjects have a- and b-wave parameters close to the median values for their age group; (c,d) the a-wave occurs within first 40 ms of the ERG response. The a-wave model (Hood and Birch 1994) fits (dashed lines) are shown.

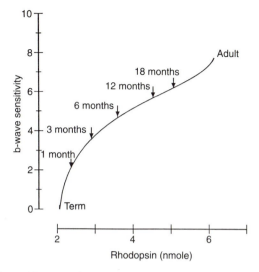

Fig. 3.6 Relationship of human rhodopsin and ERG b-wave sensitivity. The rhodopsin values are from the smooth curve shown in Fig. 3.4. The sensitivity values are taken from the growth curve fit to b-wave sensitivities (Fulton and Hansen 1993).

unlikely to explain the development of human scotopic sensitivity (Fig. 3.6). The b-wave, a proxy for the activity of second order retinal neurones, is generated proximally to the ROS and a-wave generators. Whether the lack of proportionality is caused by immaturities of phototransduction processes proximal to photoisomerization of rhodopsin, transmission from photoreceptors to second order neurones, or post-receptoral processing, remains to be discovered.

Relatively greater immaturity of rod-mediated function at near-central rather than peripheral retina accompanies delays in the anatomical development of near-central rods (Fig. 3.3; see also Hendrickson and Drucker 1992). Every 10-week-old human infant tested to date has a higher threshold at 10° than at 30°, indicating that rod-mediated visual sensitivity is less mature at 10° (Hansen and Fulton 1995a). On average the difference in infants' thresholds at 10° and 30° is 0.5 log units. Adults' thresholds at 10° and 30° are equal when tested with this procedure, and previously reported adult psychophysical thresholds at these sites are equal (Massof and Finkelstein 1979). Children with the retinal degeneration of Bardet-Biedl syndrome, which causes functional deficits across the entire retina (Jacobson *et al.* 1990; Fulton *et al.* 1993), show equal elevations of thresholds at 10° and 30° (Fig. 3.7). There is no suggestion of the infantile threshold pattern with higher thresholds at 10°. The thresholds of three out of the four children with achromatopsia show the infantile pattern with higher thresholds at 10° than 30° (Fig. 3.7).

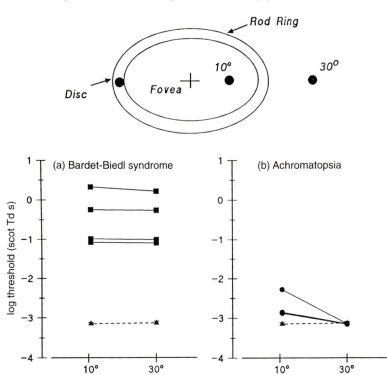

Fig. 3.7 Log thresholds within (10°) and peripheral to (30°) the rod ring are shown. Results from patients with Bardet-Biedl syndrome (squares in (a)) and achromatopsia (circles in (b)) are shown. The two thresholds of each individual are connected by a line. Mean (±1 SEM) adult thresholds are represented by the triangles in both panels.

DISCUSSION

The pattern of rod development in monkey retina has been clearly demonstrated using immunocytochemistry for rod opsin. The pattern of rho-4D2 label in monkey rods is similar to that reported for rat rods (Hicks and Barnstable 1987) with cell membrane labelling preceding ROS appearance by some days. Immunocytochemical labelling indicates a somewhat different rod developmental sequence than that reported earlier for humans (Hendrickson and Drucker 1992). Rho-4D2 staining for opsin in monkey retina follows a generalized central-to-peripheral pattern for both rod cell membrane and ROS labelling, consistent with the pattern of rod post-mitotic appearance (LaVail *et al.* 1991). This suggests that the morphological appearance of ROS on near-central rods may have been missed in the F24–26 week human retina, or that the monkey and the human have a different pattern of development. Given the sensitivity of immunocytochemistry, we favour the former conclusion. However, consistent with the earlier work on human retina, once ROS form in the monkey rod ring, these grow very rapidly to become the longest ROS before and just after birth. It is curious that both primates show a similar pattern of rod ring development, because monkey foveal development is much more advanced that that of the human at birth (Yuodelis and Hendrickson 1986; Hendrickson 1992).

Proportionality of the amplitude of the saturated a-wave and ROS length in human development is consistent with results obtained from infant rats over the course of ROS development (Fulton *et al.* 1995). The development of sensitivity of the human rod photoresponse, derived from a-wave analyses, is more problematic. At age 10 weeks human rod sensitivity (Fulton and Hansen 1992) is close to that predicted by rhodopsin content. This leads us to suggest that immaturities of the processes involved in activation of phototransduction, sited in the ROS themselves, are critical controllers of the developmental increase in scotopic sensitivity.

The present authors suspect that rhodopsin concentration is the limiting factor because other enzymes in the activation and deactivation of photo-transduction appear to reach adult levels, at least in rats and mice, before rhodopsin content (Bowes *et al.* 1988; Broekhuyse and Kuhlman 1989; Cantera *et al.* 1990; Farber *et al.* 1988; Ho *et al.* 1986; Lee *et al.* 1990). For instance, out of the principal proteins involved in the activation of phototransduction, the concentrations of G-protein (Bowes *et al.* 1988) and phosphodiesterase (Farber *et al.* 1988) are 50% of the adult value when the photo-sensitive molecule, rhodopsin, is only 20–25% of adult values (Fulton *et al.* 1995). The postu-lated immaturity in activation of phototransduction does not deny devel-opmental changes in transmission from rod photoreceptors to second-order neurones, or post-receptoral processing, a role in controlling infants' scotopic performance.

The growth of ROS length in the near-central posterior pole region is de-layed relative to ROS growth in more peripheral retina; however, eventually both regions have equal ROS lengths (see Fig. 3.3). Additionally, the parafoveal rod cells as well as cones migrate toward the foveal centre (Diaz-Araya and Provis 1992; Packer *et al.* 1990), so that from around term into early adulthood, the packing density of the near-central rods continues to increase slightly (Packer *et al.* 1990). Both factors could contribute to the late maturation of near-central rod performance (Fulton *et al.* 1991*a*). Psychophysical thresholds for small stimuli in the near-central retina (10° eccentricity) and peripheral to the rod ring (30° eccentricity) may be functional correlates of rod cell development. Data from patients (see Fig. 3.7) suggest that, among retinal disorders of early onset, achromatopsia may alter the course of near-central rod development.

For the thresholds at 30°, the difference between normal infants and adults is about 0.5 log unit (Hansen and Fulton 1995*a*), the same as the infant–adult difference in sensitivities for full-field stimuli. Possibly the infant–adult sensitivity difference at 30° as well as at 10° can be accounted for by rhodopsin in developing ROS and consequent low quantum catch (Fulton *et al.* 1991*b*). However, post receptoral immaturities (Hansen *et al.* 1992; Hansen and Fulton 1994) cannot be excluded as contributors to the >1 log unit infant–adult difference in psychophysical thresholds.

In summary, even after term, monkey and human infants' rod cell structure and function are immature, with ROS and rod-mediated vision showing greater immaturity in near-central compared with more peripheral retina. The rod cell's physical immaturities, as described in this chapter, may account for many of the characteristics of the scotopic responses observed in electroretinographic and psychophysical studies of young human infants. A receptoral contribution to the control of sensitivity does not exclude developmental changes in transmission from photoreceptors to second-order neurones and receptive field properties as other determinants of infants' scotopic sensitivity (Fulton *et al.* 1992; van Coevorden *et al.* 1992; Hansen and Fulton 1994, 1995*b*).

ACKNOWLEDGEMENTS

Supported by EY05329, the Hearst Foundation and the Massachusetts Lions Eye Research Fund, Inc. (AF, RH); EY01208 and EY04536 and Research to Prevent Blindness, Inc. (AH). ED is a Medical Student Fellow of the Northwest Lions Sight Conservation Foundation. The technical assistance of Andra Erickson and the cooperation of the staff of the Regional Primate Research Center at the University of Washington is gratefully acknowledged.

REFERENCES

Baylor, D. A., Lamb, T. D., and Yau, K.-W. (1979). The membrane current of single rod outer segments. *Journal of Physiology (London)*, **288**, 589–611.

Bowes, C., van Veen, T., and Farber, D. B. (1988). Opsin, G-protein and 48-k Da protein in normal and *rd* mouse retinas: developmental expression of mRNAs and proteins and light/dark cycling of mRNAs. *Experimental Eye Research*, **47**, 369–90.

Breton, M. E., Schueller, A., Lamb, T., and Pugh, E. N. Jr (1993). Analysis of ERG a-wave amplification and kinetics in terms of the G-protein cascade of phototransduction. *Investigative Ophthalmology and Visual Science*, **35**, 295–309.

Broekhuyse, R. M. and Kuhlmann, E. D. (1989). Assay of S-antigen immunoreactivity in mammalian retinas in relation to age, ocular dimension and retinal degeneration. *Japanese Journal of Ophthalmology*, **33**, 243–50.

Brown, A. M. (1986). Scotopic sensitivity of the two-month-old human infant. *Vision Research*, **26**, 707–11.

Cantera, R., von Schantz, M., Chader, G. J., Ehinger, B., Sanyal, S., and van Veen, T. (1990). Postnatal development of photoreceptor-specific proteins in mice with hereditary retinal degeneration. *Experimental Biology*, **48**, 305–12.

Curcio, C. and Hendrickson, A. (1991). Organization and development of the primate photoreceptor mosaic, Vol. 10. In *Progress in Retinal Research*, (ed. N. N. Osborn, G. J. Chader), pp. 90–120. Pergamon Press, Oxford.

Curcio, C., Sloan, K., Kalina, R., and Hendrickson, A. (1990). Human photoreceptor topography. *Journal of Comparative Neurology*, **292**, 497–523.

Diaz-Araya, C. and Provis, J. M. (1992). Evidence of photoreceptor migration during early foveal development: A quantitative analysis of human fetal retina. *Visual Neuroscience*, **8**, 505–14.

Farber, D. B., Park, S., and Yamashita, C. (1988). Cyclic GMP-phosphodiesterase of rd retina: biosynthesis and content. *Experimental Eye Research*, **46**, 363–74.

Fulton, A. B. and Hansen, R. M. (1992). The rod sensitivity of dark-adapted human infants. *Current Eye Research*, **11**, 1193–8.

Fulton, A. B. and Hansen, R. M. (1993). Testing the possibly blind infant. In *The eye in infancy*. 2nd edn (ed. S. Isenberg), pp. 547–54. Mosby, St Louis.

Fulton, A. B., Dodge, J., Hansen, R. M., Schremser, J.-L., and Williams, T. P. (1991*a*). The quantity of rhodopsin in young human eyes. *Current Eye Research*, **10**, 977–82.

Fulton, A. B., Hansen, R. M., Yeh, Y.-L., and Tyler, C. W. (1991*b*). Temporal summation of dark adapted 10-week-old infants. *Vision Research*, **31**, 1259–69.

Fulton, A. B., Hansen, R. M., and Glynn, R. J. (1993). Natural course of visual functions in the Bardet-Biedl syndrome. *Archives of Ophthalmology*, **111**, 1500–6.

Fulton, A. B., Hansen, R. M., and Findl, O. (1995). The development of the rod photoresponse from dark adapted rats. *Investigative Ophthalmology and Visual Science*, **36**, 1038–45.

Hansen, R. M. and Fulton, A. B. (1981). Behavioral measurement of background adaptation in human infants. *Investigative Ophthalmology and Visual Science*, **21**, 625–9.

Hansen, R. M. and Fulton, A. B. (1993). Development of scotopic retinal sensitivity. In *Early visual development, normal and abnormal* (ed. K. Simons), pp. 130–42. Oxford University Press, New York.

Hansen, R. M. and Fulton, A. B. (1994). Scotopic center surround organization in 10-week-old infants. *Vision Research*, **94**, 621–4.

Hansen, R. M. and Fulton, A. B. (1995*a*). Dark adapted thresholds at 10- and 30-deg. eccentricities in 10-week old infants. *Visual Neuroscience*, **12**, 509–12.

Hansen, R. M. and Fulton, A. B. (1995*b*). The VEP thresholds for full-field stimuli in dark adapted infants. *Visual Neuroscience*, **12**, 223–8.

Hansen, R. M., Fulton, A. B., and Harris, S. J. (1986). Background adaptation in human infants. *Vision Research*, **26**, 771–9.

Hansen, R. M., Hamer, R. D., and Fulton, A. B. (1992). The effect of light adaptation on scotopic spatial summation in 10-week-old infants. *Vision Research*, **32**, 387–92.

Hansen, R. M., Petersen, R. A., and Fulton, A. B. (1993). Retinopathy of prematurity, even if mild, perturbs development of scotopic thresholds. *Investigative Ophthalmology and Visual Science*, **34** (suppl.), 1446.

Hargrave, P. A. and McDowell, J. H. (1992). Rhodopsin and phototransduction: a model system for G-protein-linked receptors. *Federation Experimental Biology (FASEB) Journal*, **6**, 2323–31.

Hendrickson, A. (1992). A morphological comparison of foveal development in man and monkey. *Eye*, **6**, 136–44.

Hendrickson, A. and Drucker, D. (1992). The development of parafoveal and mid-peripheral human retina. *Behavioural Brain Research*, **49**, 21–31.

Hendrickson, A. and Kupfer, C. (1976). The histogenesis of the fovea in the macaque monkey. *Investigative Ophthalmology and Visual Science*, **15**, 746–56.

Hicks, D. and Barnstable, C. J. (1987). Different rhodopsin monoclonal antibodies reveal different binding patterns on developing and adult rat retina. *Journal of Histochemistry and Cytochemistry*, **35**, 1317–28.

Ho, A. K., Somers, R. L., and Klein, D. C. (1986). Development and regulation of rhodopsin kinase in rat pineal and retina. *Journal of Neurochemistry*, **46**, 1176–9.

Hoglund, G., Nilsson, S. E., and Schwemer, J. (1982). Visual pigment and visual receptor cells in fetal and adult sheep. *Investigative Ophthalmology and Visual Science*, **23**, 409–18.

Hood, D. C. and Birch, D. G. (1990a). The a-wave of the human electroretinogram and rod receptor function. *Investigative Ophthalmology and Visual Science*, **31**, 2070–81.

Hood, D. C. and Birch, D. G. (1990b). A quantitative measure of the electrical activity of human rod photoreceptors using electroretinography. *Visual Neuroscience*, **5**, 379–87.

Hood, D. C. and Birch, D. G. (1990c). The relationship between models of receptor activity and the a-wave of the ERG. *Clinical Visual Science*, **5**, 293–7.

Hood, D. C. and Birch, D. G. (1994). Rod estimation in retinitis pigmentosa: estimation and interpretation of parameters derived from the rod a-wave. *Investigative Ophthalmology and Visual Science*, **35**, 2948–61.

Jacobson, S. G., Borruat, F.-X., and Apathy, M. S. (1990). Patterns of rod and cone dysfunction in Bardet-Biedl syndrome. *American Journal of Ophthalmology*, **109**, 676–88.

Lamb, T. D. and Pugh, E. N. Jr (1992). A quantitative account of the activation steps involved in phototransduction in amphibian photoreceptors. *Journal of Physiology (London)*, **449**, 719–58.

LaVail, M. M., Rappaport, D. H., and Rakic, P. (1991). Cytogenesis in the monkey retina. *Journal of Comparative Neurology*, **309**, 86–114.

Lee, R. H., Lieberman, B. S., and Lolley, R. N. (1990). Retinal accumulation of the phosducin/$T_{\beta\gamma}$ and transducin complexes in developing normal mice and in mice and dogs inherited retinal degeneration. *Experimental Eye Research*, **51**, 325–33.

Massof, R. W. and Finkelstein, D. (1979). Rod sensitivity relative to cone sensitivity in retinitis pigmentosa. *Investigative Ophthalmology and Visual Science*, **18**, 263–72.

Molday, R. S. and MacKenzie, D. (1983). Monoclonal antibodies to rhodopsin characterization, cross-reactivity and application as structure probes. *Biochemistry*, **22**, 653–60.

Packer, O., Hendrickson, A. E., and Curcio, C. A. (1990). Developmental redistribution of photoreceptors across the *Macaca nemestrina* (pigtail macaque) retina. *Journal of Comparative Neurology*, **298**, 472–93.

Powers *et al.* (1979).

Powers, M. K., Schneck, M. S., and Teller, D. Y. (1981). Spectral sensitivity of human infants at absolute visual threshold. *Vision Research*, **21**, 1005–16.

Pugh, E. N. Jr and Lamb, T. D. (1993). Amplification and kinetics of the activation steps in phototransduction. *Biochimica et Biophysica Acta, Reviews on Bioenergetics*, **1141**, 111–49.

Teller, D. Y. (1979). The forced choice preferential looking method: a psychophysical technique for use with human infants. *Infant Behavior and Development*, **2**, 135–53.

van Coevorden, R. E., Breton, M. E., and Quinn, G. E. (1992). Changes in ERG a-wave maximum velocity in the developing infant eye. *Investigative Ophthalmology and Visual Science*, **33** (suppl.), 1409.

Wetherill, G. B. and Levitt, H. (1966). Sequential estimation of points on a psychometric function. *British Journal of Mathematical and Statistical Psychology*, **18**, 1–10.

Yuodelis, C. and Hendrickson, A. E. (1986). A qualitative and quantitative analysis of the human fovea during development. *Vision Research*, **26**, 847–56.

4

Assessing dimensionality in infant colour vision

Kenneth Knoblauch, Michelle Bieber, and John S. Werner

INTRODUCTION

Since the human visual system continues to mature and to be influenced by the visual environment over at least the first 2 years of life, the practical benefit of studies of infant vision will be in the development of screening tools for the early identification of visual deficits that might be correctable with early intervention. Along these lines, some recent studies have demonstrated with great success techniques for screening infant visual acuity (Teller *et al.* 1986; Vital-Durand and Hullo 1990). It would be of similar value to devise a screening test for infant colour vision. Since the trichromacy of normal adult colour vision requires three classes of functioning cone photoreceptors in the retina, as well as integrity of the parvocellular stream of the visual pathway from retina through the lateral geniculate nucleus to the cortex (Kaplan *et al.* 1988; Lennie and D'Zmura 1988; Shapley 1990), colour vision testing would be a valuable tool for screening for defects in this portion of the developing visual system. Such a test would be of use in the assessment of residual function in infants with partial vision or other disabilities, as well as in identifying the approximately 8% of males who inherit an abnormality of one of the longer wavelength-sensitive cone photopigment genes that result in a red–green colour defect. While tests for screening infant colour have been proposed recently (Pease and Allen 1988; Mercer *et al.* 1991), several factors may make them more difficult to interpret than equivalent adult tests. In this chapter, some of these difficulties shall be reviewed and preliminary data using techniques aimed toward ameliorating them will be presented.

NON-PARAMETRIC TESTING: MINIMAL TESTS OF COLOUR VISION

A minimal test of infant colour vision requires demonstrating the ability to discriminate at least one pair of lights solely on the basis of the differences in their spectral distributions. To rule out discriminations that might be based on a brightness cue, the intensity of one of the lights must be varied over the course of the test. If the infant can discriminate successfully between the pair of lights over the full range of intensities tested and if the step size is sufficiently small to adequately sample this range, then the hypothesis that a single photopigment mediates vision is rejected. Peeples and Teller (1975) showed in this fashion that 2-month-old infants can discriminate a long-wavelength light from a broad-band white. Note that success on this test provides no evidence of the identity nor the exact number of the discriminating mechanisms. Thus, Peeples and Teller's result proves the vision of 2-month-old infants to be at least dichromatic.

Normal adult colour vision is trichromatic, however. One minimal test of trichromacy requires showing that an individual can discriminate any monochromatic light from a given broad-band light, in other words a **neutral-point test**. This test requires two degrees of freedom since both the wavelength and the intensity of the monochromatic light must be varied to test for the existence of a discrimination failure. Thus, if the minimal test of colour vision—what might be called a test for a **brightness match**—requires n intensity levels to be tested, then a neutral-point test would require nm stimuli to be tested, where m is the number of wavelengths examined. Teller and co-workers (1978) investigated the ability of 2-month-old infants to discriminate between various coloured test lights and a broad-band background illuminant. Because of the multiplicative increase in the number of stimuli that need to be tested in this type of experiment, and also the limited time available with each infant, they had to evaluate different wavelength regions with different infants. Interestingly, they found that 2-month-old infants failed to discriminate certain of their test lights (appearing yellowish-green and mid-purple to a normal adult) from their broad-band comparison (a yellowish-white provided by tungsten illumination). This result might seem to indicate that, at 2 months, colour vision is only dichromatic; however, a few caveats should be noted.

First, ordinarily discrimination failures give a clue to the identity of the underlying mechanisms. In the case of the brightness match, the relative intensities of the two lights in the test at the discrimination failure provide a measure of the spectral sensitivity of the substrate mechanism. In the case of a neutral-point match, the wavelengths at which discrimination failures occur provide information about the directions in colour space along which the lights are equated for the spectral sensitivities of the two receptor types. To interpret these, however, requires that these spectral sensitivities be known or, equivalently, that the results be plotted in a chromaticity diagram based on these spectral sensitivities. The colour confusions shown by infants in the experiment by Teller *et al.* do not lie on a common line when plotted in the CIE chromaticity diagram. This diagram, however, is based on the spectral sensitivities of the adult observer and those of the infant may differ systematically (described later). Second, to be rigorous, this test requires the comparison of monochromatic and broad-band lights. Most of the lights that Teller *et al.* tested and all of the ones for which discrimination failures occurred were removed from the spectrum locus. This is also true of the test proposed by Mercer *et al.* (1991), which is based on neutral-point discriminations. As Teller *et al.* have observed, poor overall chromatic contrast sensitivity instead of the absence of a specific class of receptors would yield similar results (see also Banks and Bennett 1988).

Another difficulty arises in interpreting these types of infant colour vision tests. The neutral-point match is a sufficient test for trichromacy in adults because stimulus size, fixation and intensity level can be strictly controlled. In infant testing, large stimuli must be used; even with the most rigorous of care, fixation is at best weakly controlled; in addition, the intensity ranges over which infant vision have been examined tend to be at the low-photopic or high-mesopic levels. All of these conditions favour the contribution of the rod photoreceptors. Thus, failure to discriminate in a neutral-point test could result if infants used rods and one class of cone photoreceptors. Passing this test could result with rods and two classes of cones. Given the increase in the parameter space necessary to test even a neutral-point match in infants, the requirements of the next level of testing—a test for pairs of spectral lights that match a broadband light or a **complementary-pair test**—are out of the question with existing methods.

PARAMETRIC TESTING: RECEPTOR ISOLATION

The discrimination tests described above are non-parametric in the sense that they can be used to infer the dimensionality of colour discrimination with no assumptions about the spectral sensitivities of the underlying photoreceptors. The cost of this distribution-free approach is that the number of conditions that need to be tested grows geometrically with the number of photoreceptor classes for which one would like to find evidence.

Alternatively, one can consider a parametric approach. It is parametric in the sense that specific assumptions are made about the infant photoreceptor spectral sensitivities. Such assumptions allow, in principle, the construction of stimuli that drive the responses of one class of receptors in isolation, by holding the output of the others constant. This technique has been variously termed 'silent substitution', 'spectral compensation' and 'receptor isolation' (Estévez and Spekreijse 1982; Shapley 1990) but it has been only partially exploited in infant colour-vision testing (Hamer *et al.* 1982; Packer *et al.* 1984; Varner *et al.* 1985).

For example, Hamer *et al.* (1982) examined infants in the age range 1–3 months for discrimination failures between a 589 nm light and either a 550 nm or a broad-band long wavelength light (dominant wavelength 633 nm). In this region of the spectrum, the foveal vision of normal adults is dichromatic because the short-wavelength-sensitive (S) cones have a negligible sensitivity and discrimination is mediated by only the middle- (M) and long- (L) wavelength-sensitive cones (known as M-cones and L-cones). In principle, with only two cone classes, the ratio of two lights can be adjusted to equate the quantum catch for one of them so that the response is mediated by the other.

Hamer *et al.* tested a range of ratios that included ones that would be silent for M- and L-cones. Therefore, from the ability of 3-month-old and most 2-month-old infants to discriminate between these lights, one might argue that these infants have functioning M- and L-cones. As these investigators acknowledge, however, under their conditions, they could not exclude a response based on one cone type and the rods.

Is it likely that rods contribute a significant signal for wavelengths from the long wavelength portion of the spectrum? In Fig. 4.1(a) is shown data that the authors collected with the Visually Evoked Potential (VEP) from an adult protanope (aged 40) in response to square-wave flicker (7.5 Hz) between pairs of monochromatic lights equated for the Smith and Pokorny (1975) M-cone fundamental. The field was a disk of 6° diameter rear-projected on a dark surround and freely viewed with central vision. Its mean intensity was increased continuously over a 30-s period, while a vector voltmeter extracted the phase independent amplitude of the fundamental response (using a 4-s time constant). Since a protanope lacks L-cones, the field should appear steady and the VEP should show no response. For the 645/590 pair (solid line), the amplitude of the fundamental is low and does not increase over the range of luminances allowed by the optical system. However, for the 550/590 pair (dotted line) the amplitude of the fundamental begins to rise near a mean luminance of $1.0 \, cd/m^2$. That this response is caused by rods is suggested by the fact that the observer described the field as steady but experienced strong flicker in the surrounding field, presumably from scattered light whose modulation was not equated for the rods. Although obtained from an adult, this result is also consistent with those of Clavedetscher *et al.* (1988; see also Brown 1990) who found that discrimination behaviour of infants for wavelengths less than 540 nm followed the scotopic spectral sensitivity curve, which is mediated by the rod photoreceptors. For purposes of comparison, the horizontal bar in the upper right of the figure indicates the luminance range within which most studies of infant colour vision have been performed.

Given that three potential receptor classes can contribute to a discrimination, varying the ratio of two lights can only silence one of them. To make a stimulus that silences two receptor classes in order to isolate the third requires three lights. For example, the normal Rayleigh match for diagnosing red–green colour defects in adults uses a mixture of 545 nm and 670 nm matched against a 589 nm comparison. A normal trichromat produces a unique mixture to match the comparison that equates the quantum catch across the two fields for both the M- and L-cones. If a third receptor class were active, it would, in general, be stimulated differentially by the two fields and no such match would be possible.

The authors have been using a three-primary stimulus in this fashion to silence two classes of photoreceptor simultaneously. In our stimulus, a mixture of 540 nm and 610 nm is flickered against a 570 nm stimulus. The ratio of the mixture and the intensity of the 570 nm stimulus are adjusted in different conditions to isolate either the Smith and Pokorny L- or M-cones or the rods as

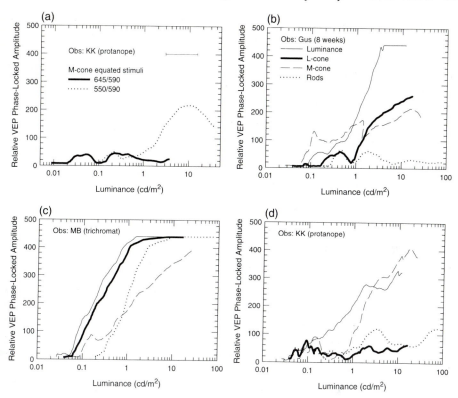

Fig. 4.1 Relative VEP phase-locked amplitude as a function of mean luminance of a square-wave flickering stimulus (7.5 Hz). (a) Responses from a protanope to counterphase flicker of pairs of lights (wavelengths indicated in legend) that are equated for M-cone response. Each curve is the average of 4 records. (b) Responses from an 8-week-old male to square-wave alternation of a mixture of 540 and 610 nm against 570 nm and to luminance flicker (570 nm). The number of records averaged for each curve are as follows: Luminance (1), L-cone isolation (2), M-cone isolation (3), rod isolation (4). (c) Responses from an adult trichromat to luminance and receptor-isolating stimuli as in (b). Conditions are indicated by the legend from (b). Each curve is the mean of 5–6 records. (d) Responses of protanope to luminance and receptor-isolating stimuli. Conditions are indicated by the legend from (b). Each response is the mean of 4–6 records.

defined by the scotopic luminous efficiency function, V'_λ (Wyszecki and Stiles 1982). In Fig. 4.1(b) the VEP responses obtained from an 8-week-old male infant to each of these isolation conditions and to pure luminance flicker are shown. The response to luminance flicker of the 570 nm stimulus alone (thin solid line) is robust. Smaller but significant responses are given to the L- and M-cone islolating conditions (thick solid and dashed lines, respectively). No discernible response is evident under rod isolation (dotted line). Although little of generality should be concluded from the records of a single infant, the results are consistent with other studies that begin to show evidence for a chromatic response in infants by 8 weeks of age (Brown and Teller 1989; Morrone *et al.* 1990). Such a chromatic response in this portion of the spectrum requires the presence of both L- and M-cones, which this infant's responses seem to indicate are present. The lack of rod response with our 6° field is consistent with the findings of Yuodelis and Hendrickson (1986) of an enlarged rod-free area in infants. Our data should be interpreted with some caution on this point, however, as we find individual differences in the rod response among adults (as discussed later).

A disadvantage of this approach is that there is no independent criterion in the data to show that the stimuli have actually isolated the mechanism in question. There are several indirect tests that one can perform, however, to satisfy oneself of the isolation efficiency of a stimulus. First, individuals with normal colour vision should respond robustly to each of the stimuli. In Fig. 4.1(c) is shown data from an adult trichromat (female, age 22 years) for each of the isolating conditions and luminance flicker. Compared with the infant's response, a robust response is seen in each condition. Interestingly, in this observer the rod isolation condition (dotted curve) produces a strong response. As with the protanope for bichromatic flicker (Fig. 4.1(a)), she described the flicker in this condition as occurring outside the 6° stimulus in the periphery. No such peripheral flicker was seen by any of the adult observers for the other isolating conditions, indicating the efficacy of the nulling of rods for these stimuli. The lateral displacement of the response to the M-cone isolating stimulus along the luminance axis probably reflects the fact that the M-cone stimulus produced a lower cone contrast (0.23) than the L-cone stimulus (0.37).

Second, individuals without a particular mechanism (e.g. colour defective individuals) ought to be unresponsive under conditions that isolate the mechanism they lack. As an example of this test, the data in Fig. 4.1(d) from the protanope of Fig. 4.1(a) under each of the isolating conditions is shown. This individual gives a robust response to both the luminance and M-cone isolating stimuli (thin solid and dashed lines, respectively). In addition, a weak response is evident under conditions of rod isolation (dotted curve). A considerably stronger response (not shown) was observed for this condition with peripheral fixation. Most importantly, however, the response to L-cone modulation (thick solid curve) is negligible. This result should be compared with the responses shown in Fig. 4.1(a), which compensated for the response of only one of the three classes of photoreceptors active in this spectral region. The authors have also tested a deuteranopic observer, who produced results converse to those of the protanope in that the M-cone response was negligible and the L-cone response was robust. Ultimately, it must be shown that these stimuli serve to similarly identify colour-defective infants.

Third, one should be able to evaluate the significance of residual contrast in the putatively silenced mechanisms under hypotheses that the spectral sensitivities on which one has based the design of the stimuli are in error. For example, while it is reasonable to assume that the photopigments mediating infant vision are the same as those found in the adult, the spectral sensitivities of the photoreceptors containing these pigments as measured at the cornea are likely to differ from those of adults. Three factors that will produce such differences are lower absorption in the lens (Werner 1982) and macular pigment (Bone *et al.* 1988) and the shorter outer segments of infant cones (Abramov *et al.* 1982). Shorter cone outer segments result in a lower optical density of cone photopigment, which, in turn, yields spectral sensitivities slightly narrower than those of adults (Wyszecki and Stiles 1982).

For wavelengths greater than about 540 nm, the variations of lens and macular pigment density among observers are likely to be negligible. Thus, variance in these two factors should be insignificant in our results. Since the validity of the calculation of a receptor-isolating stimulus depends on accurate knowledge of the spectral sensitivity of the silenced photoreceptors, the change in spectral sensitivity of the cones from optical density factors ought to be more critical.

The effects of differences in optical density can be evaluated in several different ways. First, consider that the Smith and Pokorny fundamentals as tabulated represent the spectral sensitivities for adult foveal vision. To calculate the effectiveness of foveally presented stimuli requires no additional assumptions. To make similar calculations under conditions of reduced optical density (e.g. for stimuli presented to peripheral vision or probably for infant vision) requires that the peak optical densities of the foveal cones are known (or assumed) and that absorption of light by the photopigments in cones obeys the Beer-Lambert law (Wyszecki and Stiles 1982), which relates absorption and optical density to the concentration of the photopigment and length of the cone outer segment. The greater the optical density assumed in the fovea, the narrower will be the spectral sensitivity in the periphery or an equivalent low optical density condition. The limiting low density spectral sensitivity for a given peak foveal optical density is called the extinction spectrum. If the foveal peak optical density is sufficiently high, stimulus conditions that are equated for two receptor classes in the fovea will not be equated for the extinction spectrum. The three panels of Fig. 4.2(a) show for the wavelength triple that was used (540, 570, 610 nm) how receptor contrast of the cone extinction spectra and the rods will vary for each receptor-isolating condition as a function of the peak foveal cone density if the stimuli are equated for pairs of the tabulated spectral sensitivities (foveal M and L for cones; V'_λ for rods). Owing to the short cone outer segments in the infant retina and in the adult periphery, it is assumed that the cone extinction spectra better approximate to spectral sensitivities in these conditions. In this calculation, the rod spectral sensitivity was assumed to be unchanged, since rod outer segment length is unlikely to vary with eccentricity—although it differs between infant and adult (Hendrickson and Drucker 1992).

For each isolating condition, as the optical density assumed in the fovea increases, the contrast for the extinction spectra of cone classes assumed to be nulled increases from zero to contrasts on the order of 0.1 over the range examined in the figure. Since the rod optical density does not change, the rod contrast (dotted line in right panel; at contrast of zero in left and middle panels) is invariant. To gauge the effectiveness of this residual contrast, the Weber fraction, as estimated from increment thresholds mediated by L cones (Wyszecki and Stiles 1982), is shown as a dot–dash line spanning the three panels—the value for the M cones is quite similar. The dot–dash line restricted to the right panel indicates the optimal Weber fraction for rods (Wyszecki and Stiles 1982). The proximity of this value to the computed rod contrast under our rod-isolation condition (right panel, dotted line) may account for the variation among adults that is seen in the rod response. The rapid growth of contrast in the putatively nulled receptor classes suggests that if the foveal cones have a peak optical density greater than about 0.2, then peripherally presented stimuli (and, by analogy, stimuli presented to an infant) may no longer effectively isolate a single receptor class.

The data in Fig. 4.2(b) support this suggestion. A protanopic observer viewing centrally a 6° field was presented with the L-cone isolating stimuli equated for the rods and the M-cone extinction spectrum as a function of the peak optical density assumed for foveal M-cones. For each stimulus, the observer rated the salience of the flicker on a 10-point scale, where 1 indicated no flicker and 10 indicated very strong flicker. Each stimulus was presented three times, with the order randomized. None of the stimuli appeared to flicker very strongly, since values as great as the scale maximum were never recorded in the data. By the time the assumed peak optical density reached about 0.2, the observer reliably could detect flicker in the stimulus.

While this demonstration shows the psychophysical consequences of incorrect assumptions about photopigment optical density, is such residual contrast sufficient to drive the VEP? In Fig. 4.2(c) VEP records from the same protanopic observer with each of the L-cone isolating stimuli of Fig. 4.2(b) are shown. For values of assumed peak optical density in the range 0.0–0.2, the curves appear quite flat. In the range 0.3–0.5, a small signal might have been recorded but the record for 0.6 is no different from the low density conditions. These data suggest that over the reasonable range of cone optical densities that one might assume for human vision, an incorrect assumption is not likely to lead to incorrectly concluding from VEP data that a protanope has an L-cone response.

While the above tests and analyses bolster confidence in the isolation techniques, the most direct test that can be performed is to demonstrate that the response to an isolation stimulus has the spectral sensitivity assumed for the isolated class of receptors. This can be done by varying the wavelength of one of the components of the isolation stimulus in such a fashion as to vary the receptor contrast of the stimulus. The displacement of the VEP record along the luminance axis would then generate a spectral sensitivity. Alternatively, the efficiency of adapting fields of various wavelengths can be gauged for a particular receptor class by determining the radiance of the field that displaces the response to the isolating stimulus a fixed amount along the luminance axis (Estévez *et al.* 1975). This procedure would also generate a spectral sensitivity. In either case, given the number of stimuli that would be required for a

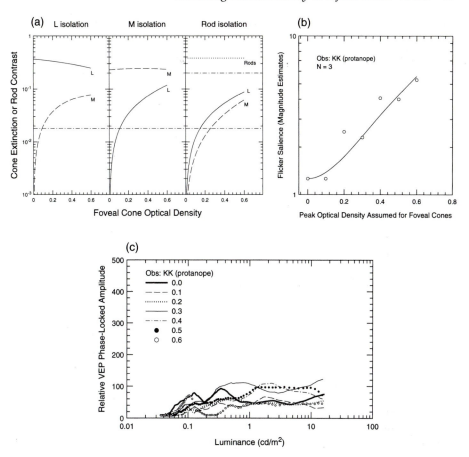

Fig. 4.2 (a) Calculated receptor contrasts to 100% modulation of a mixture of 610 and 540 nm against 570 nm adjusted for foveal L-cone isolation (left panel), foveal M-cone isolation (middle panel) and rod isolation (right panel) as a function of peak optical density of the foveal cones when sensitivity is determined by the cone extinction spectra and the rods. (b) Magnitude estimates of salience of flicker reported by a protanope in response to L-cone isolating stimuli that were calculated based on V'_λ and the M-cone extinction spectrum as a function of the peak optical density of the foveal M-cones. Each point is the geometric mean of three estimates. The curve is the best-fitting parabola. (c) VEP records from a protanope for the range of L-cone isolating stimuli in (b).

rigorous result, it is unlikely that one would be able to test more than one receptor class in a given infant at a given age. This situation may be sufficient for validating the isolation procedure, however.

An obvious extension of the above procedures is to introduce a fourth stimulus that would allow one to create stimuli that would null the response of three receptor classes simultaneously. In this way, the measurements would permit a more systematic study of the S-cones. Using chromatic adaptation to minimize the response of the other receptor classes, Volbrecht and Werner (1987) demonstrated the presence of an S-cone signal in the VEP records of infants as young as 4 weeks old. The use of receptor isolating stimuli would in principle facilitate identification of such signals. Individual differences in the optical density of the lens (Werner, 1982) would probably complicate such investigations, however.

In this chapter, several methods for testing infant colour vision and some factors that complicate the efficient implementation of these methods have been reviewed. The use of receptor-isolating stimuli remains a promising approach for screening infants but much more data using these procedures need to be collected to make a convincing story. The conservative assessment at this juncture would be that an efficient screening test for infant colour vision remains an elusive goal.

ACKNOWLEDGEMENT

Experimental work was conducted with the support of NIH grant HD19143.

REFERENCES

Abramov, I., Gordon, J., Hendrickson, A., Hainline, L., Dobson, V., and La Boissiere, E. (1982). The retina of the newborn human infant. *Science*, **217**, 265–7.

Banks, M. S. and Bennett, P. J. (1988). Optical and photoreceptor immaturities limit the spatial and chromatic vision of human neonates. *Journal of the Optical Society of America A*, **5**, 2059–79.

Bone, R. A., Landrum, J. T., Fernandez, L., and Tarsis, S. L. (1988). Analysis of the macular pigment by HPLC: Retinal distribution and age study. *Investigative Ophthalmology and Visual Science*, **29**, 843–9.

Brown, A. M. (1990). Development of visual sensitivity to light and colour vision in human infants: a critical review. *Vision Research*, **30**, 1159–88.

Brown, A. M. and Teller, D. Y. (1989). Color opponency in 3-month-old human infants. *Vision Research*, **29**, 37–45.

Clavedetscher, J. E., Brown, A. M., Ankrum, C., and Teller, D. Y. (1988). Spectral sensitivity and chromatic discriminations in 3- and 7-week-old human infants. *Journal of the Optical Society of America A*, **5**, 2093–105.

Estévez, O. and Spekreijse, H. (1982). The 'silent substitution' method in visual research. *Vision Research*, **22**, 681–91.

Estévez, O., Spekreijse, H., Van den Berg, T. J. T. P., and Cavonius, C. R. (1975). The spectral sensitivities of isolated human color mechanisms determined from contrast evoked-potential measurements. *Vision Research*, **15**, 1205–12.

Hamer, R. D., Alexander, K. R., and Teller, D. Y. (1982). Rayleigh discriminations in young human infants. *Vision Research*, **22**, 575–87.

Hendrickson, A. and Drucker, D. (1992). The development of parafoveal and mid-peripheral human retina. *Behavioural Brain Research*, **49**, 21–31.

Kaplan, E., Shapley, R. M., and Purpura, K. (1988). Color and luminance contrast as tools for probing the primate retina. *Neuroscience Research*, **8** (suppl.), S151–65.

Lennie, P. and D'Zmura, M. (1988). Mechanisms of colour vision. *CRC Critical Reviews in Neurobiology*, **3**, 333–400.

Mercer, M. E., Courage, M. L., and Adams, R. J. (1991). Contrast/color card procedure: a new test of young infant's color vision. *Optometry and Vision Science*, **68**, 522–32.

Morrone, M. C., Burr, D. C., and Fiorentini, A. (1990). Development of contrast sensitivity and acuity of the infant colour system. *Proceedings of the Royal Society of London*, **242**, 134–9.

Packer, O., Hartmann, E. E., and Teller, D. Y. (1984). Infant color vision: the effect of test field size on Rayleigh discriminations. *Vision Research*, **24**, 1247–60.

Pease, P. L. and Allen, J. (1988). A new test for screening color vision: concurrent validity and utility. *American Journal of Optometry and Physiological Optics*, **65**, 729–38.

Peeples, D. R. and Teller, D. Y. (1975). Color vision and brightness discrimination in two-month-old human infants. *Science*, **189**, 1102–3.

Shapley, R. M. (1990). Visual sensitivity and parallel retinocortical channels. *Annual Review of Psychology*, **41**, 635–58.

Smith, V. C. and Pokorny, J. (1975). Spectral sensitivity of the foveal cone photopigments between 400 and 500 nm. *Vision Research*, **15**, 161–71.

Teller, D. Y., Peeples, D. R., and Sekel, M. (1978). Discrimination of chromatic from white light by two-month-old human infants. *Vision Research*, **18**, 41–8.

Teller, D. Y., MacDonald, M. A., Preston, K., Sebris, S., and Dobson, V. (1986). Assessment of visual acuity in infants and children: the acuity card procedure. *Developmental Medicine and Child Neurology*, **28**, 779–89.

Varner, D., Cook, J. E., Schneck, M. E., MacDonald, M. A., and Teller, D. Y. (1985). Tritan discriminations by 1- and 2-month-old human infants. *Vision Research*, **25**, 821–31.

Vital-Durand, F. and Hullo, A. (1990). Cinq cents examens d'acuité visuelle du nourrisson avec les Cartes d'Acuité de Teller. *Ophtalmologie*, **4**, 208–11.

Volbrecht, V. J. and Werner, J. S. (1987). Isolation of short-wavelength-sensitive cone photoreceptors in 4–6-week-old human infants. *Vision Research*, **27**, 469–78.

Werner, J. S. (1982). Development of scotopic sensitivity and the absorption spectrum of the human ocular media. *Journal of the Optical Society of America*, **72**, 247–58.

Wyszecki, G. and Stiles, W. S. (1982). *Color science: concepts and methods, quantitative data and formulae*, (2nd edn.). Wiley, New York.

Yuodelis, C. and Hendrickson, A. (1986). A qualitative and quantitative analysis of the human fovea during development. *Vision Research*, **26**, 847–55.

5

Spatial and temporal properties of infant colour vision

David C. Burr, M. Concetta Morrone, and Adriana Fiorentini

INTRODUCTION

Information processing for colour vision starts in the retinal photoreceptors and proceeds through the inner retina, the lateral geniculate nucleus, and visual cortex. At the photoreceptor level, the spectral composition of light is analysed with three cone types with different absorption spectra, as suggested by the trichromatic theory of Young and Helmholtz. However, at the next retinal stages and at all subsequent sites, colour information is processed by cells organized into colour-opponent receptive fields, as suggested by the Hering opponent theory of colour vision (Hurvich and Jameson 1957). In this chapter, some of the evidence for development of these mechanisms will be reviewed, a few recent experiments from our laboratory will be described in detail.

When studying the development of colour vision in infants, it is useful to try and distinguish between possible neonatal immaturities at a pre-receptor or receptor levels and immaturities of the post-receptoral level, either retinal or more central. In Chapter 4, Knoblauch *et al.* discuss several techniques for testing infant colour vision at the receptor level, using receptor-isolating stimuli. They also review briefly the psychophysical studies on infant hue discrimination, showing that infants younger than 2 months are either unable to discriminate between equiluminant lights differing in spectral composition, or that discrimination performance is very poor and limited to very large stimuli (see also Teller and Bornstein 1987; Brown 1990). In this chapter recent studies of infant colour vision development aimed at elucidating the role of post-receptoral neural mechanisms will be concentrated upon.

PSYCHOPHYSICAL STUDIES OF INFANT COLOUR VISION

The Hering theory on colour-opponent neural channels was based largely on the observation that yellow is a unique chromatic sensation, and that it is not experienced perceptually as a synthesis of red and green. For normal adults there are four unique hues: blue, green, yellow and red; each is localized in a precise region of the spectrum. The spectral locations of the unique hues for adult subjects have been estimated by Boynton and Gordon (1965) by 'colour naming'. While it is impossible to ask an infant directly to 'name' colours, habituation techniques have been applied to estimate the colours perceived by infants as being in the same class. These studies suggest that 4-month-old infants categorize spectral hues similarly to adults (Bornstein *et al.* 1976; for a review of more recent hue-categorization experiments in infants, see Teller and Bornstein 1987). If the results of colour naming in adults reflect the functional properties of colour opponent cells (De Valois 1973), then the experiments with infant hue categorization suggest that colour-opponent mechanisms are present in 4-month-olds, with properties at least qualitatively similar to those of adults.

Psychophysical evidence suggesting the presence of red–green colour opponent channels in 3-month-olds was first provided by Brown and Teller (1989), who demonstrated the 'Sloan' notch in the spectral sensitivity curve of infants in the yellow region (580 nm) of the spectrum, where adults also show a notch when tested under the same adaptation conditions. Their findings are well explained by a colour opponent model based on the spectral curves of adult pigments of long- (L-) and medium- (M-) wavelength cones.

All psychophysical experiments on colour discrimination in young infants agree that when colour discrimination is possible, it requires very large stimuli. Packer *et al.* (1984) found that 1-month-olds could discriminate a 650 nm field from a 589 nm surround if the field diameter was 4° but that they could not make the discrimination for 2° stimuli. They also found that 3-month-olds discriminate fields of 2°, but not 1° diameter. On the basis of a habituation experiment, Adams *et al.* (1990) claim that even newborns can discriminate red (peak at 650 nm) and green (peak at 540 nm) stimuli from white equated in luminance, provided that the stimulus size is at least 8°. However, these latter findings are based on group averages and it is uncertain whether they can be interpreted as a successful discrimination under equiluminant conditions for single infants (Brown 1990).

VISUAL-EVOKED POTENTIALS

The dependence of infant colour discrimination upon stimulus size suggests that, in order to evaluate quantitatively the development of sensitivity to colour contrast, it is important to explore the role of the spatial and temporal characteristics of the stimulus. So far, this has not been performed in a very systematic fashion with psychophysical techniques. However, the visual-evoked potential (VEP) technique lends itself readily to studying infant vision, and this technique has been applied recently to study the development of colour vision (Morrone *et al.* 1990, 1993; Fiorentini *et al.* 1992; Allen *et al.* 1993;

Rudduck and Harding 1993). In the remainder of this chapter we discuss in some detail some of these results.

For the experiments to be described, the stimuli were red–green tartan patterns (resembling a defocused checkerboard), made by summing vertical with horizontal sinusoids on the screen of a high-resolution monitor (full details are given in Morrone *et al.* 1993). The relative strength of red (R) and green (G) luminances could be varied without varying mean luminance by varying the *colour ratio* (R/R+G) of the stimulus in a similar way to that described by Mullen (1985). When the colour ratio was 0 or 1, the stimulus was only modulated in luminance (green–black or red–black). For intermediate ratios, there was also a red–green chromatic modulation and, at some ratios (0.5 for most adults), the pattern is equiluminant, having contrast only in chromaticity. As detailed in the chapter by Knoblauch *et al.*, modulating two lights out of phase at appropriate intensities will silence one class of photo-receptor. For our red–green stimuli the colour ratios to silence the photo-receptors were 0.45 for the long-wave (L-) cones and 0.7 for the medium-wave (M-) cones. At 0.82 both the short-wave (S-) cones and the rods should be silent but, as the wavelength of the stimulus was mainly above 500 nm, neither of these receptors responded well at any colour ratio.

In general, the spatial frequency of the stimulus was very low, often 0.1 cycles/degree. The reason for this was to minimize possible chromatic aberrations (see Flitcroft 1989), that could create spurious luminance contrast, giving an artefactual response to chromatic stimuli. This is a particular problem with young infants, who exhibit a continuous variability in accommodation (see Chapter 8), that would serve to bring either the red or green patterns more into focus. For moderate and high spatial frequencies, the variation in focus would systematically vary the effective contrast of the red and green components, so the stimulus would seldom be really equiluminant. However, although this effect may become significant around 1 cycle/degree (see Morrone *et al.* 1993), it should be negligible at 0.1 cycles/degree.

How the amplitude and phase of the VEP of an adult observer (3500 weeks) varied with colour ratio is shown in Fig. 5.1. VEPs were measured under two experimental conditions, for stimuli of 6 Hz, 90% contrast, and 7.5 Hz, 30% contrast. Under both conditions, there was a strong VEP response at all colour ratios, indicating that stimuli of both luminance contrast and colour contrast can elicit VEPs, and that the VEP technique is appropriate for chromatic stimuli. Both curves are symmetrical around the equiluminant point (evaluated by psychophysical means, indicated by arrows), with an amplitude maximum at equiluminance in one condition, and a minimum in the other. Maxima at equiluminance were generally observed with stimuli of low temporal frequency and high contrast, whereas minima occurred at high temporal frequency and low contrast. At sufficiently high temporal frequencies, the response disappeared completely at equiluminance.

Examples of typical VEP response curves as a function of colour-ratio at 8.5 and 22 weeks for two different infants are shown in Fig. 5.2(a,c) (open symbols

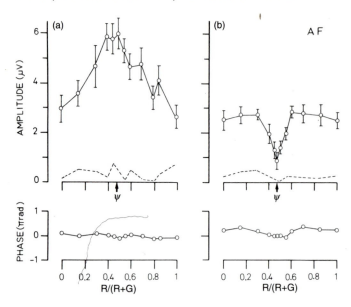

Fig. 5.1 Amplitude and phase recorded from an adult observer as a function of colour ratio of the tartan pattern. Colour ratio 0.5 refers to equiluminant red–green patterns, while ratios 0 and 1 are pure luminance patterns (green–black or red–black). The arrow indicates the point of equiluminance assessed by psychophysical means for this observer. The broken line shows the estimate of noise, and the error bars ±1 SE of the variation in amplitude (phase error was less than symbol size). For the curve (a) temporal frequency was 6.2 Hz and contrast 90%, and for (b) 7.5 Hz and 30%. Spatial frequency was 1 cycle/degree in both conditions. In both examples the amplitude curves are symmetrical about equiluminance, in one case with a local maximum and the other a local minimum. (Reprinted from Morrone *et al.* 1993.)

only). As with the adult, both curves are symmetrical about a colour ratio near 0.5 (average equiluminance for adults). However, at 8.5 weeks, there was no response at this colour ratio, suggesting that the infant lacked the neural mechanisms to respond to purely chromatic stimuli of that spatial frequency (0.4 cycles/degree). This result has recently been replicated independently by Rudduck and Harding (1993), with transient VEPs.

A cortical response at all colour ratios requires at least two types of photoreceptors, together with neural mechanisms that combine the response in appropriate ways. As the null response of the VEP does not correspond to the silent substitution point of any of the cones or the rods (already discussed), it could not result simply from the dysfunction of one or more classes of photoreceptors, nor does it suggest that rods are playing a major role. The null response occurs at the colour ratio where the L- and M-cones should modulate by the same amount but with opposite phase. Any mechanism that simply summed the M- and L-cone output should not respond at this colour ratio: a response there requires mechanisms that combine L- and M-cone signals in

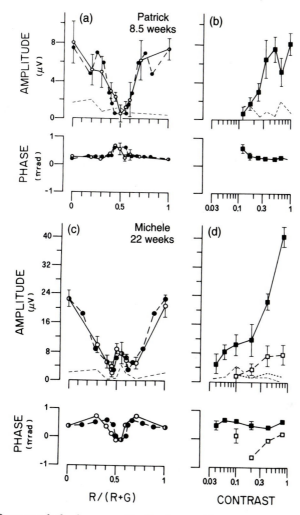

Fig. 5.2 (a,c) Open symbols show amplitude of second-harmonic modulation of visual-evoked potentials as a function of the ratio of red-to-total mean luminance for two infants, at 8.5 and 22 weeks. The error bars show the standard error of the mean, and the dashed lines show the amplitude of the second harmonic of VEPs averaged at 1.1 times stimulus rate (both measures giving an indication of signal reliability). (b,d) Contrast response curves for stimuli modulated in luminance contrast (red–black, colour ratio 1: filled symbols) or chromatic contrast (red–green, colour ratio 0.5: open symbols). For (a) and (b) spatial frequency was 0.4 cycles/degree, temporal frequency 3 Hz and contrast 0.95; for (c) and (d) spatial frequency was 1 cycle/degree, temporal frequency 5 Hz and contrast 0.3. Each colour ratio can be considered to be the sum of luminance- and chromatic-contrast: luminance-contrast is maximal at colour ratios 0 and 1 and scales linearly to zero at equiluminance, while chromatic-contrast is maximal at equiluminance and scales linearly to zero at ratios 0 and 1. For each colour ratio, the responses measured to pure luminance and pure chromatic patterns of appropriate contrast, from (b) and (d), were summed vectorially and plotted as the filled symbols in (a) and (c). In (a) only the luminance response was considered, as there was no response to pure chromatic-contrast. (Reprinted from Morrone *et al.* 1993.)

different ways, such as the chromatic opponent mechanisms described for primate retina and cortex.

The fact that the equiluminance point for infants (as judged by the point of symmetry of the amplitude curve) was very similar to those of adults agrees well with previous evidence based on the motion-null technique of Anstis and Cavanagh (1983). The red–green ratio to produce a motion-null in drifting patterns (as judged by direction of optokinetic nystagmus) was the same for 1–3-month-old infants as for adults (Maurer *et al.* 1989; Teller and Lindsey 1989). All these results reinforce the suggestion that the spectral sensitivity V(λ) of infants in the medium and long wavelength region of the spectrum is adult-like.

As Banks and his colleagues have clearly argued (Banks and Bennett 1988; Allen *et al.* 1993), the lack of response at equiluminance is insufficient by itself to prove the absence of chromatic mechanisms. Owing to their broad and largely overlapping spectral sensitivity curves, chromatic stimuli modulate cones less effectively than luminance stimuli, by about a factor of three for the M-cones and a factor of seven for the L-cones. The reduced amplitude of modulation should increase thresholds (by a factor of five according to Allen *et al.* 1993), so the lack of response at equiluminance may result merely from the lower effective contrast. However, the contrast response curve to luminance stimuli (Fig. 5.2(b)) shows that this is unlikely. The response to luminance patterns remained strong at contrasts down to at least 0.14, a factor of seven. Clearly, the lack of response at equiluminance does not result solely from the lower effective cone contrast of the chromatic stimuli.

Further evidence for the lack of a chromatic response is given by the fact that the amplitudes and phases at all colour ratios can be predicted by the response to pure luminance contrast. The filled circles on the colour ratio curve of Fig. 5.2(a) are responses to pure luminance contrast, taken from the data of Fig. 5.2(b) at appropriate contrasts (luminance contrast is maximum at colour ratios 0 and 1, and scales linearly to 0 at equiluminance). Both the amplitude and phase of the responses to luminance contrast follow closely the colour-ratio functions, suggesting that the luminance response is sufficient to explain the data at all colour ratios.

In Fig. 5.2(c) (open symbols only) are shown VEPs from a 22-week-old infant to low contrast 1 cycle/degree patterns, as a function of colour ratio. At this age, there was a reliable response at all colour ratios, including the equiluminance point (ratio 0.5). Under these particular conditions, the minimal amplitude was not at equiluminance but at colour ratios either side of equiluminance; this did not occur under all conditions but only at certain contrasts and spatial and temporal frequencies (Morrone *et al.* 1993). Note that, despite the secondary minima in the amplitude response, the phase was minimal at equiluminance. This was a general trend observed under all conditions in infants over about 10 weeks of age, implying longer response latencies at equiluminance (discussed later).

The filled symbols of Fig. 5.2(c) show the responses predicted from the contrast response curves of Fig. 5.2(d). Here the prediction is not based on the response to luminance alone but on the combined response to luminance and chromatic contrast (chromatic contrast is maximal at equiluminance and scales to zero at the extremes). For each colour ratio, the responses from Fig. 5.2(d) at appropriate luminance and colour contrasts were added *vectorially* (taking account of both amplitude and phase), and plotted as the filled symbols. The predictions from the response to pure luminance and pure colour follow closely those measured as a function of colour ratio, including the secondary peak at equiluminance with the minima on either side. The reason for the local minima is that the phases of the luminance and colour response are different, so they tend to annul each other at that ratio. The fact that the response as a function of colour ratio can be well predicted from the contrast response curves to pure luminance and pure colour contrast suggests that the two responses are functionally independent, and sum at the electrode.

The VEP studies have shown that the response of infants to chromatic patterns is highly dependent on contrast and spatial frequency (Morrone *et al.* 1993). For example, during the same session that the data of Fig. 2(a) was recorded at 0.4 cycles/degree, there was a good response at 0.1 cycles/degree. However, a week earlier, there was no response whatsoever at any spatial or temporal frequency (down to 1 Hz, 0.05 cycles/degree). Fig. 5.3 shows how contrast sensitivity and acuity to both luminance and colour patterns improve with age. Before 4–7 weeks (varying from infant to infant) there was no response to chromatic stimuli of 0.1 cycles/degree, even at 95% contrast (Fig. 5.3(a)). Contrast sensitivity to luminance stimuli was between 5 and 8 over that period. Both chromatic and luminance sensitivity increased with age (chromatic sensitivity more quickly than luminance sensitivity) to asymptote near adult levels around 6 months of age.

Fig. 5.3(b) shows the improvement in acuity with age. When the VEP to chromatic stimuli began to appear, acuity was around 0.1 cycles/degree, while the acuity for luminance stimuli at this age was around 2 cycles/degree, 20 times higher. Chromatic acuity increased more rapidly than luminance acuity over the first 20 weeks, to approach adult levels by about 6 months. This result agrees well with the psychophysical evidence discussed previously (Packer *et al.* 1984; Adams *et al.* 1990), that showed that when young infants can make colour discriminations, they can do so only for very large (i.e. low spatial frequency) stimuli.

While the acuity and contrast sensitivity (at 0.1 cycles/degree) provide a good indication of the resolution limits of luminance and chromatic patterns, a more complete description is provided by the contrast sensitivity functions of Fig. 5.4. The filled symbols indicate luminance contrast and open symbols colour contrast, with the last point on each graph showing spatial acuity. Both curves improve rapidly with age, in both sensitivity and resolution, while those for equiluminant stimuli improve more rapidly than to luminance stimuli.

While the acuity and contrast sensitivity (at 0.1 cycles/degree) provide a good indication of the resolution limits of luminance and chromatic patterns, a more complete description is provided by the contrast sensitivity functions

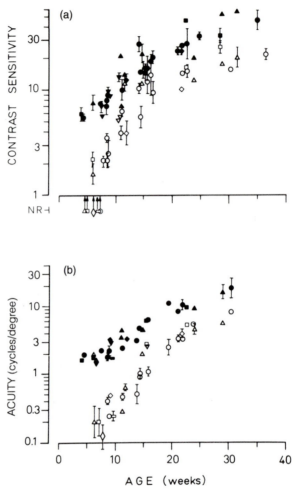

Fig. 5.3 (a) Development of contrast sensitivity (the inverse of contrast threshold) for chromatic stimuli (open symbols) and luminance stimuli (filled symbols). The different symbol types refer to longitudinal measurements of the eight infants. Contrast sensitivity was estimated by measuring VEP amplitudes as a function of contrast, fitting with a third-order polynomial and extrapolating to zero response. In adults, this technique gives estimates of contrast sensitivity that coincide closely with those measured psychophysically (Campbell and Maffei 1970; Fiorentini et al. 1991). The arrows below the abscissa indicate the latest recording session at which no response could be elicited by chromatic stimuli at 90% contrast. Spatial frequency was always 0.1 cycles/degree, and temporal frequency varied with age, chosen to yield maximal response to chromatic stimuli: 2 Hz from 4–7 weeks, 3 Hz from 7–20 weeks, and 5 Hz thereafter. Both chromatic and luminance sensitivities increased with age, fairly rapidly up to 15 weeks, and more slowly thereafter. (b) Development of acuity for chromatic and luminance stimuli (open and closed symbols, respectively), estimated by extrapolating amplitude *versus* spatial frequency functions to zero response. Contrast was always 0.9, and temporal frequency varied with age. (Reprinted from Morrone et al. 1990.)

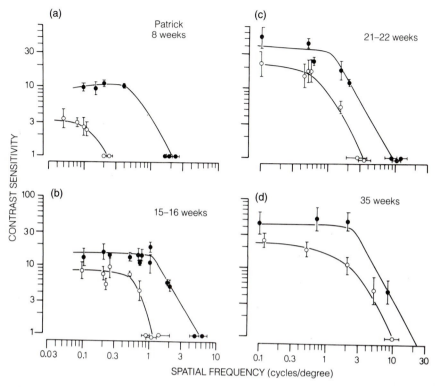

Fig. 5.4 Contrast sensitivity estimated from VEPs as a function of spatial frequency for an infant at ages of 8 (a), 15–16 (b), 21–22 (c) and 35 (d) weeks. Filled circles refer to luminance patterns, and open circles to equiluminant red–green patterns. The temporal frequency was 3 Hz for (a) and (b) and 5 Hz for (c) and (d). Vertical bars (for contrast sensitivity data) and horizontal bars (for acuity data) indicate standard error. To appreciate how the data scales with age in both sensitivity and resolution, photocopy the figure onto three transparencies, and try to superimpose the data at the four ages by vertical and horizontal translation (translation on logarithmic axes corresponds to multiplicative scaling in sensitivity and resolution). It is possible to align all the luminance data, or all the colour data but not both with the same translation, showing that development proceeds at different rates for luminance and colour. (Reprinted from Morrone *et al.* 1993.)

of Fig. 5.4. The filled symbols indicate luminance contrast and open symbols colour contrast, with the last point on each graph showing spatial acuity. Both curves improve rapidly with age, in both sensitivity and resolution, while those for equiluminant stimuli improve more rapidly than to luminance stimuli.

At all ages, contrast sensitivity curves to luminance patterns (for both monkeys and infants) can be well fitted by a single function that simply scales in sensitivity and in resolution as the infant matures (Movshon and Kiorpes 1988; see also Chapter 1 by Kiorpes, this volume). The contrast sensitivity functions can also be fitted by a single function scaled in sensitivity and in resolution. This is true both for luminance contrast sensitivity (confirming the

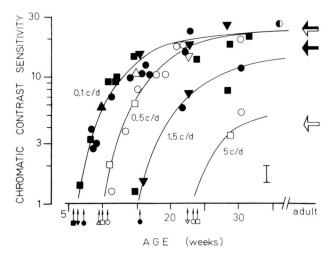

Fig. 5.5 Development of contrast sensitivity for red–green patterns of four different spatial frequencies. The different symbols refer to longitudinal measurements of different infants, and adult values are indicated by the arrows on the right. The arrows below the abscissa indicate, for each spatial frequency, the last recording session at which no response could be elicited by chromatic stimuli at 100% contrast. The vertical bar is the average standard error of the experimental points. (Reprinted from Morrone *et al.* 1993.)

result of Movshon and Kiorpes) and for chromatic senstivity. However, the degree by which the chromatic sensitivity functions need to be scaled is greater than that needed to scale the luminance sensitivity functions, both in sensitivity and in resolution. Using the technique suggested in the figure caption, it is possible to align the luminance curves of all ages, or the colour curves of all ages, but not both simultaneously, since the colour curves require more translation than the luminance curves. This is perhaps the strongest evidence that chromatic vision in infants does not arise solely from reduced cone contrast (as suggested by Allen *et al.* 1993), as this would result in parallel improvement for the sensitivity for luminance and colour.

Fig. 5.5 summarizes how chromatic contrast sensitivity at various spatial frequencies increases with age. At 0.1 cycles/degree, contrast sensitivity was nearly adult-like by 15–20 weeks, before there was any response at 5 cycles/ degree. The curves at all spatial frequencies have similar form, simply shifted along the age abscissa and in absolute sensitivity. That is to say, 10–15 weeks after a response at a certain spatial frequency first appears (at maximal contrast), sensitivity asymptoted to near adult levels.

All the experiments discussed so far have investigated the spatial properties of infant colour vision. However, a complete description of colour vision should also include an analysis of its temporal characteristics. The authors have studied the development of the temporal properties of colour vision, by measuring both steady-state VEPs (as a function of temporal frequency) and transient VEPs (Fiorentini *et al.* 1992). Up to about 10 weeks, both luminance and chromatic curves are low-pass as a function of temporal frequency. After 10 weeks, the luminance function becomes progressively more band-pass, while the colour function remains low-pass.

The major difference in development was observed in the response latency. Fig. 5.6 shows examples of **transient evoked potentials** measured in response to abruptly reversing patterns. The traces on the left were measured soon after the response to chromatic patterns appeared at 8 weeks, and those at the right 13 weeks later. At 8 weeks, the latencies for both luminance and chromatic patterns are long, about 200 ms (similar to that previously described for luminance patterns: Sokol and Jones 1979; Moskovitz and Sokol 1980; Fiorentini and Trimarchi 1992). At 21 weeks, the latencies to both patterns had decreased but that to luminance more so than that to colour. The latency for the luminance response was about 110 ms, and that for the colour response 150 ms. Both these estimates are similar to those obtained with adults (Fiorentini *et al.* 1991).

Response latency can be estimated quite accurately from the rate at which the phase of the steady-state VEP decreases with temporal frequency (see Fiorentini and Trimarchi 1992; Porciatti *et al.* 1992 for procedural details).

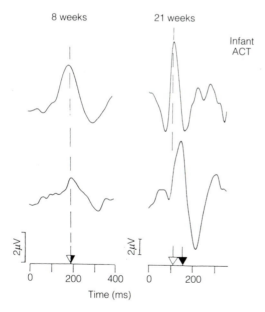

Fig. 5.6 Examples of transient evoked potentials in response to abrupt contrast-reversal of luminance patterns (upper traces) and colour patterns (lower traces): 0.3 cycles/degree, 0.5 Hz, 95% contrast. At 8 weeks of age the major positive peak in both traces shows a similar delay, of nearly 200 ms. At 21 weeks the latency to luminance contrast has decreased to about 110 ms, whereas that to colour contrast remains relatively longer, about 150 ms. This difference is preserved in adults.

Fig. 5.7 shows how estimates of response latency for luminance and chromatic modulation decrease with age. At the earliest age, both luminance and colour estimates were about 250 ms, then decreased rapidly. After about 10 weeks the curves begin to diverge, as the latencies for luminance stimuli decreased more rapidly than those to chromatic stimuli. By about 25 weeks, the latencies approached adult levels. The difference in response latency occurs at a similar age to that when the temporal frequency tuning to luminance contrast but not colour contrast becomes progressively more band-pass, suggesting that the two measures may reflect similar processes.

CONCLUSION

Taken together, the results of the experiments reported here suggest that colour vision develops relatively late in infants, then matures rapidly. The behavioural studies have shown that infants are either unable to make hue discriminations, or require very large fields in order to do so (Packer *et al.* 1984; Adams *et al.* 1990). This observation finds strong physiological parallels in the fact that no evoked potentials can be recorded in infants younger than 7 weeks (Morrone *et al.* 1990; Rudduck and Harding 1993); and once the response appears, it occurs only for very low spatial frequencies and high contrasts (Figs 5.3–5.5).

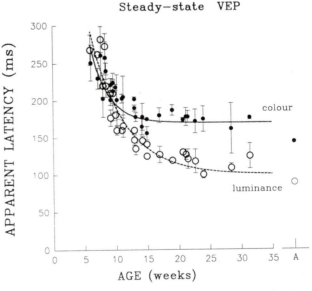

Fig. 5.7 Latency of steady-state VEPs, estimated from the rate at which phase decreases with temporal frequency. Up to about 10 weeks, the latencies are very similar for luminance and colour. Thereafter the curves separate to asymptote around 100 ms for luminance and 160 ms for colour near adult levels.

The strongest evidence for different developmental courses for sensitivity to luminance contrast and colour contrast is given by the contrast sensitivity curves of Fig. 5.4. The curves for both luminance and colour contrast steadily improve in both sensitivity and resolution but at different rates. At 8 weeks, the curves for luminance and colour sensitivity are quite distant, then steadily converge with age. The factors limiting chromatic sensitivity are clearly different from those limiting luminance sensitivity.

The only data that would seem to run contrary to these generally agreed findings are those of Allen *et al.* (1993), who reported visual evoked potentials to chromatic stimuli of 0.8 cycles/degree in a few young infants, including a 2-week-old. This result is certainly difficult to reconcile with the lack of response observed by Rudduck and Harding (1993) and by us (even at 0.1 cycles/degree: Fig. 5.3), and with the psychophysical data showing that chromatic discriminations are not possible with small stimuli at this age. As mentioned earlier, it is possible that in very young infants, spontaneous changes in accommodation may change the effective contrast of red and green patterns at moderate spatial frequencies, creating a luminance artefact at all colour ratios (see Morrone *et al.* 1993). Of course one cannot be certain that this is the explanation for the discrepancy but since the vast bulk of psychophysical and electrophysiological data would suggest separate development of luminance and colour vision, some caution should be exercised in interpreting the data of Fig. 5 of Allen *et al.*, pooled between subjects with possibly different equiluminant points.

Given the evidence for normal photoreceptor function of young infants (summarized in the chapter by Knoblauch *et al.*), it would seem that the development in chromatic acuity most probably reflects maturation in the organization of receptive fields of neurones responding to chromatic stimuli. The temporal properties of the VEP, particulaly the latencies, also suggest separate development of luminance and colour vision. The latencies to both colour and luminance increase with age but at a different rate (Figs 5.6 and 5.7), suggesting different maturation of their respective generators.

It is tempting to speculate whether the evidence for separate development of luminance and colour processing may have implications for the development of the anatomically separate M- and P-pathways (see Shapley and Perry 1986; Kaplan *et al.* 1990 for review). The M-pathway, comprising the large-bodied fast-conducting retinal and geniculate neurones has a more phasic and faster response than the P-pathway (Maunsell and Gibson 1992; Nowak *et al.* 1994) but is thought not to respond well to purely chromatic stimuli (Merigan 1989). Both the M- and P-pathway respond to luminance stimuli and could therefore both contribute to the VEP response to luminance stimuli. Furthermore, the latency of the response within a single P-ganglion cell of an adult monkey is faster for luminance than for chromatic stimuli (Benardete and Kaplan 1993), which could explain, at least in part, the differences observed with the cortical VEP. It is therefore possible that the lack of response at equiluminance before 7 weeks of age could reflect lack of the chromatic function of the

P-pathway, while the luminance vision is mediated by the same P-pathway and/or by the M-pathway, with a possible contribution from subcortical pathways (Atkinson 1984). The greater rate of improvement in response latencies for luminance stimuli may suggest that the M-pathway becomes progressively more phasic with age, at a greater rate than the P-pathway. Whatever the physiological generators of the VEP response and the different rates of development of M- and P-pathways, the results reviewed in this chapter would suggest that the sensitivity, resolution and temporal properties of chromatic vision develop at a different rate from those of luminance vision.

REFERENCES

Adams, R. J., Maurer, D., and Cashin, H. A. (1990). The influence of stimulus size on newborn's discrimination of chromatic from achromatic stimuli. *Vision Research*, **30**, 2023–30.

Allen, D., Banks, M. S., Norcia, A. M., and Shannon, L. (1993). Does chromatic sensitivity develop more slowly than luminance sensitivity? *Vision Research*, **33**, 2553–62.

Anstis, S. and Cavanagh, P. (1983). A minimum motion technique for judging equiluminance In *Colour vision*, pp. 155–66 (ed. J. D. Mollon and L. T. Sharpe), Academic Press, London.

Atkinson, J. (1984). Human visual development over the first six months of life: a review and a hypothesis. *Human Neurobiology*, **3**, 61–74.

Banks, M. S. and Bennett, P. J. (1988). Optical and photoreceptor immaturities limit the spatial and chromatic vision of human neonates. *Journal of the Optical Society of America*, **A5**, 2059–79.

Benardete, E. A. and Kaplan, E. (1993). Spatiotemporal dynamics of P-cells and their cone inputs. *Society of Neuroscience*, (Abstract), **19**, 13.8.

Bornstein, M. H., Kessen, W., and Weiskopf, S. (1976). Color vision and hue categorization in young human infants. *Journal of Experimental Psychology*, **2**, 115–29.

Boynton, R. M. and Gordon, J. (1965). Bezold-Bruecke hue shift measured by color-naming technique. *Journal of the Optical Society of America*, **55**, 78–86.

Brown, A. M. (1990). Development of visual sensitivity to light and color vision in human infants: a critical review. *Vision Research*, **30**, 1159–88.

Brown, A. M. and Teller, D. Y. (1989). Chromatic opponency in 3-month-old human infants. *Vision Research*, **29**, 37–45.

Campbell, F. W. and Maffei, L. (1970). Electrophysiological evidence for the existence of orientation and size detectors in the human visual system. *Journal of Physiology (London)*, **207**, 635–52.

De Valois, R. L. (1973). Central mechanisms in colour vision. In *Handbook of sensory physiology*, Vol. 7, (ed. R. Jung). Springer, Berlin.

Fiorentini, A. and Trimarchi, C. (1992). Development of temporal properties of pattern electroretinograms and visual evoked potentials in infants. *Vision Research*, **32**, 1609–21.

Fiorentini, A., Burr, D. C., and Morrone, M. C. (1991). Spatial and temporal characteristics of colour vision: VEP and psychophysical measurements. In *From pigment to perception: advances in understanding visual processing.* pp. 139–50. (ed. A. Valberg and B. B. Lee). Plenum Press, Berlin.

Fiorentini, A., Morrone, M. C., and Burr, D. C. (1992). Development of temporal properties of pattern visual evoked potential to equiluminant stimuli in infants. *Investigative Ophthalmology and Visual Science*, **33**, 3293.

Flitcroft, D. I. (1989). The interactions between chromatic aberration, defocus and stimulus chromaticity: implications for visual physiology and colorimetry. *Vision Research*, **29**, 349–60.

Hurvich, L. M. and Jameson, D. (1957). An opponent-process theory of color vision. *Psychological Review*, **64**, 384–404.

Kaplan, E., Lee, B., and Shapley, R. M. (1990). New views of primate retinal function. *Prog. Retinal Res*, **9**, 273–336.

Maunsell, J. H. R. and Gibson, J. R. (1992). Visual response latencies in striate cortex of the macaque monkey. *Journal of Neurophysiology*, **68**, 1332–44.

Maurer, D., Lewis, T. L., Cavanagh, P., and Anstis, S. (1989). A new test of luminous efficiency for babies. *Investigative Ophthalmology and Visual Science*, **30**, 297–304.

Merigan, W. H. (1989). Chromatic and achromatic vision of macaques: role of the P pathway. *Journal of Neuroscience*, **9**, 776–83.

Morrone, M. C., Burr, D. C., and Fiorentini, A. (1990). Development of infant contrast sensitivity and acuity to chromatic stimuli. *Proceedings of the Royal Society B*, **242**, 134–9.

Morrone, M. C., Burr, D. C., and Fiorentini, A. (1993). Development of infant contrast sensitivity to chromatic stimuli. *Vision Research*, **33**, 2535–52.

Moskovitz, A. and Sokol, S. (1980). Spatial and temporal interaction of pattern-evoked cortical potentials in human infants. *Vision Research*, **20**, 699–707.

Movshon, J. A. and Korpes, L. (1988). Analysis of the development of spatial contrast sensitivity in monkey and human infants. *Journal of the Optical Society of America*, **A/5**, 2166–72.

Mullen, K. T. (1985). The contrast sensitivity of human colour vision to red–green and blue–yellow gratings. *Journal of Physiology, (London)*, **359**, 381–400.

Nowak, L. G., Munk, M. H. J., Chounlamountri, N., and Bullier, J. (1994). Temporal aspects of information processing in area V1 and V2 of the macaque monkey. In *Oscillatory event-related brain dynamics*, pp. 85–98 (ed. C. Pantev, Th. Elbert and B. Lutkenhoner), Plenum Press, New York.

Packer, O., Hartmann, E. E., and Teller, D. Y. (1984). Infant colour vision: the effect of test field size on Rayleigh discriminations. *Vision Research*, **24**, 1260–84.

Porciatti, V., Burr, D. C., Morrone, M. C., and Fiorentini, A. (1992). The effects of ageing on the pattern electroretinogram and visual evoked potential in humans. *Vision Research*, **32**, 1199–1209.

Rudduck, G. A. and Harding, G. F. A. (1993). The development of the chromatic transient VEP. *Investigative Ophthalmology and Visual Science (Suppl.)*, **34 (1)**, 1355.

Shapley, R. and Perry, H. (1986). Cat and monkey retinal ganglion cells and their visual functional roles. *Trends in Neuroscience*, **5**, 229–35.

Sokol, S. and Jones, K. (1979). Implicit time of pattern evoked potentials in infants: an index of maturation of spatial vision. *Vision Research*, **19**, 747–55.

Teller, D. Y. and Bornstein, M. H. (1987). Infant color vision and color perception. In *Handbook of perception*, pp. 185–236 (ed. P. Salapatek and L. B. Cohen), Academic Press, New York.

Teller, D. Y. and Lindsey, D. T. (1989). Motion nulls for white versus isochromatic gratings in infants and adults. *Journal of the Optical Society of America*, **6A**, 1945–54.

6

Development of visual motion processing

John R. B. Wattam-Bell

INTRODUCTION

Motion is perhaps the most fundamental visual dimension. It provides one of the richest and least ambiguous sources of information about the contents and layout of the environment, and about the observer's own movement within it. Hence it is not surprising that, unlike other visual dimensions such as colour and stereopsis, motion sensitivity is apparently present in all visual systems, from the most primitive to the most advanced. Horridge (1984) has argued that from an evolutionary point of view, detection of relative motion is the primary method of segmenting the visual scene, and that object vision emerges in higher animals as an elaboration of this basic mechanism.

This suggests that motion might play a fundamental role in the development of vision, and that motion sensitivity might be one of the first visual functions to appear. The commonplace observation that newborns readily attend to moving visual stimuli might suggest that motion sensitivity is already quite mature at birth. However, the ability to distinguish between moving and stationary stimuli, which is implied by this observation, may reflect sensitivity to temporal modulation rather than motion as such; infants readily show a visual preference for dynamic stimuli that do not move, such as full-field flicker (Regal 1981). Full use of motion information requires sensitivity to speed and direction, and is it generally thought that the first stage of motion analysis consists of more-or-less local estimates of these basic quantities by directionally selective mechanisms. These low-level mechanisms provide the foundation for more global perceptual processes, and insight into their development will provide an important first step towards a full understanding of the development of visual motion processing.

Sensitivity to direction (usually discrimination between opposite directions) is a specific and robust criterion that has been used widely in psychophysical and physiological studies of motion mechanisms. Most of the evidence for direction discrimination in infants comes from experiments using one of three measures of performance: eye movements; visual-evoked potentials; and preferential looking.

EYE MOVEMENTS

Observation of smooth eye movements that track a moving visual stimulus offers an indirect method of assessing motion processing. One variety of smooth eye movement—optokinetic nystagmus (OKN), which is elicited by large- or full-field motion—can be seen at birth (Kremenitzer *et al.* 1979). The direction of OKN matches that of the stimulus, which implies that directional motion mechanisms are present in the newborn visual system. At first, monocular OKN (mOKN) shows a marked horizontal asymmetry; it is readily elicited by temporal-to-nasal motion but hardly at all in the opposite direction. Symmetrical responses start to appear at around 2 months (Atkinson and Braddick 1981; Naegele and Held 1982), initially for low stimulus velocities, and only later at high velocities (Mohn 1989). Neurophysiological studies in other species suggest that OKN is mediated by the nucleus of the optic tract (NOT). At birth, the neurones of each NOT are driven only by a direct input from the contralateral eye, and their responses exhibit the same directional asymmetries as mOKN (Hoffmann and Schoppmann 1981). Later, an indirect pathway via visual cortex to NOT develops, leading to binocular and directionally symmetrical responses, and it is this development that is thought to underlie the emergence of symmetrical mOKN (Hoffman 1987). In this view, OKN is at first a purely subcortical reflex, and it seems unlikely that the directional mechanisms involved could play any direct part in perception; cortical directional mechanisms are presumably required for this, and it seems that the development of these is also responsible for the emergence of symmetrical OKN. Moreover, the results of Mohn (1989) suggest that the development of cortical directionality follows a low to high velocity sequence.

Recently, this picture of the development of OKN has been called into question. The VEP studies of Norcia *et al.* (1991), which are discussed later, and recent observations on hemispherectomized infants (Braddick *et al.* 1992; see also the chapter by Braddick, Atkinson and Hood in this volume), suggest that the cortex may be involved in OKN at an earlier stage than is implied by the development of symmetrical responses, and that part of the early OKN asymmetry is caused by directional asymmetries in cortical motion processing. However, it is still unclear whether these mechanisms are functional at birth, or whether there is an initial period during which control of OKN is essentially subcortical.

Functionally, OKN serves to stabilize the gaze by countering the average motion across large regions of the visual field. The tracking of relatively small, isolated targets, on the other hand, is reckoned to be the domain of smooth pursuit. Of course in the case of an isolated target against a homogenous background this distinction is not necessarily clear-cut. However, a mature pursuit system can be expected to track targets against a textured background, when the net large-field motion, at least on the retina, is in the opposite direction to the motion of the pursued object.

In adults, the generation of smooth pursuit involves cortical pathways (Lisberger *et al.* 1987), and developmental studies might therefore be expected to shed light on the emergence of cortical motion mechanisms. Unfortunately there is disagreement about when smooth pursuit is first seen. Some studies have suggested that very young infants use saccadic eye movements to track isolated targets, and that smooth pursuit is not seen before about 8 weeks of age (Dayton *et al.* 1964; Aslin 1981). Others have reported brief periods of pursuit in younger infants (Kremenitzer *et al.* 1979; Roucoux *et al.* 1983; Hainline 1985). It may be that, in these cases, the optokinetic system was responsible. Alternatively, the failure to find pursuit before 8 weeks may be because of the use of inappropriately high stimulus velocities; Roucoux *et al.* (1983) and Hainline (1985) reported that the maximum velocity that will elicit pursuit increases during development, while Shea and Aslin (1990) found that in 7–11-week-olds, pursuit velocity was low and largely independent of target velocity and was therefore least accurate at high target velocities. It is quite possible that this reflects an underlying sensory limitation—the absence of cortical motion mechanisms sensitive to high velocities.

Neither the OKN nor the smooth pursuit results provide a clear answer to the question of whether cortical directionality is present at birth. However, they do suggest that, at first, cortical directionality only operates at relatively low velocities, and that its upper velocity limit increases with age. Is the same true for the perception of motion? This is not necessarily the case; the cortical mechanisms involved in eye movement control may not be the same as those responsible for perception. Even if there is a common substrate of cortical directional mechanisms, the pathways involved must diverge at some later point, and the velocity limits on smooth eye movements may be imposed after this.

VISUAL-EVOKED POTENTIALS

Visual-evoked potentials (VEPs) offer a fairly direct way of assessing sensory function. It is probable that VEPs are dominated by activity in cortical visual areas (in particular V1 and V2); hence they provide a measure of cortical as opposed to subcortical function. One useful approach in developmental work is to design VEP stimuli that are specific to the sensory dimension of interest—those that will only elicit a response if cortical mechanisms of the required selectivity are present. In this vein, Wattam-Bell (1991) measured direction-specific motion VEPs in infants. The stimulus was a random-dot pattern that oscillated vertically, its direction reversing four times per second. Now, direction reversals in an otherwise unchanging pattern could generate responses in mechanisms that are insensitive to direction. To eliminate these, the random-dot pattern was replaced by a new, uncorrelated pattern each time the direction reversed, producing incoherent 'jumps'. These jumps will themselves elicit a non-specific response. To allow the jump and direction-specific responses to be isolated from each other, a second set of jumps was introduced mid-way between reversals. Hence, in the final stimulus, the four direction reversals per second were embedded in a sequence of eight jumps per second. The steady-state VEP was analysed for components at the jump frequency (8 Hz), and also at the direction reversal frequency (4 Hz). The latter component can only arise from mechanisms that are selective for the direction of motion.

A group of longitudinally tested infants first showed a statistically significant direction reversal component in the VEP at a median age of 74 days when the velocity was 5°/s, while for a velocity of 20°/s the onset age was significantly later at 89 days. In adults, the direction reversal component has a larger amplitude at 20°/s that at 5°/s. Thus its development is not simply a matter of a uniform increase in VEP amplitude; instead it implies that the development of cortical directionality starts at low velocities and spreads to progressively higher velocities as the infant matures, which agrees with the conclusion drawn from the OKN results discussed above. Hence the first appearance of the motion VEP at 10 weeks does not necessarily mark the onset of cortical directionality; test velocities below 5°/s might well give directional responses at an earlier age.

Norcia *et al.* (1991) have described a different type of motion VEP. They recorded responses to oscillatory displacements (90° phase shifts) of a vertical grating. With monocular viewing, young infants' VEPs showed a prominent first harmonic component, that is a left/right directional asymmetry. The phase of this component was reversed between the two eyes, implying that the under-lying asymmetry is between the nasal and temporal directions, as is the case for monocular OKN. The VEP asymmetry declines with age but persists for longer at high rates of oscillation, which matches the more prolonged mOKN asymmetries at high velocities reported by Mohn (1989). All this suggests that at least part of the asymmetry of mOKN is a result not of an absence of cortical control but of directional asymmetries in cortical motion processing. Whether this is true at birth remains unclear, although recently Brown *et al.* (1993) have reported VEP asymmetries in infants as young as 3 weeks.

PREFERENTIAL LOOKING

Upper velocity thresholds

Wattam-Bell (1992*a*) has systematically explored the development of sensitivity to direction of motion in behavioural experiments, which, like the VEP study described above, used drifting random-dot patterns that periodically reversed direction. A 10° wide vertical strip of the pattern, which appeared on either the left or right of the midline, moved at the same speed as the rest of the pattern but always in the opposite direction, that is it moved upwards when the background moved down, and *vice versa*. Adults could easily detect the strip, since it appeared clearly segregated from the background. When tested with forced-choice preferential looking (FPL), infants also proved capable of detecting it,

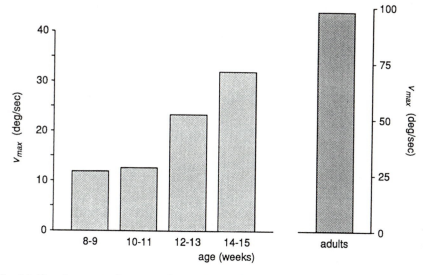

Fig. 6.1 Development of upper velocity thresholds (v_{max}) for discrimination of direction of motion in random-dot patterns. Note the change of scale between infant and adult data. From Wattam-Bell (1992*a*).

which implies that they could discriminate between the opposite directions of motion in the stimulus, since this was the only cue available. The experiments went on to measure upper velocity thresholds (v_{max}) for this discrimination. The results, illustrated in Fig. 6.1, show the same pattern as the eye movement and VEP data discussed above: v_{max} for direction discrimination increases with age.

In the stimulus used for this experiment, motion was sampled temporally; it consisted of a sequence of discrete displacements at the frame rate of the video monitor (20 ms interval) and velocity was varied by varying the size of these displacements. With apparent motion stimuli of this kind, adults' performance is limited by displacement size rather than velocity (Baker and Braddick 1985; Snowden and Braddick 1989); making the interval between displacements longer than 20 ms produces a proportionate reduction in v_{max} and thus a constant maximum displacement limit (d_{max}). Wattam-Bell (1992*a*) found that the same was true for infants who were older than about 12 weeks; changing the displacement interval from 20 ms to 40 ms produced a two-fold reduction in v_{max} in other words, no change in d_{max}. Younger infants, on the other hand, gave the opposite result: v_{max} remained constant and d_{max} increased.

Thus in older infants, as in adults, v_{max} reflects an underlying spatial limit, which implies that the rise in v_{max} (i.e. d_{max}) between 12 weeks and adulthood results from an increase in the spatial range or scale over which motion mechanisms operate. This is the opposite of the coarse-to-fine development of lower velocity thresholds (see later discussion). There is not necessarily a contradiction here. Motion processing may begin operating over medium spatial scales, and development may involve simultaneous medium-to-fine and

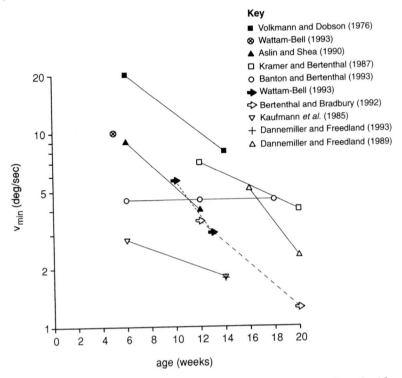

Fig. 6.2 Development of lower velocity thresholds (v_{min}). The data plotted with arrows and broken lines involved tasks that required direction discrimination, while the remainder involved discrimination between moving and static patterns.

medium-to-coarse progressions. It would be interesting to know whether motion processing is unique in this, or whether it is also true for other visual functions.

While it is likely that development of spatial characteristics plays a part in the rise in v_{max} before 12 weeks, the results obtained from younger infants in the displacement interval experiment indicate that an additional process is involved: an improvement in the temporal properties of motion mechanisms (i.e. a narrowing of temporal scale, or increase in upper temporal frequency limit). This temporal maturation appears to be largely complete by 12 weeks and is reminiscent of the rapid development of sensitivity to high temporal frequencies that has been observed in several studies (Moskowitz and Sokol 1980; Regal 1981; Hartmann and Banks 1992).

Lower velocity thresholds

The majority of FPL studies on low-level motion processing in infants have concentrated on lower velocity thresholds (v_{min}). Fig. 6.2 gives a summary of results from several of these. One striking aspect of these data is the wide variation between studies in the estimated value of v_{min} at any given age. Despite this, all but one of the studies in which different age groups were tested agree in finding a decrease in v_{min} with age. The one exception (Banton and Bertenthal 1993) was not strictly an FPL experiment, since the response criterion was the direction of tracking (smooth or saccadic) elicited by full-field motion; possible implications of this result are discussed later.

Most of the experiments summarized in Fig. 6.2 measured thresholds for discrimination between moving and stationary patterns. In principle, sensitivity to the direction of motion is not necessary for this kind of task, so it is by no means certain that motion mechanisms are involved. However, Aslin and Shea (1990) found that v_{min} did not change when they altered the spatial frequency of their square-wave stimuli; thresholds were determined by velocity, not temporal frequency. Likewise, by varying temporal frequency, Dannemiller and Freedland (1993) showed that infants' detection of standing wave motion is based on velocity rather than amplitude. This invariance of v_{min} with changing stimulus parameters certainly suggests that motion mechanisms are involved (although this is not a foolproof criterion; as was seen above, it does not hold for upper velocity thresholds). In addition, the studies of Bertenthal and Bradbury (1992) and Wattam-Bell (1993), whose results are plotted in Fig. 6.2 with arrows and broken lines, used tasks that require direction discrimination; they also found that v_{min} decreased with age. The tasks were quite similar in these two experiments: discrimination of a random-dot pattern containing regions moving in opposite directions, from a uniformly-moving pattern, although Bertenthal and Bradbury's stimulus contained modulations of speed as well as direction.

The directional v_{min} data of Wattam-Bell (1993) shown in Fig. 6.2 came from an experiment that measured both v_{min} and v_{max} in each subject. Fig. 6.3 shows the full results of this experiment, and provides a useful summary of the picture so far. The development of directional motion processing is characterized by an expanding velocity range, and this expansion results from a simultaneous decrease in v_{min} and increase in v_{max}. This picture raises several interesting questions. One concerns the implications of this expanding velocity range for motion processing in younger infants; possible alternatives are illustrated by the broken lines in Fig. 6.3, and this issue will be taken up in a later section. Another concerns the development of motion sensitivity at intermediate velocities, away from upper and lower thresholds.

Intermediate velocities

It is tempting to assume that the development of velocity thresholds represents specific improvements at the extremes of the velocity range, for example the emergence of mechanisms sensitive to low and high velocities. However, this is not the only possibility: diverging thresholds could also arise from a uniform increase in sensitivity throughout the velocity range. This idea can be

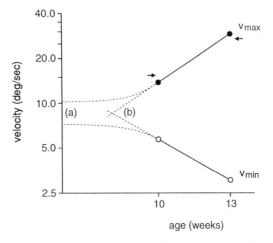

Fig. 6.3 Development of directional v_{min} and v_{max} between 10 and 13 weeks. Note that the backwards extrapolations from the data (broken lines) are purely illustrative. The arrows show mean v_{max} values obtained from infants of the same age by Wattam-Bell (1992a). From Wattam-Bell (1993).

understood by analogy with the development of acuity and contrast sensitivity. Improvements in contrast sensitivity are well documented, and a uniform increase in contrast sensitivity across all spatial frequencies will, by itself, increase acuity. The question is whether this alone is sufficient to account for the observed improvement in acuity, or whether an additional more specific process needs to be invoked, such as the emergence of mechanisms with small receptive fields, or at least an above-average increase in their sensitivity.

In the motion domain, the obvious way to approach this issue is to measure sensitivity to motion at intermediate velocities. A way of doing this was introduced by van Doorn and Koendrink (1982a,b). The idea is to degrade the coherent motion of a random-dot pattern by the addition of incoherent motion (i.e. a spatiotemporally uncorrelated pattern, like 'snow' on an untuned television; van Doorn and Koendrink achieved this by varying the relative contrast of superimposed coherently and incoherently moving patterns. More recently, several studies (Williams and Sekuler 1984; Newsome and Pare 1988) used a different approach in which the relative numbers of coherently and incoherently moving dots are varied and sensitivity is given by the coherence threshold—the smallest percentage of coherently moving dots for which subjects can perform the chosen task (this is an inverse measure of sensitivity).

This latter approach was used by Wattam-Bell (1994) to measure coherence thresholds in infants at a velocity of 8°/s. This was an FPL experiment, and used a direction discrimination task that was essentially the same as that used in the experiments described above. The infants (11–15-week-olds) showed poor sensitivity, with coherence thresholds of around 50 per cent under conditions for which an adult subject's threshold was 5–7 per cent. Moreover,

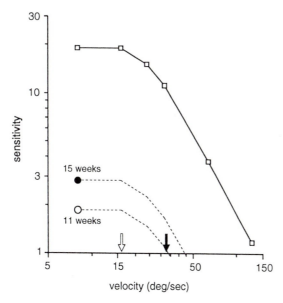

Fig. 6.4 Sensitivity [100/(percentage coherence threshold)] *vs.* stimulus velocity for an adult subject (open squares). The circles show mean sensitivity of 11-week (open circles) and 15-week (filled circles) infants at a velocity of 8°/s. The broken curves are vertically (but not horizontally) displaced versions of the adult sensitivity curve. The arrows show mean v_{max} at 11 weeks (open) and 15 weeks (filled) obtained by Wattam-Bell (1992a). From Wattam-Bell (1994).

within the group of infants coherence thresholds decreased significantly with age.

These results indicate that motion sensitivity improves with age at intermediate velocities. This must play a significant role in the development of velocity thresholds but the question remains as to whether it is sufficient to account for the latter. In the case of v_{max}, the data plotted in Fig. 6.4 suggest that it may not be the case. This shows the 'motion-sensitivity function' (i.e. inverse coherence threshold *vs* velocity) for an adult subject. When this is shifted down —simulating a uniform reduction in sensitivity—to meet measured sensitivities of 11- and 15-week-olds at 8°/s, the resulting intercepts with the velocity axis lie some distance above the values of v_{max} measured by Wattam-Bell (1992a) in infants of the same ages. This discrepancy is larger for the younger infants, and suggests that the improvement in sensitivity at high velocities is greater than at intermediate velocities, which, in turn, implies that there is some specific process, in addition to a uniform increase in motion sensitivity, involved in the development of v_{max}. This is most likely to be the emergence of motion mechanisms with large receptive fields, as already discussed. However, this can only be a tentative conclusion at present, since it is based on a comparison of data from different experiments, and thus different groups of infants.

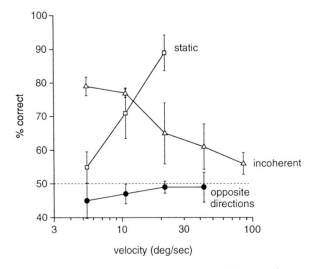

Fig. 6.5 Mean (±1 SE) FPL performance of 3–6-week-olds as a function of stimulus velocity for discrimination between opposite directions ('opposite directions'), between moving and static patterns ('static'), and between coherent and incoherent motion ('incoherent'). From Wattam-Bell (1992*b*; 1993).

THE ONSET OF DIRECTIONALITY

The divergence of direction discrimination velocity thresholds during development raises questions about motion processing in younger infants. Two possi bilities are illustrated by the alternative ways of extrapolating back from the data to younger ages shown in Fig. 6.3. In the first, v_{min} meets v_{max}, so that there is some age before which infants are insensitive to direction at any velocity while in the second the thresholds do not meet—from birth, infants can dis criminate opposite directions of motion, although only over a relatively narrow range of velocities.

Wattam-Bell (1992*b*; 1993) examined this question in experiments on younger infants. When tested with FPL, 3–6-week-olds gave no evidence of direction discrimination, producing chance performance at all velocities tested (Fig. 6.5 filled circles). However, they did better in two control conditions, involving discrimination of a coherently moving target from a static background, and from an incoherently moving background. In principle, at least, neither of these controls requires sensitivity to direction, and the infants' good performance in them implies a quite specific deficit in direction discrimination. Either 3–6 week-olds are not sensitive to direction at all, of if they are, it is only over a range of velocities that is substantially narrower than the 2:1 ratio between adjacent test velocities.

These findings were confirmed in habituation-recovery experiments. This technique has the advantage that, unlike FPL, it does not rely on an intrinsic preference to demonstrate discrimination between two stimuli. The infants were habituated to uniform motion—a random-dot pattern in which all the dots moved in the same direction—and then tested with a pattern segregated into regions, which moved in opposite directions. The 3–5-week-olds showed no evidence of habituation recovery to the test pattern, although they did when tested with the control discriminations used in the FPL experiments. In contrast, a slightly older group of infants (6–8-week-olds) showed habituation recovery in the direction discrimination condition.

Thus the habituation results suggest that sensitivity to direction emerges at about 7 weeks of age. Alternatively, it may be that the younger infants are sensitive to direction, but are unable to use it as a cue for segregation. To test this, a second habituation experiment examined absolute direction discrimination (leftwards *vs* rightwards uniform motion). Again, 3–5-week-olds showed no sign of discrimination but, surprisingly, neither did 6–8-week-olds. The unidirectional motion used in this experiment inevitably elicited intermittent tracking eye movements that were not present in the previous experiment (in the latter, tracking was inhibited by periodic reversals in the direction of motion, which cannot be used when testing absolute direction discrimination), and these may have disrupted discrimination in the older infants. In adults, direction discrimination is not generally disrupted by smooth tracking; this must reflect the ability of the visual system to combine information about eye movements with measures of retinal image motion, and it is quite possible that this process is not yet functional at 6–8 weeks. However, although intermittent tracking might cause considerable variations in retinal speed, it will have much less effect on retinal direction, which should therefore remain a fairly consistent cue for discrimination. It may be, then, that perceptual discrimination of direction first emerges for relative motion, as was present in the segregated pattern of the previous experiments. This certainly makes sense in the context of the use of motion in perception; it is relative motion that provides information about the layout of the environment. Uniform motion, on the other hand, is more relevant for the control of eye movements (particularly OKN). Indeed, while the 6–8-week-olds showed no evidence for perceptual discrimination of absolute direction, they produced appropriate oculomotor responses. A similar dichotomy is also apparent in the v_{min} data plotted in Fig. 6.2; whereas Banton and Bertenthal (1993) found no change in v_{min} between 6 and 18 weeks for ocular tracking of uniform motion, the FPL experiments, most of which used relative motion (moving regions presented against either a stationary or oppositely directed background), showed a substantial decrease in v_{min} during this period.

MOTION CUES IN PERCEPTION

The discussion so far has been cast in terms of the properties of low-level local motion mechanisms. These form only the first stage of motion analysis; further, more global processes are involved in the use of motion for perception. Perhaps the most basic of these is image segmentation; motion information can, by itself, support the perceptual grouping of regions sharing a common motion, and the detection of boundaries between regions of different motion. There is evidence for this kind of processing in quite young infants; indeed, the experiments described in the previous section suggest that the earliest evidence for motion sensitivity is to be found with stimuli containing cues for segmentation, although these experiments do not themselves prove that infants can use these cues for image segmentation. However, Kaufmann-Hayoz *et al.* (1986) have shown that 3-month-olds can detect motion-defined contours and are sensitive to the two-dimensional shape of objects defined by them. Likewise, 4-months-olds can group the spatially separated parts of a partially occluded object which share a common motion (Kellmann and Spelke 1983), although Slater *et al.* (1990) found no evidence of this grouping process in newborns. These studies suggest that the basic processes of segmentation are functional by 3–4 months, although both involved movement against a stationary background and it would be interesting to know whether this conclusion holds for the more general case of a moving background.

In these studies, the objects moved uniformly—that is, all parts moved with the same velocity. Non-uniformities in an object's motion (or at least in its two-dimensional projection on the retina) can also provide shape information, in other words 'structure-from-motion'. Here the picture with infants is not so clear. At 3 months, infants can distinguish between rigid and non-rigid motion of an object (Gibson *et al.* 1979), and Arterberry and Yonas (1988) have shown that 4-month-olds are capable of quite subtle shape discrimination in three-dimensional structure-from-motion displays using random-dot patterns. Somewhat paradoxically, Spitz *et al.* (1992) found that infants are apparently unable to extract two-dimensional structure from non-uniform motion (rotation or expansion in random-dot patterns) until around 7 months. This contrasts with reports that the blink response elicited by an approaching (i.e. expanding) visual input emerges at about 2–3 months (van Hof-van Duin and Mohn 1986) and can sometimes be seen in infants as young as 1 month of age (Yonas and Granrud 1985). However it is obviously desirable to establish an optical blink reflex as early as possible, and it may be a rather specialized system that is largely independent of more general motion processing.

CONCLUSIONS

It is natural to think of visual motion analysis as hierarchical, with local, low-level measurements providing the input to later stages that perform more global operations such as image segmentation. It is also natural to assume a similar hierarchy for development. However, it is doubtful how far low-level motion mechanisms either function or develop independently of feedback from later stages. Directional responses can be recorded in the visual cortex of newborn kittens (Albus and Wolf 1984), and the results of Brown *et al.* (1993) suggest that the same may be true for humans, but it is by no means certain that from the outset these mechanisms are functional in the sense of being able to support perceptual discriminations. In the cat (and no doubt in the human) there is a sensitive period for directionality in which adequate visual experience is required for normal maturation of responses (Daw and Wyatt 1976). It seems likely that a structured visual input—one containing the kind of global patterns that are reckoned to be the domain of later stages in the motion processing hierarchy—is necessary here and that, for example, spatiotemporal noise (which contains all possible speeds and directions of motion but has no structure) would not be adequate.

Thus behavioural measures of the onset of directionality may depend on later stages of the motion processing system attaining at least a degree of competence. The results described above suggest an onset age of about 6–8 weeks. In the last section it was seen that fairly soon after this infants are capable of quite sophisticated motion-based perceptual discriminations. Most of these experiments have been carried out on infants aged 3 months or more. Further work is needed to determine just how rapidly such abilities emerge, and the extent to which they are constrained by factors such as the limited velocity range of developing low-level motion mechanisms. There is not necessarily a simple relationship here; this chapter has deliberately taken a somewhat narrow view of motion processing, one based on the low-level directional mechanisms of the short-range or first-order system (Braddick 1974). This system is undoubtedly of major importance in adult vision but there are other possibilities. For example, directional selectivity is not necessarily required for motion-based segmentation; in the real world relative motion generally involves differences in speed, which could be detected with an array of non-directional spatiotemporally tuned mechanisms, although it is not clear whether such mechanisms make a significant contribution to motion processing in adults or infants. Nevertheless, alternatives to first-order motion exist in adult vision: the long-range (Braddick 1980) and second-order (Chubb and Sperling 1988) processes (which may or may not be distinct entities) can support the perception of motion but may have limited use in motion-based functions such as image segmentation or control of eye movements. Little is known about the development of these alternative processes, although some preliminary experiments on infants' detection of second-order motion are described in the chapter by Braddick *et al.* in this volume.

ACKNOWLEDGEMENTS

This work is supported by the Medical Research Council. I would like to thank Jan Atkinson, Ol Braddick and the staff of the Visual Development Unit for their help and encouragement.

REFERENCES

Albus, K. and Wolf, W. (1984). Early postnatal development of neuronal function in the kitten's visual cortex: a laminar analysis. *Journal of Physiology (London)*, **348**, 153–8.

Arterberry, M. E. and Yonas, A. (1988). Infants' sensitivity to kinetic information for three-dimensional object shape. *Perception and Psychophysics*, **44**, 1–6.

Aslin, R. N. (1981). The development of smooth pursuit in human infants. In *Eye movements: cognition and visual perception,* (ed. R. A. Monty and J. W. Senders), Erlbaum, Hillsdale, New Jersey.

Aslin, R. N. and Shea, S. L. (1990). Velocity thresholds in human infants: implications for the perception of motion. *Developmental Psychology*, **26**, 589–98.

Atkinson, J. and Braddick, O. J. (1981). Development of optokinetic nystagmus in infants: an indicator of cortical binocularity? In *Eye movements: cognition and visual perception*, (ed. D. F. Fisher, R. A. Monty, and J. W. Senders), Erlbaum, Hillsdale, New Jersey.

Baker, C. L. and Braddick, O. J. (1985).Temporal properties of the short-range process in apparent motion. *Perception*, **14**, 181–92.

Banton, T. and Bertenthal, B. I. (1993). Sensitivity to global motion in 6- to 18-week-old infants. *Investigative Ophthalmology and Visual Science*, **34** (suppl.), 1357.

Bertenthal, B. I. and Bradbury, A. (1992). Infants' detection of shearing motion in random-dot displays. *Developmental Psychology*, **28**, 1056–66.

Braddick, O. J. (1974). A short-range process in apparent motion. *Vision Research*, **14**, 519–27.

Braddick, O. J. (1980). Low-level and high-level processes in apparent motion. *Philosophical Transactions of the Royal Society B*, **290**, 137–51.

Braddick, O. J., Atkinson, J., Hood, B., Harkness, W., Jackson, G., and Varga-Khadem, F. (1992). Possible blindsight in infants lacking one cerebral hemisphere. *Nature*, **360**, 461–3.

Brown, R. J., Norcia, A. M., Hamer, R. D., Wilson, J. R., and Boothe, R. G. (1993). Development of motion processing mechanisms in monkey and human infants. *Investigative Ophthalmology and Visual Science*, **34** (suppl.), 1356.

Chubb, C. and Sperling, G. (1988). Drift-balanced random stimuli: a general basis for studying non-Fourier motion perception. *Journal of the Optical Society of America*, **A5**, 1986–2007.

Dannemiller, J. L. and Freedland, R. L. (1989). The detection of slow stimulus movement in 2–5-month-olds. *Journal of Experimental Child Psychology*, **47**, 337–55.

Dannemiller, J. L. and Freedland, R. L. (1993). Motion-based detection by 14-week-old infants. *Vision Research*, **33**, 657–64.

Daw, N. W. and Wyatt, H. J. (1976). Kittens reared in a unidirectional environment: evidence for a critical period. *Journal of Physiology (London)*, **257**, 155–70.

Dayton, G. O., Jones, M. H., Steele, B., and Rose, M. (1964). Developmental study of coordinated eye movements in the human infant. II. An electrooculographic study of the fixation reflex in the newborn. *Archives of Ophthalmology*, **71**, 871–5.

Gibson, E. J., Owsley, C. J., Walker, A., and Megaw-Nice, J. (1979). Development of the perception of invariants: substance and shape. *Perception*, **8**, 609–19.

Hainline, L. (1985). Oculomotor control in human infants. In *Eye movements and human information processing,* (ed. R. Groner, G. W. McConkie, and C. Menz), Elsevier, Amsterdam.

Hartmann, E. E. and Banks, M. S. (1992). Temporal contrast sensitivity in human infants. *Vision Research*, **32**, 1163–8.

Hoffmann, K.-P. (1987). The influence of visual experience on the ontogeny of the optokinetic reflex in mammals. In *Adaptive processes in visual and oculomotor systems*, (ed. F. L. Keller and D. J. Zee), Pergamon, Oxford.

Hoffmann, K.-P. and Schoppmann, A. (1981). A quantitative analysis of the direction specific response of neurons in the cat's nucleus of the optic tract. *Experimental Brain Research*, **42**, 146–57.

Horridge, G. A. (1984). The evolution of visual processing and the construction of seeing systems. *Proceedings of the Royal Society B*, **230**, 279–92.

Kaufmann, F., Stucki, M., and Kaufmann-Hayoz, R. (1985). Development of infants' sensitivity for slow and rapid motions. *Infant Behaviour and Development*, **8**, 89–95.

Kaufmann-Hayoz, R., Kaufmann, F., and Stucki, M. (1986). Kinetic contours in infants' visual perception. *Child Development*, **57**, 292–9.

Kellmann, P. J. and Spelke, E. S. (1983). Perception of partly occluded objects in infancy. *Cognitive Psychology*, **15**, 483–524.

Kramer, S. J. and Bertenthal, B. I. (1989). Infants' sensitivity to motion in random-dot kinematograms. *Investigative Ophthalmology and Visual Science*, **30** (suppl.), 312.

Kremenitzer, J. P., Vaughan, H. G., Kurtzberg, D., and Dowling, K. (1979). Smooth-pursuit eye movements in the newborn infant. *Child Development*, **50**, 442–8.

Lisberger, S. G., Morris, E. J., and Tychsen, L. (1987). Visual motion processing and sensory-motor integration for smooth pursuit eye movements. *Annual Review of Neuroscience*, **10**, 97–129.

Mohn, G. (1989). The development of binocular and monocular optokinetic nystagmus in human infants. *Investigative Ophthalmology and Visual Science*, **40** (suppl.), 49.

Moskowitz, A. and Sokol, S. (1980). Spatial and temporal interaction of pattern-evoked cortical potentials in human infants. *Vision Research*, **20**, 699–708.

Naegele, J. R. and Held, R. (1982). The post-natal development of monocular optokinetic nystagmus in infants. *Vision Research*, **22**, 341–6.

Newsome, W. T. and Pare, E. B. (1988). A selective impairment of motion processing following lesions of the middle temporal visual area (MT). *Journal of Neuroscience*, **8**, 2201–211.

Norcia, A. M., Garcia, H., Humphrey, R., Holmes, A., and Orel-Bixler, D. (1991). Anomalous motion VEPs in infants and in infantile esotropia. *Investigative Ophthalmology and Visual Science*, **32**, 436–9.

Regal, D. M. (1981). Development of critical flicker frequency in human infants. *Vision Research*, **21**, 549–55.

Roucoux, A., Culée, C., and Roucoux, M. (1983). Development of fixation and pursuit eye movements in human infants. *Behavioural Brain Research*, **10**, 133–9.

Shea, S. L. and Aslin, R. N. (1990). Oculomotor responses to step-ramp targets by young human infants. *Vision Research*, **30**, 1077–92.

Slater, A., Morison, A., Somers, M., Mattock, A., Brown, E., and Taylor, D. (1990). Newborn and older infants' perception of partly occluded objects. *Infant Behavior and Development*, **13**, 33–49.

Snowden, R. J. and Braddick, O. J. (1989). Extension of displacement limits in multiple-exposure sequences of apparent motion. *Vision Research*, **29**, 1777–88.

Spitz, R. V., Stiles, J., and Siegel, R. M. (1992). Infant use of relative motion as information for form: evidence of spatio-temporal integration of complex motion displays. *Perception and Psychophysics*, In press.

van Doorn, A. J. and Koendrink, J. J. (1982*a*). Temporal properties of the visual detectability of moving spatial white noise. *Experimental Brain Research*, **45**, 179–88.

van Doorn, A. J. and Koendrink, J. J. (1982*b*). Spatial properties of the visual detectability of moving spatial white noise. *Experimental Brain Research*, **45**, 189–95.

van Hof-van Duin and Mohn, G. (1986). The development of the visual threat response in human infants. *Behavioural Brain Research*, **20**, 154.

Volkmann, F. C. and Dobson, V. (1976). Infant responses of ocular fixation to moving visual stimuli. *Journal of Experimental Child Psychology*, **22**, 86–99.

Wattam-Bell, J. (1991). Development of motion-specific cortical responses in infancy. *Vision Research*, **31**, 287–97.

Wattam-Bell, J. (1992*a*). The development of maximum displacement limits for the discrimination of motion direction in infancy. *Vision Research*, **32**, 621–30.

Wattam-Bell, J. (1992*b*). Are one-month-old infants motion-blind? *Perception*, **21**, A2.

Wattam-Bell, J. (1993). One-month-old infants fail in a motion direction discrimination task. *Investigative Ophthalmology and Visual Science*, **34** .(suppl.), 1356.

Wattam-Bell, J. (1994). Coherence thresholds for discrimination of motion direction in infants. *Vision Research*, **34**, 877–83.

Williams, D. W. and Sekuler, R. (1984). Coherent global motion percepts from stochastic local motions. *Vision Research*, **24**, 55–62.

Yonas, A. and Granrud, C. E. (1985). The development of sensitivity to kinetic, binocular and pictorial depth information in human infants. In *Brain mechanisms and spatial vision*, (ed. D. J. Ingle, M. Jeannerod, and D. N. Lee), Martinus Nijhoff, Dordrecht.

Part II
Refraction and resolution

When the science of infant vision is applied to assessing children who may have visual disorders, the most common starting point is to ask about the child's acuity, or resolution of vision, and the refractive state of the child's eyes. These questions are closely linked. However, they have to be asked separately, because refractive error is only one of the possible constraints on visual resolution in the developing visual system, and conversely significant refractive errors would not necessarily be detected in young infants by their effects on acuity.

Several of these chapters are concerned with the techniques of refracting the eyes of infants. Thorn, in Chapter 7, explains why there are still controversies about the choice of retinoscopic methods, and with Gwiazda and Held, in Chapter 8, explores the specific technique of 'near retinoscopy'. Chapter 7 also introduces photo- and video-refractive methods, results from which are presented in more detail in Chapter 10 by Atkinson and Chapter 11 by Angi and Pilotto.

The importance of testing infants' refraction at an early age is that refractive errors may have long term correlates and consequences. These are the subject of Chapters 9–11. In particular, it may be possible to detect conditions whose optical correction can reduce later problems of amblyopia and strabismus. The case for screening populations of infants for refractive errors rests on this possibility, which can only be investigated by large-scale, long-term programmes of the type described in Chapters 10 and 11. For screening to become widespread, it is not simply a question of establishing scientific relationships. Clinicians need to be convinced that the methods have satisfactory specificity and sensitivity, that the costs of screening are commensurate with its benefits, and that the methods and protocols are applicable in everyday clinical practice, as well as in the hands of the few specialist teams who have pursued them so far.

As well as addressing some of these issues, Chapter 10 points out the different requirements of screening large populations in whom most children will be normal, compared with assessing more fully those children in whom visual disability is already known or suspected. In between these two cases comes the visual investigation of children who are 'at risk' for visual problems for various reasons. In Chapter 12, van Hof-van Duin and Pott describe the use of acuity testing with a specific group who are at risk because of their birth history. Vital-Durand, Ayzac and Pinzaru (in Chapter 13) look at a broader group of children and ask 'What can we regard as risk factors that increase the likelihood of a child having a visual problem?'

7

Basic considerations when refracting infants

Frank Thorn

INTRODUCTION

Parents and teachers remember how their eye doctor placed lenses in front of their eyes and asked them to say which lens enabled them to see most clearly. Since this is a process based on subjective judgement and an oral report by the patient, these people wonder how a refractionist can determine the best lens for an infant. Conceptually, the basic optical methods used to perform an 'objective' refraction are simple. However, these elementary optical procedures are not always simple to implement and are invariably affected by the conditions under which they are used. This chapter is written to help the professional who works with infants but who does not perform eye examinations, to understand the procedures and problems encountered while refracting an infant. The author has tried to explain the basic procedure in as simple a manner as possible. The discussion of the six conditions, under which refractions can be performed and which affect the results of the refraction, involves a more complex analysis than the basic refractive procedure.

An older child or adult views the world through the optics of the eye (the cornea, pupil, and crystalline lens). Through a carefully designed series of eyeglass lens changes and answers to questions about clarity of vision, an examiner can determine the eyeglass lens characteristics that are best for the patient. The actual eyeglass prescription is typically based on this *subjective* manifest reaction, that is, the maximum plus (or minimum minus) lens power that allows the patient to see distant objects clearly under natural viewing conditions. It must be emphasized that what the patient sees is far more important for prescribing corrective lenses than what the examiner measures with an autorefractor or retinoscope, although the instrument measurements can provide the refractionist with very useful information. Ultimately, a patient's final refractive correction is determined by the most positive spherical lens correction combined with the astigmatic correction that provides a patient with the most acute and comfortable vision possible. An eyeglass prescription may also include adjustments for several factors such as interocular differences in refraction (anisometropia), accommodation and convergence problems, and simply the comfort of the patient when wearing the correction.

The most widely used 'objective' refracting device is the retinoscope. It is objective only in the sense that the patient's subjective impressions are not used. However, the retinoscopist must make a complex series of subjective decisions. How the retinoscope works will be explained in the following section. The less widely used autorefractors use variations on the same optical principles employed by the retinoscope.

WHAT IS RETINOSCOPY?

What is actually measured?

Most children and young adults can change the optical focus of their eyes so that they can view clearly both distant mountains and a book held near the face. To focus on a near object, the ciliary muscle within the eyes must contract, thus altering the shape of the crystalline lens so that the lens is more spherical; to focus on a distant object, the ciliary muscle must relax, thus putting pressure on the lens that causes it to flatten. This combination of ciliary muscle and crystalline lens action is the basis for accommodation. Most young people use reflex accommodation to produce clear vision over a wide range of distances.

The basic measure of refraction is the ophthalmic lens power that allows a person to see clearly at long distances with a relaxed ciliary muscle. With this lens power in front of the eye, the ciliary muscle that controls lens shape can remain relaxed when a person looks into the distance and requires the least amount of contraction when the person focuses on near objects. With this correction a person can focus on the greatest range of distances from near to far and will usually experience the greatest degree of comfort when looking at the world.

If a person cannot see clearly at distance with a completely relaxed ciliary muscle, the condition is defined as myopia or nearsightedness. When focused at the furthest possible distance, the eyes' optics are too strong for the length of the eye; thus, a 'minus' (concave) lens must be prescribed to reduce the effective strength of the eyes' optics. Conversely, if a person must accommodate to see clearly at distance, his or her condition is defined as hyperopia or farsightedness. If the hyperopia is so great that it is difficult for the person to accommodate enough to see clearly and comfortably into the distance, 'plus' (convex) lenses may be prescribed to enhance the effective optical power of the eye. People also start wearing convex lenses after 40 years of age. These are worn only for reading and other near work because the accommodative apparatus becomes increasingly less effective with age. This condition, known as presbyopia, occurs independently of the refractive errors that cause nearsightedness or farsightedness.

An informal demonstration

To demonstrate how retinoscopy works, the author will ask the readers who have never performed a refraction to try the following experiment. Sit near your window and watch people walking by across the street. Now, hold your arm out straight in front of you, form a circle between your thumb and first finger, and look though the circle to watch people walk by. Obviously, everyone will be standing upright and walking in the same direction in which they would be moving if you were not looking through the circle made by your fingers (Fig. 7.1(a)). If you then take off your regular eyeglasses, or put on your reading glasses or a friend's glasses, the pedestrians will be blurred but they will still appear to stand upright and walk in the expected direction.

Next, hold a ×2 or ×3 magnifying glass (+4.00 or +6.00 dioptre lens) at arm's length and look at the pedestrians through it. You will see that the pedestrians now appear upside down and backwards and therefore appear to walk in a direction opposite to normal viewing (Fig. 7.1(c)). If you are young and are able to accommodate or if you are older and wearing your reading glasses, the upside-down pedestrians will look clear. If you are older and not wearing your reading glasses, the pedestrians will be blurred but they will still appear to be upside down and walking in the wrong direction. The reason the pedestrians appear upside down and backwards is because the magnifier has created an image of the pedestrians in front of you. That image is inverted, just as the image formed by a camera lens on a sheet of film is inverted. When you look at pedestrians through the magnifying glass, you actually look at the inverted image formed between the magnifier and your eye. As a result of this inversion, everyone appears to be walking in the wrong direction.

If you use a weaker lens, such as those in your reading glasses (+1.50 to +2.50 dioptres if you do not have a significant refractive error), and hold it at the correct distance from your eye, the pedestrians will appear to be coloured flashes of light (Fig. 7.1(b)). You cannot judge if a pedestrian is upright or inverted, nor if the person is walking toward the left or the right. This occurs when the plus lens is at the precise distance that causes the pedestrians' images to be formed at your cornea. You can even measure the power of the lens by finding the exact distance the lens must be held from your eye for it to cause the pedestrians to appear as totally blurred flashes. The reciprocal of this distance measured in metres defines the power of the lens in dioptres. For example, if a lens exactly 0.5 m from your eye totally blurs a pedestrian's image, then the power of the lens must be +2.00 dioptres.

Using a retinoscope

In principle, this is all that an ophthalmologist or optometrist does when performing retinoscopy. The examiner sits 0.5 m or 0.66 m from the patient (depending on the length of the examiner's arms) and sweeps a streak of light projected by the retinoscope across the patient's eye. Most of the streak passes across the outer surface of the eye but part is projected through the pupil onto

(a)

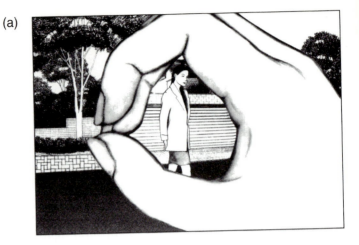

(b)

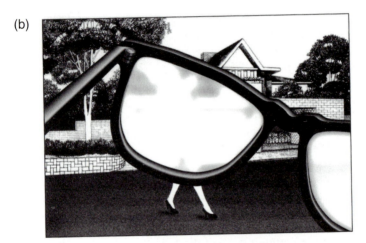

(c)

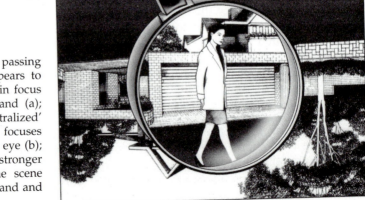

Fig. 7.1 How a passing street scene appears to you when it is in focus beyond your hand (a); when it is 'neutralized' by a lens that focuses the scene at the eye (b); and when a stronger lens focuses the scene between your hand and your eye (c).

the retina. The examiner looks through a peephole in the retinoscope that aligns his or her sight with the projected streak of light. The part that passes through the pupil always moves in the same direction as the streak moving across the eye's outer surface; however, the streak within the pupil may appear to the examiner to move in the opposite direction if the patient's eye is focused in front of the examiner.

Now, think of the streak moving on the retina as analogous to the pedestrians walking on the pavement. The combined cornea/lens optical system of the patient's eye is like the circle formed by your thumb and finger or the reading lens or the magnifier that you held in your hand while looking at the pedestrians. If the patient is focused in the distance behind the examiner, the examiner will see a blurred streak within the pupil moving in the same direction as the streak that moves across the surface of the eye. This is called 'with' motion (Fig. 7.2(a)). If the patient is focused closer so that the image of the retina is in front of the examiner, the examiner sees an inverted streak moving in the opposite direction within the patient's pupil (Fig. 7.2(c)). The streak movement in the opposite direction is called an 'against' motion.

The task for the retinoscopist is to find the lens that causes the image of the streak within the patient's pupil to be focused at the retinoscopist's cornea when the patient's accommodation is fully relaxed. The retinoscopist recognizes that the image is focused at his or her own cornea when he or she can no longer see a streak moving within the patient's pupil in either the 'with' or 'against' direction. Instead, there is simply a bright flash filling the pupil when the streak passes across it. This is called the 'neutralization' point (Fig. 7.2(b)).

The examiner may determine the lens that precisely 'neutralizes' the retinoscopy motion by trying different lenses. This is not a random search for the correct lens. Instead, an experienced retinoscopist can look at the direction and speed of motion as well as the amount that the streak appears to be blurred when a lens is placed in front of the patient's eye. The examiner then estimates the strength of the lens needed to produce 'neutralization'. If the retinoscope and the examiner's eye are 0.5 m from the patient's eye and a +2.00 lens placed in front of the patient's eye 'neutralizes' the motion of the streak, then the patient must be focused at infinity. This would suggest that the patient has no refractive error. If an examiner with longer arms sat so that the retinoscope was 0.66 m from the same patient's eye, a +1.50 dioptre lens would 'neutralize' the motion of the streak. In all cases, the retinoscopist must subtract the strength of the lens that offsets the 'working distance' from the value of the lens actually found to 'neutralize' the motion of the streak in order to calculate the strength of the lens that focuses the patient's eye at infinity.

Autorefractors all use a variation on the optical principles just described. As an example, the new VIVA Videorefractor (Fortune Optical) has been specially designed to refract infants and young children (Angi and Pilotto 1994). It uses the principle of static retinoscopy but with a stable light source that is located off-axis rather than a moving on-axis light source. Note that there are two

(a)

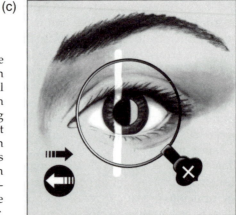

(b)

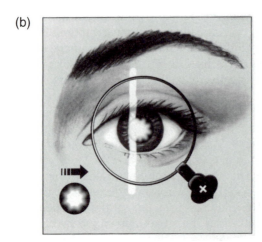

(c)

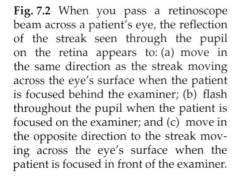

Fig. 7.2 When you pass a retinoscope beam across a patient's eye, the reflection of the streak seen through the pupil on the retina appears to: (a) move in the same direction as the streak moving across the eye's surface when the patient is focused behind the examiner; (b) flash throughout the pupil when the patient is focused on the examiner; and (c) move in the opposite direction to the streak moving across the eye's surface when the patient is focused in front of the examiner.

differences: stable light source and off-axis location. First let us consider the stable source. Think back to your observations of the pedestrians. If they only walked from the right side into the circle formed by your fingers and stopped immediately, they would appear to be located at the right side of the circle. If you were looking through the magnifying glass that turned them around, they would appear to be located upside down at the left side of the magnifier. Thus, if you simply aimed your light source so that it entered the pupil at the right pupillary border, you could estimate the refractive error based on the location of the image in the pupil rather than the direction of movement. Since it is very difficult to aim a beam of light at the edge of the pupil, this is really not a practical procedure. However, the concept of using retinal image position rather than movement can be made practical.

The VIVA Videorefractor actually uses infrared lights that are located to the side of an infrared camera. This is unlike the retinoscope for which the examiner's line of sight is perfectly aligned with the instrument's light source. Thus, the VIVA is classified as an off-axis refractor. When a patient looks at a scene, its image is projected upside down and backwards on the retina. When a patient looks at the VIVA infrared video camera, the retinal image of an infrared light located to one side of the video camera is located near the opposite edge of the pupil. Therefore the autorefractor can either estimate the position of the infrared light source within the pupil or move the infrared light sideways, closer or further away from the camera, until the image is perfectly centred within the pupil (it could actually fill the pupillary aperture if the eye were focused near the camera).

The VIVA Videorefractor locates its infrared light sources just to the side of the camera for relatively precise measurements of low refractive errors, while lights further to the side of the camera are used to estimate roughly high refractive errors. If the patient focuses behind the camera, the image of the infrared light will appear to be at the opposite edge of the pupil from where the infrared light is actually located; if the patient focuses in front of the camera, the image of the infrared light will appear to be on the same side of the pupil as the infrared light source because the video camera is actually capturing the inverted image of the retinal illumination that is projected in front of the eye. The exact amount of the displacement relative to the eccentricity of the light source determines the amount of the eye's defocus. This technique cannot provide optical information as precise as the retinoscope but it is very fast and truly objective. However, it is subject to all the factors that may influence or confuse accurate retinoscopy.

Factors that can confuse the retinoscopist

There are several confounding factors that confuse the examiner during retinoscopy and most other types of refraction. For example, owing to ocular aberrations, precise 'neutralization' is sometimes impossible so that the retinoscopist can only bracket the 'neutralization' point, finding a highly blurred 'with' motion with one lens and highly blurred 'against' motion with a lens that has a slightly more plus power. Often, the exact refractive error is slightly different at the centre of the pupil than in its periphery so that the examiner sees blurred streaks moving simultaneously in opposite directions rather than seeing a perfect 'neutralization'. The retinoscopist must make a judgement based on this 'scissors' motion. An autorefractor would record slightly different locations for several different images being focused through different places within the pupil and would be programmed to use the average of these positions.

The most troublesome problem for the retinoscopist may be the patients who do not fully relax their accommodation or who continually change their accommodative state. Cycloplegic drugs are often used to immobilize the accommodative apparatus in an attempt to eliminate this problem. With older children and adults, patients may be asked to look at a distant target with a lens that has the most plus value through which the patients can see clearly at distance, placed in front of the eye viewing the target. Some examiners then use a slightly stronger plus lens in the belief that 'fogging' the eye may relax the patient's accommodation even more. Unwanted accommodation may reduce the maximum plus value of the 'neutralization' point if neither cycloplegic drops nor maximum plus lenses can be used. Often, the retinoscopist can see changing amounts of 'with' and 'against' motion during a continuous period of looking through the retinoscope. The 'neutralization' lens used during the moments when accommodation is most relaxed should be used to estimate refractive error. Autorefractors do not make these judgements and thus may miss the full refractive error of a patient with unsteady accommodation.

REFRACTION CONDITIONS

Different measurement conditions

Cycloplegic drugs relax accommodation during a refraction. How does this accommodative state relate to the most relaxed state that a person can actually use during normal viewing? Can autorefractors that require a person to look into an instrument actually relax accommodation and thus achieve refractive measurements similar to those found when looking into the distance? Can plus lenses, which are meant to relax accommodation when placed in front of the eyes, relax accommodation as effectively as when a patient looks into the real distance? When trying to judge the validity of a measurement technique, these questions are often more important than the hardware that is used. Retinoscopes, autorefractors, and photorefractors are all well-designed optical instruments (although they may differ in precision); however, they are designed to be used in different ways and require different modes of viewing by patients. These different modes often produce different refractive error measurements.

There are six possible viewing conditions that can be used during a refraction. They are by no means equivalent but they are all used in one procedure or another and are as follows.

(1) A patient's accommodation is immobilized by an anticholinergic drug;
(2) A patient looks at a *distant* target through the maximum plus (or least minus) lens that allows clear or slightly blurred vision;
(3) A patient looks at a *near* target through the maximum plus (or least minus) lens that allows clear or slightly blurred vision;
(4) A patient simply focuses on a distant target (without the use of lenses);
(5) A patient simply focuses on a near target (without the use of lenses);
(6) A patient has nothing to focus on, as in darkness.

Procedure 1 is designed to measure refractive error with the accommodative apparatus as relaxed as is biologically possible.

Procedures 2 and 3 measure refractive error when the eye's accommodative apparatus is believed to be relaxed to its natural physiological limit.

With procedures 4–6 it is less certain what is measured.

In this section each of these six refracting conditions will be discussed, with an emphasis on how the testing condition can affect refractive measurements.

Cycloplegic refractions

A cycloplegic refraction is often considered the 'gold standard' of refractions. It is easy to perform because the accommodative system is immobilized so that there is almost no variability in focus and the crystalline lens within the eye approaches its absolute minimum refractive power. The problem with this measurement is that, in real life, it is often impossible for the lens shape to relax this much. Thus, this is not the functional refractive error of the eye and is not the appropriate measurement for prescribing corrective lenses. It is not a 'gold standard' for this purpose.

Many refractionists have pointed out the problems and limited application of cycloplegic refractions. Michaels (1975) in his popular text on refraction states that:

Cycloplegia is not always complete, not always equal, and not always properly timed. The increased aberrations, reduced depth of focus, altered accommodation—convergence, spurious off-axis measurements, … are the price paid for immobilizing the ciliary muscle and dilating the pupil. Moreover, few people would wear a lens prescribed only from cycloplegic measurements very long or very comfortably. Cycloplegics are indicated because it is occasionally difficult to refract without them and, more importantly, because the information provided adds to our diagnostic data. The question is not whether to use cycloplegics but when.

Michaels continues, 'Cycloplegia is not synonymous with validity' and 'One must not conclude that cycloplegic and noncycloplegic refraction always give the same information'.

Infants are difficult to refract so it is common practice to use cycloplegics in order to obtain more reliable results. However, this refraction does not necessarily provide the most valid refractive error measurement (i.e. the best measurement of an infant's ability to focus the image of a distant object on the retina). Since the effect of cycloplegic drugs can vary from one person to another, residual accommodation after cycloplegia can be as high as 1–2 dioptres in adults. Good procedure calls for this residual accommodation to be ascertained just prior to refraction through the use of such tests as dynamic retinoscopy or the accommodative push-up technique. If such levels of residual accommodation are found, further instillation of cycloplegia is indicated. Unfortunately, these procedures are difficult or impossible with infants, even though infants are known to be especially resistant to the effect of cycloplegic drugs. Even with good cycloplegia the refraction of an infant may entail significant variability because of ever-changing fixation eye movements.

Distance (manifest) refraction with corrective lenses

The most common type of 'objective' non-cycloplegic refraction is a manifest refraction using a retinoscope. The examiner performs retinoscopy on one eye while the patient looks at a distant pattern with the other eye through a lens that is just convex enough to slightly blur vision. Maximum relaxation of accommodation is assumed to have occurred in both eyes under this viewing condition owing to consensual accommodation. Thus, the eyes' focus should approach that of the eyes' 'true' functional refractive limit. In fact, calculations based on this 'objective' manifest refraction normally approximate the correction given in an eyeglass prescription. However, as noted before, the actual eyeglass prescription for older children and adults is typically based on the *subjective* manifest refraction.

Although the manifest refraction is our 'gold standard' for prescribing glasses, there are inherent problems in this technique. Since the purpose of accommodation is to use the eye's optics to make images clear, it is often assumed that accommodation is controlled by optical blur; however, the controls are much more complex than this. Proximity cues (the knowledge of distance based on any information available in the testing room) allow a patient to judge the actual distance of a test pattern. This knowledge may contradict the information provided by the optical blur cues from the maximum plus lens for image clarity. Thus, the patient may focus at a distance that is based on a compromise between these conflicting distance cues (optical blur vs. other cues for distance). This can produce significant underestimation of hyperopia. Since the fixation target is seen at 3–6 m rather than 'real' infinity, this may also bias the response of emmetropes in a slightly myopic direction. These factors differ from person to person but these are the same factors that people face when wearing glasses in the real world. Consequently, the refractionist can feel safe prescribing the most comfortable, most plus lenses determined under precisely the same conditions in which they will be worn in daily life.

The individual differences involved in a manifest refraction as well as the individual differences involved in a cycloplegic refraction cause the cycloplegic to vary significantly from the manifest refraction for many patients. However, only the manifest subjective refraction provides a valid general standard for prescribing lenses.

Unfortunately, it is impossible to lure an infant into focusing onto a distant target while an examiner just 0.5 m away flashes a bright light into the infant's eyes. As a result, the best 'gold standard' (the manifest refraction) cannot be used with infants.

Refraction during near viewing with corrective lenses

In this procedure a person focuses on a near target either monocularly or binocularly through relatively strong plus lenses. The problems involving conflicting distance cues just described for distant viewing are generally worse when testing with a near target. In addition, the distance cues used for testing with near viewing are no longer closely related to real-world conditions. Thus, when an individual peers into an instrument to fixate on a small target presented within it at optical infinity, 'instrument myopia' is likely to occur. As a result, non-cycloplegic refractions taken with automatic refractors must be considered nothing more than an initial estimate that can be used as a reference point for starting a distance refraction. Similarly, a patient may actually have normal visual acuity when instruments such as the B & L Ortho-Rater, the Titmus Vision Tester, and the Keystone Telebinocular show reduced visual acuity. The visual reduction measured with these instruments may simply be a result of the subject's inability to focus properly with the conflicting distance cues inherent in this type of instrument. The Canon R-1 Autoref with its see-through infrared reflecting window is the only auto refractor that allows patients to look directly through a window at a distant target in the room rather than at a target within the instrument.

The near viewing technique seems to be more feasible than distance retinoscopy with infants. Dynamic retinoscopy is a form of retinoscopy in which the patient fixates on an object attached to the retinoscope. These objects have included everything from a page of text with a hole in the middle for the retinoscope to a bell that attaches to the retinoscope and rings each time the retinoscope moves. The technique is generally used to measure where a person focuses when viewing a near target. It is used routinely by many optometrists to measure the accommodative accuracy of young school-age children and even pre-school children when they look at a near target. Haynes *et al.* (1965) used one type of dynamic retinoscopy to measure the accommodation of infants. Infants looked at a test pattern while the examiner performed retinoscopy through a hole in the test pattern and briefly placed correcting lenses before the infants' eyes. This study showed that infants less than 3 months old tended to over-accommodate. During the first month of life this over-accommodation often exceeded 3 or 4 dioptres.

Dynamic retinoscopy can probably be adapted to perform refractions on infants. To do this, an illuminated pattern would be mounted on the retinoscope to induce the infant to accommodate to the examiner's working distance (perhaps 0.5 m) and then plus lenses would be placed before the infant's eyes to relax accommodation until the infant could no longer reduce accommodation. The resulting measurement would be analogous to that of some autorefractors. However, all the problems inherent in the use of the autorefractor with adults would be expected to occur for infants, with the additional problem that infants tend to over-accommodate sporadically and unpredictably to near targets.

Distant viewing without corrective lenses

Manifest refraction must be measured with a corrective lens in front of the eye that is *not* being measured; thus a patient focusing on a distant target will fully relax accommodation in this fixating eye and consensual accommodation will cause the accommodation of the other eye, which is being measured, to relax also. It is surprising how often this essential step is ignored. This procedural error can just as easily confound the results of examinations using autorefractors as those using retinoscopy. For example, the Canon R-1 Autoref is commonly used in experiments on accommodation and accommodative tonus. Since Canon R-1 measurements can often be difficult to make when lenses are worn in front of the eyes, investigators tend to avoid their use (Owens *et al.* 1991; Chiu *et al.* 1993). This can lead to some bewildering results. When groups of normal adults in these experiments were refracted with the Canon R-1, they looked at distant targets that were 4 m or 6 m away. Using this procedure, virtually no hyperopia was found. One must assume that this lack of hyperopia is a result of measurement error from hyperopic subjects accommodating to see the target clearly. The existence of a measurement error was confirmed when the room lights were turned off in order to determine where the eye focused without a fixation target (tonic accommodation). Some subjects actually showed a significant decrease in their refractive status (i.e. a negative tonic accommodation). This, of course, is a logical impossibility since by definition the refractive error is measured when accommodation is as relaxed as possible. These measurements simply cannot be made accurately without corrective lenses.

Near viewing without corrective lenses

Dynamic retinoscopy is rarely performed without using lenses to find refractive or accommodative errors. Legend has it that Copeland, the designer of the Copeland retinoscope, could walk in front of an audience and 'accurately' perform retinoscopy on each person in the front row without using lenses and barely even breaking stride. Today few of us are legends. However, dynamic retinoscopy can often avoid the use of lenses by moving the retinoscope nearer or further away from the patient and by changing the position of the light source within the retinoscope. Brookman (1983) has used these tricks to measure infantile accommodation with dynamic retinoscopy without lenses.

On-axis photorefraction has been designed as a screening technique and, like dynamic retinoscopy, defies some of the constraints for normal refractive technique. The infant or child is induced to fixate on a toy or pattern near the photorefractor, which is located just 0.75 m or 1.5 m away from the subject. Since neither lenses nor cycloplegia are used, hyperopic and emmetropic children can accommodate toward the target, thus reducing the measured amount of hyperopia. Knowing this, those who use this photorefractive technique do not claim to be performing a refraction but instead describe their measurement as the 'optical focus' of a child who is fixating on the target.

Even the most sophisticated of these instruments (Howland and Howland 1974; Howland and Sayles 1987) do not have the accuracy of a retinoscope or many autorefractors. Nevertheless, the procedure is very fast and easily used with infants and young children (Atkinson *et al.* 1984; Howland and Sayles 1987). Cycloplegic refractive error estimates are derived from photorefractive optical focus measurements either by using an empirically based regression equation or by dividing the population of optical focus measurements into putative hyperopes, emmetropes, and myopes. Although ophthalmologists and optometrists may find these estimates to be 'inaccurate', the technique appears to provide valuable screening information (Atkinson *et al.* 1984).

Viewing no focusing target in darkness (near retinoscopy)

It is relatively easy to perform the near retinoscopy procedure with infants and young children. The examiner simply turns off the lights, attracts the attention of the infant to the retinoscope light, and places lenses in front of one eye while covering the other eye. There is nothing else for the infant to look at than the retinoscope beam so it is easy to attract its attention. The lenses can often be sneaked in front of the eye being examined while the hand holding the lens can be placed in front of the other eye without the infant reacting. Astigmatism and anisometropia are readily measured. However, the interpretation of the spherical correction measured by near retinoscopy is not straightforward.

It was once thought that when a person is deprived of a fixation target on which to focus (as in darkness) the eye would 'relax' to its least accommodating state and thus provide an approximation to the manifest refractive state. Mohindra (1975, 1977*a*, *b*) used this principle to develop 'near retinoscopy' as a quick and easy screening technique for young children before tonic accommodation was accepted as a basic optical property of the eye (Leibowitz and Owens 1975; 1978). Mohindra found in a group of older children and young adults that near retinoscopy provided refractive error measurements that differed from traditional manifest refraction measurements by approximately −0.75 dioptres. This finding indicates that the subjects looking at the retinoscope in the dark actually accommodate by an average of 0.75 dioptres. Thus, Mohindra made a purely empirical +0.75 dioptres correction in her measurements to estimate manifest refractive error. This correction is implemented when the retinoscopist corrects for the 0.5 m working distance by subtracting

+1.25 dioptres from the neutralization lens rather than the optically appropriate +2.00 dioptres. It is important to note that Owens *et al.* (1980) have since shown that a retinoscopic beam does not provide an adequate accommodative cue for adults so that near retinoscopy measurement provides one type of measurement of dark focus (refractive error plus tonic accommodation) rather than the refractive error itself. Early studies that required co-operating adults to make fine, difficult judgements about the relative position or movement of a target in an optometer, showed a mean relaxation state (tonic accommodation level) of approximately +1.5 dioptres with great individual variations (Leibowitz and Owens 1975; 1978). However, recent studies using objective optical measurements (primarily with the Canon R-1 Autoref) show that the average tonic or resting accommodation level is between +0.50 dioptres and +0.75 dioptres and rarely exceeds +1.25 dioptres when a subject relaxes and looks into darkness (Gwiazda *et al.* 1991; Chiu *et al.* 1993). Thus, near retinoscopy appears to provide a good estimate of dark focus and thus an indirect estimate of the refractive state of older children and adults to within ±0.50 dioptres.

However, we cannot be certain that infants looking at a bright light in a dark room are performing the same as co-operative children and adults. If they tend to accommodate more with more variability than older children as Haynes *et al.* (1965) suggested, then a greater correction for tonic accommodation may be appropriate when calculating the spherical refractive correction. This will be discussed further in the following chapter.

The new VIVA Videorefractor used by Angi and Pilotto (see Chapter 11) requires infants to look at flickering red LEDs 1 m away from them. It is unlikely that these LEDs are adequate accommodative targets. Thus, this photorefractor may employ a viewing condition that is very similar to that used in near retinoscopy.

CONCLUSIONS

Retinoscopy was designed to provide an objective starting point for a refraction and to provide information supplementary to a full subjective refraction. It was not intended to provide a precise refractive measurement for prescribing eyeglasses. If examiners expect this kind of precision, they will be disappointed. If an examiner prescribes eyeglasses based on these measurements, patients will be even more disappointed. However, when examining infants one must rely on retinoscopy or other objective procedures intended to replace them. As accurate as these methods may be, one must not expect to precisely reflect the eyeglass prescriptions that would best suit infants if the infants could actually tell us how the world looked through lenses.

Many instruments are now available for objectively measuring refractive errors. Since all are based on the same optical principles, one should at first glance expect all of them to provide the same refractive error measurements with perhaps different amounts of precision. However, the instruments require patients to view fixation targets under many different conditions. Without cycloplegic drugs, the accommodative control mechanisms will respond differently under these different conditions and the resulting refractive error measurements will differ. This is not a great problem if we understand the sources of variance, control them as well as possible, and appreciate the nature of the errors still likely to occur with a given method. With this proviso, clinical measurements of great value will be obtained. Cycloplegic drugs will allow more reliable refractive errors but provide us with a different set of unknowns. One cannot be certain that cyloplegia is complete, and if it is complete one cannot be certain that an infant can actually relax accommodation this much. Cycloplegia also has very limited application when trying to screen large numbers of children inexpensively and quickly.

Most of the refractive instruments available at this time require more co-operation than infants can provide. Only photorefraction, both off-axis and on-axis, and retinoscopy, both near and dynamic, appear to be appropriate for refracting infants. Since these techniques require an infant to look at a near target or at a non-accommodative target in the dark, they can only be used to estimate an infant's manifest refractive error. However, each can do this with a precision that makes them very useful in a clinical setting. Special efforts are required for these procedures to provide data that are accurate enough for many research purposes.

ACKNOWLEDGEMENTS

I thank James P. Comerford, Jane Gwiazda, Richard Held, and Sondra Thorn for their helpful comments on the manuscript. This work was supported in part by NIH-2R01 EY 1191 and SP30-EY02621.

REFERENCES

Atkinson, J., Braddick, O. J., Durden, K., Watson, P., and Atkinson, S. (1984). Screening for refractive errors in 6–9-month-old infants by photorefraction. *British Journal of Ophthalmology*, **68**, 105–12.

Brookman, K. E. (1983). A retinoscopic method of assessing accommodative performance of young human infants. *Journal of the American Optometric Association*, **52**, 865–69.

Chiu, N., Rosenfeld, M., Ciufredda, K. J., and Duckman, R. (1993). Accommodative adaptation in infants. *Investigative Ophthalmology and Visual Science*, **34** (suppl.), 1309.

Gwiazda, J., Thorn, F. , Bauer, J., and Held, R. (1991). Tonic accommodation increases more in myopic than hyperopic children following near work. *Investigative Ophthalmology and Visual Science*, **32** (suppl.), 1125.

Haynes, H., White, B. L., and Held, R. (1965). Visual accommodation in human infants. *Science*, **148**, 528–30.

Howland, H. C. and Howland, B. (1974). Photorefraction: a technique for study of refractive state at a distance. *Journal of the Optical Society of America*, **64**, 240–9.

Howland, H. C. and Sayles, N. (1987). A photorefractive characterization of focusing ability of infants and young children. *Investigative Ophthalmology and Visual Science*, **28**, 1005–15.

Leibowitz, H. W. and Owens, D. A. (1975). Anomalous myopias and the intermediate dark focus of accommodation. *Science*, **189**, 646–8.

Leibowitz, H. W. and Owens, D. A. (1978). New evidence for the intermediate position of relaxed accommodation. *Documenta Ophthalmologica*, **46**, 133–47.

Michaels, D. D. (1975). *Visual Optics and Refraction*. Mosby, St Louis, p. 186.

Mohindra, I. (1975). A technique for infant examination. *American Journal of Optometry and Physiological Optics*, **52**, 867–70.

Mohindra, I. (1977a). Comparison of 'near retinoscopy' and subjective refraction in adults. *American Journal of Optometry and Physiological Optics*, **54**, 319–22.

Mohindra, I. (1977b). A non-cycloplegic refraction technique for infants and young children. *Journal of the American Optometric Association*, **48**, 518–23.

Owens, D. A., Mohindra, I., and Held, R. (1980). The effectiveness of the retinoscope beam as an accommodative stimulus. *Investigative Ophthalmology and Visual Science*, **19**, 942–9.

Owens, D. A., Haimes, D. J. S., and Francis, E. L. (1991). Adaptation of tonic accommodation in children. *Investigative Ophthalmology and Visual Science*, **32** (suppl.), 1125.

8

Using near retinoscopy to refract infants

Frank Thorn, Jane Gwiazda, and
Richard Held

INTRODUCTION

The MIT Infant Vision Laboratory initiated research on the development of infant vision 20 years ago. This laboratory was interested initially in the development of visual acuity and then the development of stereopsis and binocular fusion. It was immediately obvious that the laboratory could not claim that infants' visual capabilities are poorer than those of adults unless it demonstrated that poor optical focus was not limiting visual performance. Thus, it was necessary to refract the infants on the same day they were performing the experimental procedures of the laboratory, which usually involved forced-choice preferential looking.

Since the laboratory must recruit infants' parents, convince the parents to bring their infants back for several repeat visits, and test the infants' visual abilities and refractive errors during each brief visit without upsetting the infants or their parents, the choice of refractive procedures was crucial. Thus, it was decided that infants could not be sedated or forcibly held during an eye examination. Similarly, eye drops, that is cycloplegic drugs, could not be used. It would also be desirable for the infants to seem to enjoy the refractive procedure or at least not cry and withdraw during it. This is the ideal that everyone would like to have when screening infants and young children.

Investigators at the Infant Vision Laboratory decided that Mohindra's 'near' retinoscopy technique was best suited to fill these requirements. Mohindra had developed this method as a quick, non-invasive, non-threatening refractive method for mass, visual screenings of infants and young children (Mohindra 1975; 1977). The technique has met the needs of the laboratory by being non-threatening, non-invasive and highly repeatable, has been very easy to use in pre-school screenings and, as a bonus, has provided landmark data on several aspects of infantile refractive errors. Accordingly, there has been widespread interest concerning the exact procedures used in near retinoscopy.

PERFORMING NEAR RETINOSCOPY

A parent is asked to sit and hold a baby so that the baby feels comfortable and relaxed and faces toward the examiner. The exact position is unimportant because the retinoscope is so small and lightweight that the retinoscopist can readily adjust to the infant's position: sitting before one infant, kneeling before another, standing over another, and examining another while walking behind a parent who walks around the room with the infant over a shoulder. However, the retinoscopist always works with a 50 cm distance between the retinoscope and the infant's eye. If the baby is less than 4 months of age, the parent is asked to encourage the baby to suck on a bottle or a pacifier. This acts to hold the head in one position and to relax further the infant without putting it to sleep immediately. The examiner then dims the room lights, attracts the infant's attention to the retinoscope light, and places lenses in front of one eye while covering the other eye with the hand holding the lens. The retinoscope beam is the only point of illumination for the infant to look at so it is easy to attract the infant's attention. The lens can often be moved in front of the eye with such stealth that the infant does not react to it.

Occasionally, an infant sleeps or cries during an examination. Even then, it is usually possible to measure a refractive error by lifting the eyelid of the sleeping infant with our fingers or refracting the crying infant during moments when the eyes are dry. Although these are useful measurements for informing parents about their child's vision, one may lack confidence in their precision and thus not use them as experimental data.

ASTIGMATISM MEASUREMENT

Astigmatism is measured readily using near retinoscopy. In fact, infantile astigmatism data were the first refractive data to be published by this laboratory. It is almost as easy to measure astigmatism accurately in an infant with near retinoscopy as it is to measure it in an adult with normal distance retinoscopy. Astigmatism usually varies little during accommodation. Thus, whether an infant is focused at distance or near, the astigmatism is approximately the same and the near retinoscopy procedure for measuring it is the same. The examiner determines the two orthogonal meridians for which the movement of the retinoscope streak, seen through the pupil on the retina, parallels the streak moving across the eye's surface. These are defined as the major meridians of the refractive error and determine the axis of the astigmatism. Next, the retinoscopist determines the power of lenses placed in front of the eye that neutralizes the movement of the retinal reflection of the streak. These are exactly the steps that must be followed in any retinoscopic examination. The only difference with near retinoscopy is that the power of the neutralizing lenses must be determined within one or two seconds of each other two or three times so that we can be confident that an accommodative change has not occurred between the two determinations. It is easy for a retinoscopist who practices such speed to alternately confirm the neutralizing power in both major meridians two or three times within 5 s.

Near retinoscopy and photorefraction provided the first measurements of infantile astigmatism (Howland *et al.* 1978; Mohindra *et al.* 1978). The first presentation of these findings showed that more than 50 per cent of infants between 3 and 5 months of age had a significant astigmatism ($\geq$1.0 dioptres) and that more than 50 per cent of these were oriented in an against-the-rule direction. The power of the astigmatism and the proportion of infants showing an astigmatism decreased rapidly during the following 4 years. Few of those present at the 1978 session of ARVO will forget the vehemence with which several prominent paediatric ophthalmologists denounced these findings, declaring that they had performed cycloplegic retinoscopy on thousands of infants and knew that infants had very little astigmatism. Indeed, low astigmatism levels in infants was the wisdom of the day. They insisted that this report of infantile astigmatism showed how unreliable near retinoscopy was as a refracting technique. Now, of course, infantile astigmatism has been reported using numerous techniques and is universally accepted (Dobson *et al.* 1984; Gwiazda *et al.* 1984; Howland and Sayles 1984). We do not claim that the failure to observe infantile astigmatism with cycloplegic retinoscopy during the preceding decades shows that cycloplegic retinoscopy is an unreliable technique. One of the surprising findings is that general infant populations refracted in the USA have a high proportion of infants with against-the-rule astigmatism (vertical axis for minus cylindrical corrective lenses) (Dobson *et al.* 1984; 1983; Gwiazda *et al.* 1984; Howland and Sayles 1984) but Chinese infants have a high proportion of with-the-rule astigmatism. Yet, in our laboratory, the parents of both the Caucasian and Chinese infants had the same small amounts of astigmatism with a preponderance of with-the-rule astigmatism (Thorn *et al.* 1987).

MEASUREMENT OF ANISOMETROPIA

Anisometropia in a given meridian or pair of meridians is also determined easily with near retinoscopy. In this case, the retinoscopist passes the retinoscopic streak and hand-held lenses across both eyes several times within a few seconds. The procedure and rationale are similar to that for measuring astigmatic power as described above. Even if one cannot be certain of the absolute spherical refractive error of either eye, one can say with confidence whether or not the spherical error for the two eyes is the same and, if different, by approximately what amount. If it is assumed that the two eyes accommodate by approximately the same amount, then the anisometropic comparison is more accurate than the absolute spherical refractive measurement of either eye. We and others (Howland and Sayles 1987) have found little anisometropia in

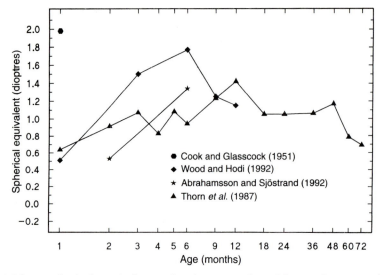

Fig. 8.1 Mean spherical equivalent refractive error data. Near retinoscopy data by Thorn (▲) from 1 to 42 months of age and distance retinoscopy from 42 to 72 months of age. Neonatal cycloplegic data using multiple instillations of atropine are from Cook and Glasscock (1951). Cycloplegic data using cyclopentolate in infants are from Abrahamsson and Sjöstrand (1992) and Wood and Hodi (1992).

infants, despite the fact that equivalent spherical refractive errors are far more variable among infants than older children.

MEASUREMENT OF EQUIVALENT SPHERICAL REFRACTIVE ERROR IN INFANTS

Retinoscopy with cycloplegia

The measurement of spherical refractive errors is the greatest problem in refracting infants with any measurement technique. Even when cycloplegia is used to paralyse the ciliary muscle, there is a doubt about the spherical refractive error. The cycloplegic refractive errors for newborn infants in the classic Cook and Glasscock study (1951) showed a mean of +2.0 dioptres of hyperopia in neonates treated with 1 drop of 1 per cent atropine instilled four times at 6-hour intervals (Fig. 8.1). Franceschetti's (1935) results using atropine with newborn infants are similar to this (+1.62 dioptres). Using two drops of cyclopentolate, Wood and Hodi (1992) and Abrahamsson and Sjöstrand (1992) have recently shown mean cycloplegic refractive errors of less than +1.00 dioptres for infants who are 1–2 months old (Fig. 8.1). In all of these studies retinoscopy was used to perform the refractions. The differences between the two pairs of cycloplegic data are problably caused by the differences in the strength of cycloplegic agents and administration procedures. The very young infants appear to be accommodating about 1 dioptre when cyclopentolate is used as the cycloplegic. As the infants become more sensitive to cycloplegia with age, their accommodation decreases and therefore hyperopia appears to increase (Wood and Hodi 1992).

Near retinoscopy and tonic accommodation

The near retinoscopy fixation target is the retinoscope beam of light but this beam does not provide an adequate stimulus for accommodation (Owens *et al.* 1980). Left without a stimulus on which to focus, infants are likely to focus near their resting state of accommodation. In older children and young adults, Mohindra has shown a consistent difference between manifest distance retinoscopy and near retinoscopy of about +0.75 dioptres. This difference is consistent with recent estimates of tonic accommodation in older children and young adults (Gwiazda *et al.* 1991).

At this time the tonic accommodation levels of infants are unknown; however, studies of infantile accommodation and studies comparing near retinoscopy to cycloplegic retinoscopy suggest that infants may have higher levels of tonic accommodation than older children.

The data of Mohindra and Molinari (1979), Borghi and Rouse (1985), Cruz *et al.* (1990), and Saunders and Westall (1992), which compare cycloplegic retinoscopy to near retinoscopy, show that a correction for accommodation of +1.25 dioptres is needed for infants older than 6 months of age rather than the +0.75 dioptre correction required for school age children and young adults. Each of these studies stresses the excellent reliability of the near retinoscopy technique and the high correlation between near retinoscopy and cycloplegic retinoscopy measurements. Others have been less successful in demonstrating reliability and good correlations when comparing near retinoscopy to cycloplegic retinoscopy measurements (Maino *et al.* 1984; Wesson *et al.* 1990). Overall, these studies indicate that in the hands of most refractionists, near retinoscopy is a useful, reliable technique for measuring refractive error.

Many years ago Santonastaso (1930) compared cycloplegic and non-cycloplegic retinoscopy in infants. His data show a mean cycloplegic refractive error of +1.0 dioptres and a mean non-cycloplegic refractive error of −7.0 dioptres during the first 15 days of life. It must be noted that Santonastaso's non-cycloplegic technique appears to be a variation of dynamic retinoscopy rather than near retinoscopy. Thus, his findings are consistent with the dynamic retinoscopy data of Haynes *et al.* (1965) and the Canon R-1 Autorefractor data of Aslin *et al.* (1990), which showed huge amounts of non-stimulus-controlled over-accommodation in infants during the first month.

Unfortunately, it is unknown how much these young infants would over-accommodate to a retinoscope light during near retinoscopy. Our observations suggest how to minimize such accommodation in young infants but these observations are inconclusive.

Observing infants' optical focus fluctuations during near retinoscopy

The scenario during near retinoscopy testing of the most difficult subjects—infants less than 2 months old—will first be described. A mother sits down, holds her infant comfortably, the room lights are dimmed, and the retinoscopist starts moving the retinoscope streak slowly back and forth across both eyes. Our examiner (FT) is a very passive retinoscopist, who uses a soothing voice and demonstrates great patience. In most cases (about 90 per cent of the young infants) the initial retinoscopic reflection shows a strong 'against' motion (i.e. the streak of light within the pupil moves in the opposite direction to the movement of the light across the surface of the eye). This means that the infant is focused in front of the retinoscope. Since the retinoscope is located 50 cm from the infant's eyes, the infant's 'against' retinoscopic motion indicates more than –2.0 dioptres of myopia to start with. Within 10–20 s most infants start to focus near the retinoscope or slightly behind it (indicating a small amount of myopia). Thereafter, unless the infant becomes excited or upset, a 'with' motion is seen (the streak within the pupil moves in the same direction as the movement on the surface of the eye). Even mild excitement such as the mother repositioning the infant, the retinoscopist starting to scan his light after a brief rest, or a loud noise in the hall can trigger renewed accommodation. If these pitfalls can be avoided, a 'with' motion is soon seen even when a +2 dioptre or +3 dioptre lens is placed before the infant's eyes. This indicates that the infant is actually hyperopic. As the infant's accommodation relaxes, plus lenses of increasing strength are placed before the infant's eyes until the retinoscopist determines the highest plus lens that can neutralize the reflex (the retinoscopic reflex appears as just a flash of light without a clear direction of motion).

This pattern of observations has many variations. The initial retinoscopic motion may be neutral or slightly 'with'. The 'with' motion (indicating hyperopia) may reach its maximum quickly, within a minute, or take several minutes to be achieved. The measurements are highly dependent on the comfort and relaxation of the infant. Drowsiness, sleep, and sucking behaviour are associated with increased amounts of hyperopia. Popping a bottle, pacifier, or thumb into an infant's mouth usually elicits an immediate and occasionally dramatic reduction in accommodation. Thus, in most cases, final measurements are taken while the infant sucks on something. Some infants show continuous cycles of accommodation; others relax and show relatively steady accommodative variation (< 1.0 dioptres).

It should be noted that near retinoscopy was initially designed to be a fast, efficient screening technique. All practitioners of the technique wait for the initial accommodative fluctuations to settle down. They then pick a specific criterion for the retinoscopic measurement that they accept for the record. Our current procedure is to wait as long as it takes for accommodation to fully relax so that our measurements approach the refractive state expected from a manifest refraction, that is, if it were possible to perform a manifest refraction on an infant.

Fig. 8.1 shows the mean near retinoscopy refractive errors measured as a function of age in our laboratory by FT. The retinoscopic measurements on children under 3.5 years are always performed in a dark room with near retinoscopy. However, measurements on children 3.5 years or older are performed in a dimly lit room using distance retinoscopy. These children look at a projected 20/40 Snellen letter while the highest plus lens that does not blur vision is held in front of the eye that is not being tested. It should be noted that the data form a smooth continuum between near retinoscopy and distance retinoscopy. This is consistent with the many studies that show that near retinoscopy provides a close approximation to non-cycloplegic retinoscopy.

REFRACTIVE DATA FROM THE INFANT VISION LAB

Our near retinoscopy data are surprisingly similar to those of Wood and Hodi (1992) and Abrahamsson and Sjöstrand (1992) although we do not show the high hyperopic peak at 3–6 months that is shown in the data of Wood and Hodi (Fig. 8.1). The near retinoscopy data show a peak at 1 year or slightly older, at which point the level of hyperopia approaches that of Wood and Hodi (1992).

Despite the differences in the mean refractive errors among the studies represented in Fig. 8.1, the distribution of refractive errors is similar in all studies, with standard deviations of ±1.50 to ±2.00 dioptres prior to 3 months of age and standard deviations approaching ±1.0 dioptres at 1 year of age. This suggests that different retinoscopic techniques may demonstrate slightly different absolute spherical refractive powers but the measurements are closely related.

When performing near retinoscopy, much accommodative fluctuation may occur even when accommodation is most relaxed. Fig. 8.2 plots two near retinoscopy measurements taken during the same time period on the same infants. One is the most plus optical focus observed with the retinoscope. This is our estimate of the manifest refractive error. It is the same as the measurements shown in the preceding figure. The lower curve represents the mean optical focus during the period when the most plus measurement was made. These measurements approach each other at about 6 months.

For infants less than 3 months of age, the accommodative system may never stabilize during near retinoscopy. Thus, the refractive error measurement and the optical focus observed most of the time by the retinoscopist can differ by significant amounts in young infants. Such variability may cause a retinoscopist not familiar with near retinoscopy to lack confidence in it. It causes the experienced near retinoscopist to be very careful in the interpretation of the refractive measurements.

For individual infants the difference between the refractive error and the most common optical focus state varies considerably (Fig. 8.3). This difference represents the difference between optical focus with the least amount of accommodation noticed and that with the usual amount of accommodation noticed

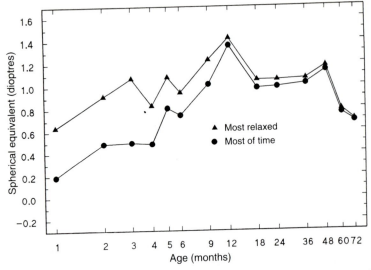

Fig. 8.2 Mean spherical equivalent refractive error (defined as the most plus lens determined by retinoscopy) by Thorn (▲) as in Fig. 8.1. The mean spherical equivalent optical focus of the same group (defined as the most commonly determined plus lens during the same time period in which the most plus determinations were made).

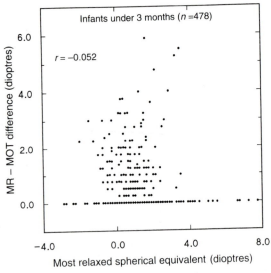

Fig. 8.3 The median level of accommodation for individual infants under 3 months of age during the period when the refractive error was being determined as a function of retinoscopically determined spherical equivalent refractive error. Note that many of the points representing 0.25 dioptres or less of accommodation represent measurements from many infants.

during the final time period when refractive measurements were actually taken. Thus, the Y axis approximates the infant's usual amount of accommodation at the time that near retinoscopy readings were taken. It is clear that this accommodation is not correlated with the most plus near retinoscopy refractive error ($r = 0.056$). That is, hyperopes and myopes show about the same amount of accommodation during near retinoscopy. The difference between the most common equivalent spherical error and the most plus equivalent spherical error rarely exceeds +1.50 dioptres (10 per cent of the time). On those very rare occasions (1 per cent of the time) when it exceeds +4.0 dioptres, the infants showed a range of accommodative fluctuations during which accommodation relaxed dramatically for just a few seconds. The maximum plus measurement was picked off during this brief relaxation period. Behaviourally, these infants are usually excited throughout the retinoscopy procedure. These two near retinoscopy measurements are taken when FT thinks that an infant's accommodation will not relax any further.

Mohindra originally designed the near retinoscopy technique as a quick, efficient screening technique. She performed the near retinoscopy in a manner appropriate for screening many infants. Her measurements (Mohindra and Held 1981) suggest that infants tend to be myopic (mean refraction = -0.70 dioptres) during the first month and continue to have refractions that are slightly myopic or emmetropic for the next 3 months. The average infant is hyperopic by 6 months of age. However, the hyperopia decreases after the first year. Mohindra's near retinoscopy measurements show developmental changes during the first year that are similar to those found in recent cycloplegic studies, while her refractive errors suggest far less hyperopia than these recent studies demonstrate (Wood and Hodi 1992; Abrahamsson and Sjöstrand 1992).

With the accommodative apparatus unparalysed, the absolute refractive error levels measured by near retinoscopy, or any refractive technique where the accommodative apparatus is in a natural state, are highly dependent on the precise manner in which the technique is implemented. We believe that Thorn's technique most closely approximates traditional refractive measurements. However, our technique is being re-evaluated because we believe that Mohindra's method of near retinoscopy may best approximate the optical focus of the eyes during states of visual alertness. This visual alertness is similar to an infant's state during preferential looking testing, during which Dr Gwiazda does her best to keep infants very alert and attentive. That is, one procedure approximates cycloplegic refractions, while the other estimates the clarity of real objects to an infant. Obviously, this second potential characteristic of near retinoscopy sets it apart from other refraction techniques.

Perhaps, the most important contribution of Mohindra's implementation of near retinoscopy is in its outstanding ability to predict the refractive errors of adolescents and young adults. Gwiazda *et al.* (1994) discuss these predictions in the following chapter. This method of near retinoscopy must accurately measure a critical aspect of refraction for these predictions to occur. It should

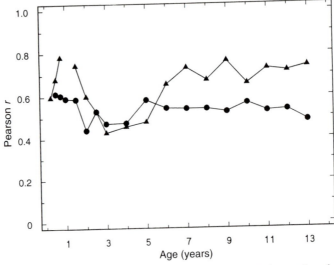

Fig. 8.4 Correlation between the refractive errors of infants 0–3 months of age (●) and 9–12 months of age (▲) determined by Mohindra's near retinoscopy *vs.* the distance retinoscopy of Thorn for the same children at later ages.

be noted that Howland and his colleagues have now roughly confirmed these predictions using non-cycloplegic photorefraction, in which infants are looking at and probably accommodating to a relatively near target (Howland *et al.* 1993).

Does the ability to predict adolescent refractive errors require the use of refractive techniques, such as near retinoscopy and photorefraction, which incorporate within them a certain amount of accommodation? The best predictions from Mohindra's near retinoscopy (Fig. 8.4) are based on the refractions of infants between 9 and 12 months, when large, uncontrollable accommodative swings are rare. This suggests that the basic refractive state plus tonic accommodation may provide the best prediction. During the past 7 years, Thorn has collected near retinoscopy data in which infantile accommodation is minimized in an attempt to approximate traditional refractive measurements. Within the next year or two, we will be able to start performing the same correlations between infantile refractive errors and the refractive errors of schoolchildren that Gwiazda *et al.* (1994) have reported, based on Mohindra's infantile near retinoscopy. This will indicate the best procedure for predicting refractive errors in children of school age. In the meantime, we invite those working in ophthalmological clinics, where paediatric patients are examined for several years, to compare the cycloplegic refractive errors of a sample of adolescents to their cycloplegically determined refractive errors in infancy in order to ascertain how well cycloplegic refractions can be used to make these predictions.

SUMMARY

Near retinoscopy has proven to be a powerful technique for measuring the optical focus of an infant's eyes. It can be used to easily and accurately measure astigmatism and anisometropia. It can be used readily to find the spherical equivalent refractive error of one infant relative to a large population of infants, similar to the use of photorefraction (Atkinson *et al.* 1984; Howland and Sayles 1987). It has the special advantage that it can be implemented to approximate refractive errors measured with traditional retinoscopy or to measure the optical focus of the attentive infant. The second of these possibilities has proven itself valuable in its ability to predict refractive errors years later during adolescence.

ACKNOWLEDGEMENTS

We thank Indra Mohindra and Mitchell Scheiman for performing the early retinoscopy measurements, Joseph Bauer for his many contributions, and James P. Comerford for his helpful comments on the manuscript. This work was supported by NIH-2R01 EY 1191 and SP30-EY02621.

REFERENCES

Abrahamsson, M. and Sjöstrand, J. (1992). Refractive changes in normal and amblyopic children. *Investigative Ophthalmology and Visual Science*, **33** (suppl.), 1338.

Aslin, R. N., Shea, S. L., and Metz, H. S. (1990). Use of the Canon R-1 autorefractor to measure refractive errors and accommodative responses in infants. *Clinical Vision Science*, **1**, 61–70.

Atkinson, J., Braddick, O. J., Durden, K., Watson, P., and Atkinson, S. (1984). Screening for refractive errors in 6–9-month-old infants by photorefraction. *British Journal of Ophthalmology*, **68**, 105–12.

Borghi, R. A. and Rouse, M. W. (1985). Comparison of refraction obtained by 'near retinoscopy' and retinoscopy under cycloplegia. *American Journal of Optometry and Physiological Optics*, **62**, 169–72.

Cook, R. C. and Glasscock, R. E. (1951). Refractive and ocular findings in newborns. *American Journal of Ophthalmology*, **34**, 1407–13.

Cruz, A. A. V., Sampaio, N. M. V., and Vargas, J. A. (1990). Near retinoscopy in accommodative esotropia. *Journal of Pediatric Ophthalmology and Strabismus*, **27**, 245–9.

Dobson, W., Fulton, A. B., and Sebris, S. L. (1984). Cycloplegic refractions of infants and young children: the axis of astigmatism. *Investigative Ophthalmology and Visual Science*, **25**, 83–7.

Franceschetti, A. (1935). Fur refraktionskurv des neugeborenen. *Klinische Monatsblatter Augenheilkunde*, **95**, 98–9.

Gwiazda, J., Scheiman, M., Mohindra, I., and Held, R. (1984). Astigmatism in children: changes in axis and amount from birth to six years. *Investigative Ophthalmology and Visual Science*, **25**, 88–92.

Gwiazda, J., Thorn, F., Bauer, J., and Held, R. (1991). Tonic accommodation increases more in myopic than hyperopic children following near work. *Investigative Ophthalmology and Visual Science*, **32** (suppl.), 1125.

Haynes, H., White, B. L., and Held, R. (1965). Visual accommodation in human infants. *Science*, **148**, 528–30.

Howland, H. C. and Sayles, N. (1984). Photorefractive measurements of astigmatism in infants and young children. *Investigative Ophthalmology and Visual Science*, **25**, 93–102.

Howland, H. C. and Sayles, N. (1987). A photorefractive characterization of focusing ability of infants and young children. *Investigative Ophthalmology and Visual Science*, **28**, 1005–15.

Howland, H. C., Atkinson, J., Braddick, O., and French, J. (1978). Infant astigmatism measured by photorefraction. *Science*, **202**, 331–3.

Howland, H. C., White, S., and Peck L. (1993). Early focusing predicts later refractive state: a longitudinal study. *Investigative Ophthalmology and Visual Science*, **34** (suppl.), 1352.

Maino, J. H., Cibis, G. W., Cress, P., Spellman, C. R., and Shores, R. E. (1984). Non-cycloplegic *vs* cycloplegic retinoscopy in preschool children. *Annals of Ophthalmology*, **16**, 880–2.

Mohindra, I. (1975). A technique for infant examination. *American Journal of Optometry and Physiological Optics*, **52**, 867–70.

Mohindra, I. (1977). A non-cycloplegic refraction technique for infants and young children. *Journal of the American Optometric Association*, **48**, 518–23.

Mohindra, I. and Held R. (1981). Refractions in humans from birth to five years. *Documenta Ophthalmologica Proceedings Series*, **28**, 19–27.

Mohindra, I. and Molinari, J. F. (1979). Near retinoscopy and cycloplegic retinoscopy in early primary grade school children. *American Journal of Optometry and Physiological Optics*, **56**, 34–8.

Mohindra, I., Held, R., Gwiazda, J., and Brill, S. (1978). Astigmatism in infants. *Science*, **202**, 329–31.

Owens, D. A., Mohindra, I., and Held, R. (1980). The effectiveness of the retinoscope beam as an accommodative stimulus. *Investigative Ophthalmology and Visual Science*, **19**, 942–9.

Santonastaso, A. (1930). La refrazione oculare nei primi anni di vita. *Annali di Oftalmologia e Clinica Oculistica*, **58**, 852–85.

Saunders, K. J. and Westall, C. A. (1992). Comparison between near retinoscopy and cycloplegic retinoscopy in the refraction of infants and children. *Optometry and Vision Science*, **69**, 615–22.

Thorn, F., Held, R., and Fang, L. L. (1987). Orthogonal astigmatic axes in Chinese and caucasian infants. *Investigative Ophthalmology and Visual Science*, **28**, 191–4.

Wesson, M. D., Mann, K. R., and Bray, N. W. (1990). A comparison of cycloplegic refraction to near retinoscopy technique for refractive error determination. *Journal of the American Optometric Association*, **61**, 680–4.

Wood, I. C. J. and Hodi, S. (1992). Refractive finding of a refractive study of infants from birth to one year of age. *Investigative Ophthalmology and Visual Science*, **33** (suppl.), 971.

9

Prediction of myopia in children

*Jane Gwiazda, Joseph Bauer, Frank Thorn, and
Richard Held*

INTRODUCTION

Children who become myopic generally do so sometime between 7 and 13 years of age. The aetiology of this school-age myopia has been debated for centuries (for a review see Curtin 1985). The latest research indicates that, although myopia has a genetic component, close-up visual activity, such as reading and playing computer games, also contributes to the genesis and progression of myopia in susceptible eyes. Recent findings from longitudinal studies of refraction indicate that it is now possible to predict whether an infant will become myopic at school age. This chapter will review some of the new findings relevant to the prediction of myopia in children.

LONGITUDINAL STUDY OF REFRACTION

Much of what we know about refractive errors in children has been obtained from cross-sectional studies, which are, for obvious reasons, easier to conduct than longitudinal studies. However, without a longitudinal study of refraction, it is impossible to know whether refractive changes in infancy are related to those that occur when the child is older. More specifically, cross-sectional data are inadequate to determine whether the infant who showed significant myopia, which was reduced or eliminated during the pre-school years, is the same child who again becomes myopic at school-age.

In the MIT Infant Vision Laboratory, we began a longitudinal study of refractive error in children 18 years ago (Gwiazda *et al.* 1993*a*). To our knowledge, this study contains the largest number of refractions of children followed from infancy into school age. We now have serial refractions numbering almost 8000 from over 400 children. Infants were recruited into our research programme by a letter sent to parents residing in the area of Cambridge, Massachusetts. Those parents who brought their babies to the laboratory for a first visit were invited to continue participation in the study, and approximately 20 per cent have returned for repeated visits at regular intervals.

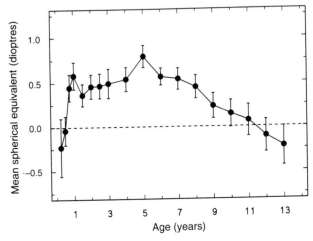

Fig. 9.1 Mean spherical equivalent refractive errors of 72 children refracted at regular intervals throughout childhood. Error bars indicate standard errors.

Methods of refraction

All of our refractions were obtained without cycloplegia (paralysis of the ciliary muscle). Near-retinoscopy, a technique in which the infant fixates the light from the retinoscope in a dark room , was used for children from birth to 3.5 years (Mohindra 1977). Non-cycloplegic distance retinoscopy, with the child fixating a letter on the Snellen eye chart, was used after 3.5 years of age.

Emmetropization

As shown in Fig. 9.1, non-cycloplegic refraction data in the first year reveal a shift from myopic readings in the early months to emmetropia by 6 months, which probably reflects improved accommodative control over this period. These data are taken from 72 children, refracted at regular intervals from birth to at least 9 years, and comprise nearly 1400 individual refractions. Contrary to the received view, this same trend has now been shown in cycloplegic refraction data, although less myopia is found in neonates when they are refracted with cycloplegia (Abrahamsson and Sjöstrand 1992; Schalij-Delfos *et al.* 1992; Wood and Hodi 1992). In a recent study using cycloplegic and non-cycloplegic retinoscopy on the same infants, the cycloplegic readings were 0.85 dioptres more hyperopic, with large variability for both techniques (Saunders and Westall 1992). These results indicate that non-cycloplegic readings include an accommodative component.

The dispersion of refractive errors, shown by the standard errors around the points in Fig. 9.1, is largest shortly after birth and smallest at 6 years. This reflects the emmetropization process (tendency for refractive errors to be reduced or eliminated) which occurs over the first 4–5 years. During this

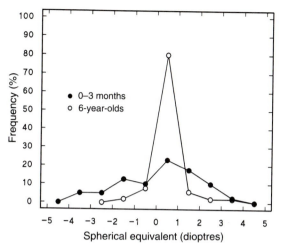

Fig. 9.2 Distribution of spherical equivalent refractive errors. (Reprinted from Gwiazda *et al.* (1993*a*) with kind permission from Elsevier Science Ltd.)

period, the refractions of most children tend to converge on emmetropia or a slight degree of hyperopia. However, the children who were myopic as infants on average never reach the same level of hyperopia as those who were hyperopic in infancy. Emmetropization occurs in most children, as shown in Fig. 9.2. The distribution of spherical equivalents (obtained by taking one-half of the cylindrical component of refraction and algebraically adding that value to the spherical component of refraction) is broad shortly after birth, with only 22 per cent showing emmetropia and the remainder showing myopia or hyperopia. By 6 years, however, the percentages are reversed, with 80 per cent of the children emmetropic.

Prediction of myopia based on infantile refractions

Our longitudinal data confirm the finding from cross-sectional studies that, after a period of emmetropization, some children start to develop myopia. We can predict with some degree of certainty which children will develop myopia by looking at their infantile refractions. Half the children with infantile spherical equivalents less than +0.50 dioptres (a cut-off value used by Hirsch, 1964, see later) are myopic at age 9 to 16 years, and that figure is likely to grow as the children age. For those children with infantile spherical equivalents of +0.50 dioptres or greater, only 20 per cent are myopic. Calculation of an odds ratio indicates that an infant with a spherical equivalent less than +0.5 dioptres is 4.2 times more likely to develop myopia between 9 and 16 years as an infant with a spherical equivalent of +0.5 dioptres or greater.

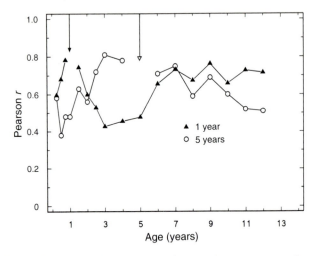

Fig. 9.3 Correlations between spherical equivalents at 1 year compared to all other ages (▲) and at 5 years compared to all other ages (○). (The *r* values for 1 year with 1 year and 5 years with 5 years have been omitted, since they are, by definition, equal to 1.0. Their locations are designated by the closed and open arrows, respectively.)

The refraction at 1 year of age has been found to afford the best prediction of later refractive error (Fig. 9.3). Correlations of spherical equivalents at 1 year with neighbouring ages are high, as expected, but are also high after 5 years (*r* = 0.65 and above). Lower values are found during the pre-school years when most children are emmetropic. Correlations at 5 years with neighbouring ages are high, as expected, but are lower in infancy and after 7 years. Based on these data and those in Fig. 9.2, it is concluded that the traditional time for a first eye screening, when a child is about to enter school, is not so likely to provide useful information about future refractive errors, including myopia, as an examination in infancy. During the pre-school years, most children's refractive errors converge on emmetropia or a small amount of hyperopia, with little indication of the wide range of refractive errors seen in infancy and later at school age.

Recently, Howland *et al.* (1993) reported similar findings from a longitudinal study conducted over 13 years using photorefraction. They found that focusing behaviour in the first 2 years predicted refractive state beyond 6 years, despite an intervening period of emmetropization. Between ages 2 and 6 years, however, it was not possible to predict later refractive state.

The notable absence of significant refractive error in 5–6-year-olds also was found in the Orinda longitudinal study of refraction in school children (Hirsch 1964). Refractions of 261 eyes at the initial screening at 5 or 6 years of age were compared with refractions from the same eyes at 13 or 14 years of age. In agreement with results from our study that it is rare to find myopia in 5–6-year-olds, only 4 out of the 261 eyes in Hirsch's study showed myopia at 5 years. By

13 years, however, 35 per cent of the eyes were myopic. Most of those who became myopic had refractions at 5 years that were greater than Plano but less than +0.50 dioptres. Conversely, most of the children who were hyperopic at 13 years had refractions at 5 years in excess of +0.75 dioptres, with half showing +1.5 dioptres or more.

These three longitudinal studies of refraction (Gwiazda *et al.* 1993a; Howland *et al.* 1993; Hirsch 1964) make it clear that the process of emmetropization results in a limited range of refractive errors between 2 and 6 years of age. As a result, only weak predictions of later refractive error can be made from a refraction at 5 years, the typical age for a first eye examination.

GENETIC FACTORS

Studies of refractive errors in parents and children, including twins, have demonstrated a significant familial incidence of myopia (for a review see Curtin 1985). Strong support for the genetic origin of refractive errors is provided by these studies, although it is unlikely that a single gene is involved. In the MIT longitudinal study of refraction, almost two-thirds of the mothers and fathers are myopic, much higher than the incidence of 25 per cent reported for adults in the USA. The high incidence of myopia in the parents provides increased chances of finding myopic children, and this has proven to be the case. When both parents of children in the longitudinal group are myopic, 42 per cent of their children aged 9–16 years are myopic. When only one parent is myopic, the incidence of myopia in the children drops to 22.5 per cent, and with neither parent myopic, the incidence is further reduced to 8 per cent.

NEAR WORK AND MYOPIA

Parents often ask if excessive reading and computer game playing and TV watching (if the child sits close to the set) will lead to nearsightedness in their children. This important question has been the subject of much debate over the years. According to Curtin (1985): 'There are few subjects in ophthalmology capable of triggering the impassioned responses, often visceral rather than cerebral, that the subject of near work and myopia genesis evokes.' Refraction data from various ethnic groups reveal an increased prevalence of myopia after the introduction of formal education. For example, in a study of Eskimos, Young and colleagues found virtually no myopia in individuals over 40 years, but a high incidence in younger subjects (Young *et al.* 1969). They attributed the increase to the introduction of compulsory schooling after World War II.

Many studies have reported an increased prevalence of myopia with years in school and with volume of near work; however, this association does not imply a cause and effect relationship (Angle and Wissman 1978; Richler and Bear 1980). One of the difficulties in collecting data is that researchers must rely on reports from children or their parents regarding the amount of near work in which they engage. In our study, a questionnaire was distributed to parents to ascertain the amount of time that their children engaged in tasks involving near work. The myopic children in our group spent, on average, 3.0 hours per day engaged in close work, while the emmetropic children spent 2.5 hours per day, a difference that was suggestive but not significant. A key question that can only be answered by a longitudinal study is whether a large volume of near work, especially in children with an accommodative deficit (see later), *precedes* the onset of myopia. By tracking refractive error, near-work habits, and accommodative functioning in individual children, we hope to determine the causal relationship between near work and school-age myopia.

ACCOMMODATIVE INSUFFICIENCY

As mentioned in this chapter, epidemiological studies have shown correlations between myopia and near visual tasks that appear to require accommodation (the ability of the ciliary muscle and the lens of the eye to adjust for near distances). Alternatively, reduced ability to accommodate for close work has been claimed to be a risk factor in the development of myopia (Avetisov 1990). How do we reconcile the assertion that intensive near work with habitual accommodation leads to myopia with evidence indicating that myopic subjects have poor accommodation? One explanation is that near work for those with reduced accommodation results in chronic blur, and that it is the blur, not the accommodative effort, that induces myopia. When susceptible children are learning to read they may be experiencing a mild form of pattern deprivation. It is possible that if at-risk children seldom engaged in close work they might not become myopic. This possibility poses a dilemma for parents and a challenge for educators and eye care professionals.

A recent study from our laboratory established that newly myopic children show a reduced range of accommodation (Gwiazda *et al.* 1993*b*). We measured the accommodative responses of 64 children to letter targets displayed at fixed distances from 4.0 m to 0.25 m and to a 4.0 m letter target optically moved over the same range through the use of negative lenses. Each child was refracted before testing and wore the best subjective refraction (most plus) to within 0.25 dioptres while viewing the targets displayed at fixed distances. For the lens series, the refractive error was used as the starting point for the added lenses. Our results indicated that myopic children accommodated significantly less than emmetropic children. They accommodated very little when lenses were used to move the target closer, which may reflect the inability of myopic eyes to use blur cues for accommodation. For the more typical viewing situation with real targets at close distances, a condition that provides proximity cues, myopic children still accommodated less than emmetropic children by a small but statistically significant amount.

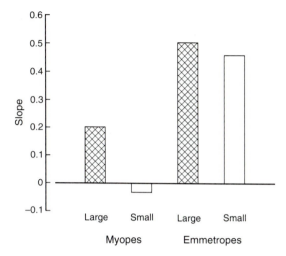

Fig. 9.4 Slopes of the accommodative response functions for myopic and emmetropic children tested with both 20/30 (small) and 20/100 (large) letters.

A recent report indicated that children with Down Syndrome showed reduced accommodation relative to a control group (Woodhouse *et al.* 1993). In agreement with our findings, within the Down Syndrome group the amplitude of accommodation was lowest for the myopic children.

It has been suggested that perhaps our subjects did not have to accommodate very much to clear the blurred targets, which contained 20/100 letters, but that with smaller letters accommodation might improve. To investigate this possibility, we measured the accommodative responses for both 20/100 and 20/30 letters in a group of 14 emmetropic children and 9 myopic children. To our surprise, it was found that with 20/30 letters accommodation for the myopic children did not improve but was worse than with the larger letters (Fig. 9.4). The slope of the accommodative response function was significantly less for small letters for the myopic children ($t = 3.3$, df $= 8$, $p = 0.01$). A related finding, that accommodation was best for intermediate spatial frequencies, was reported by Owens (1980).

METHODS FOR HALTING THE PROGRESSION OF MYOPIA

The identification of risk factors for myopia and a better understanding of underlying mechanisms may point the way to effective methods for delaying the onset or halting the progression of myopia. The most common methods that have been tried in the past are bifocals, rigid contact lenses, visual training, biofeedback, and drugs to relax accommodation (for a review see Grosvenor

1991). Most of these methods have been used on individuals who are already myopic, which means that axial elongation of the eye has occurred. Therefore it is not altogether surprising that most controlled studies show little or no reduction of myopia. However, what if we were able to identify a likely group of children at risk for myopia based on the factors already discussed? In this situation, some of the methods for myopia control could be implemented on eyes that had not yet undergone axial elongation. More research is needed to determine whether some existing methods, implemented on at-risk children, may work better than others and whether new methods involving drugs or alternate modes of presentation of reading matter may prove useful.

CONCLUSIONS

Several factors that predispose a child to developing myopia at school age have been identified. Within limits, myopia in children can be predicted from consideration of:

(1) the parents' refractions;
(2) the child's refraction in infancy; and
(3) the child's accommodative response to blur.

The incidence of myopia is highest in children with two (compared with zero or one) myopic parents. Refractive status at 1 year of age is predictive of refraction at school age, despite an intervening period, at 3–6 years, when most children have little or no refractive error. A third risk factor for myopia is based on the focusing of the child's eye in response to optically induced blur. Insufficient accommodative response to blur is found in newly myopic children and, perhaps, in those at risk for myopia. Some children who engage in extended periods of near work may also be at risk. If we can identify potentially myopic children based on the aforementioned factors, then as ameliorative measures become better understood they can be applied selectively to those children.

REFERENCES

Abrahamsson, M. and Sjöstrand, J. (1992). Refraction changes in normal and amblyopic children. *Investigative Ophthalmology and Visual Science*, **33** (suppl.), 1338.

Angle, J. and Wissman, D. A. (1978). Age, reading, and myopia. *American Journal of Optometry and Physiological Optics*, **55**, 302–8.

Avetisov, E. S. (1990). Myopia in children. In *Pediatric Ophthalmology*, (ed. D. Taylor), pp. 32–44. Blackwell, Boston.

Curtin, B. (1985). *The Myopias*. Harper & Row, Philadelphia.

Grosvenor, T. (1991). Management of myopia: functional methods. In *Refractive anomalies: research and clinical applications*, (ed. T. Grosvenor and M. Flom), pp. 345–70. Butterworth-Heinemann, Boston.

Gwiazda, J., Thorn, F., Bauer, J., and Held, R. (1993*a*). Emmetropization and the progression of manifest refraction in children followed from infancy to puberty. *Clinical Vision Science*, **8**, 337–44.

Gwiazda, J., Thorn, F., Bauer, J., and Held, R. (1993*b*). Myopic children show insufficient accommodative response to blur. *Investigative Ophthalmology and Visual Science*, **34**, 690–4.

Hirsch, M. (1964). Predictability of refraction at age 14 on the basis of testing at age 6. *American Journal of Optometry*, **41**, 567–73.

Howland, H., Waite, S., and Peck, L. (1993). Early focusing predicts later refractive state: a longitudinal study. *Investigative Ophthalmology and Visual Science*, **34** (suppl.), 1352.

Mohindra, I. (1977). A non-cycloplegic refraction technique for infants and young children. *Journal of the American Optometric Association*, **48**, 518–23.

Owens, D. A. (1980). A comparison of accommodative responsiveness and contrast sensitivity for sinusoidal gratings. *Vision Research*, **20**, 159–67.

Richler, A. and Bear, J. C. (1980). Refraction, near work, and education: a population study in Newfoundland. *Acta Ophthalmologica*, **58**, 468–78.

Saunders, K. and Westall, C. (1992). Comparison between near retinoscopy and cycloplegic retinoscopy in the refraction of infants and children. *Optometry and Visual Science*, **69**, 615–22.

Schalij-Delfos, N., Barbian, C., Wittebol-Post, D., and Cats, B. (1992). The development of myopia in premature infants with and without retinopathy of prematurity. *Investigative Ophthalmology and Visual Science*, **33** (suppl.), 1281.

Wood, I. and Hodi, S. (1992). Refractive findings of a longitudinal study of infants from birth to one year of age. *Investigative Ophthalmology and Visual Science*, **33** (suppl.), 971.

Woodhouse, J. M., Meades, J., Leat, S., and Saunders, K. (1993). Reduced accommodation in children with Down Syndrome. *Investigative Ophthalmology and Visual Science*, **34**, 2382–7.

Young, F., Leary, G., Baldwin, W., West, D., Box, R., Harris, E., and Johnson, C. (1969). The transmission of refractive errors within Eskimo families. *American Journal of Optometry*, **46**, 676–85.

10
Issues in infant vision screening and assessment

Janette Atkinson

INTRODUCTION

In this chapter, methods of infant vision testing applied in two practical contexts, screening and assessment will be considered. The demands of these two applications are quite different. Screening is the attempt to identify undetected vision problems, or their precursors, in the population as a whole. Screening has to be targeted on specific disorders for which there are clear benefits in early detection, and the methods must be appropriate, in terms of costs to the health care system and demands on families, for use with large numbers of children most of whom will turn out to be normal. Visual assessment deals with much smaller numbers of children who are already believed to have a problem with vision. The detailed nature of the problem in each case needs to be determined for purposes of diagnosis, clinical management, rehabilitation, and understanding the impact of any visual disability on everyday activities. Compared with screening, a much more intensive investigation of the individual child is possible; however, protocols must be available to cope with many different patterns of visual performance, associated with the whole range of ophthalmological and neurological disorders that may affect vision and visually guided behaviour.

SCREENING FOR STRABISMUS AND AMBLYOPIA

Strabismus and amblyopia are not necessarily the most serious childhood visual problems for the individual but they are important because they are the most prevalent in developed countries. Estimates of incidence from different studies and different populations have been quite variable; however, in the UK, 3 per cent of pre-school children would be a conservative estimate. Screening procedures vary from country to country (see reviews by Ehrlich *et al.* 1983; Hyvarinen 1988; van der Lem *et al.* 1990). Most procedures for children below 3 years of age have attempted to identify strabismus alone; at 3–5 years, orthoptic tests are commonly extended to include monocular visual acuity. (Without refractive measures, however, amblyopic and optical effects on acuity cannot be dissociated.) Variations in the criteria for strabismus and amblyopia and also in the selection of the screening population and in attendance are likely to be responsible, in part, for the variation in reported incidence; however, often the critical information is not presented explicitly in published reports. Evaluations of the efficacy of screening are usually in terms of sensitivity and specificity in detecting strabismus and amblyopia. However, identification should only be an intermediate outcome; the ultimate test of screening must be whether it leads to effective intervention.

Given these problems with the present literature on screening, a set of basic questions can be formulated:

What group should be screened, and with what tests?

Two alternative strategies have been pursued. The first is to screen subgroups thought to be at high overall risk of visual defects; the second is to screen whole population at a particular age. The former strategy may turn out to be the most cost-effective but raises problems of equity. Examples of high-risk populations might be very premature infants, those with other major congenital defects, or a significant family history of vision defects (e.g. a first degree relative with strabismus). For some at-risk groups, a single screening test may not be appropriate; the kind of battery needed to evaluate vision in the presence of major neurological handicap is discussed in a later section.

There is still some debate about what constitutes *surveillance* as opposed to *screening* in child vision. Holland and Stewart (1990) define screening as a more specific tool within more general programmes of health surveillance, to be used for particular conditions or in particular high-risk groups. In the UK, the Hall Report (Hall 1989) recommended a core programme of surveillance (including vision at ages between 21 months and 11 years) to be undertaken by primary health care teams, with no specific vision screening tests included. Visual defects were to be detected largely from parental report and family history. The effectiveness of this approach has been doubted (Bax and Whitmore 1990), and many cases of amblyopia without accompanying strabismus, most refractive error and less apparent ophthalmological defects are likely to go undetected by parents in the pre-school years.

A wide variety of pre-school screening programmes is in use in Europe (see van de Lem *et al.* 1990) but there have been few detailed measures of their effectiveness. In those evaluations that have been attempted, the screened population has often been pre-selected (McClellan 1977) or analysis has been carried out on relatively small samples (Beardsell 1989). The Hall Report (1989) doubted the value of any of the present pre-school screening schemes in the UK and recommended that they be discontinued until proven effective. Nonetheless, many clinical professionals believe that screening makes a valuable contribution to detecting vision problems at an early age.

Refraction is a measure that is now possible in early childhood and which may not only indicate present visual defect but also be predictive of amblyopia and strabismus. To date, two groups in the UK have carried out population screening programmes for infant refractive errors, aiming to assess their predictive value for later pre-school vision defects. Ingram *et al.* (1985) screened by retinoscopy, which requires extremely skilled personnel and a certain degree of co-operation on the part of the child. It is consequently costly and not optimal for widespread screening. The Cambridge programme of Atkinson *et al.* (1984; 1987; Atkinson 1993) has used isotropic photorefraction, carried out by trained orthoptists, a method that has been validated previously against retinoscopy both by Atkinson *et al.* and independently by Spanish and Russian clinical groups (Castenera de Molina *et al.* 1989; Somov 1989). Compared with retinoscopy, isotropic photorefraction requires less highly trained personnel and less co-operation on the child's part; it is therefore a relatively robust and inexpensive method.

Both studies have shown a high predictive value for identifying children at risk of strabismus and amblyopia from their cycloplegic refraction. The Cambridge study is described more fully later. Several other studies have attempted to identify amblyopia precursors (Castenera de Molina *et al.* 1989; Angi 1992). Several different photo- and videorefractive instruments, based on related optical principles, are available either commercially or in prototype form and are now being compared (Braddick and Atkinson 1984; Howland 1991). The value of this approach can only be realized if treatment of refractive precursors reduces the incidence of long-term visual defects.

How significant are the defects, if not successfully treated, in causing visual disability and wider developmental problems?

There are few measures of the degree of disability likely to evolve from a particular visual defect, or detailed accounts of the extent of disability with increasing age. For example, it is unlikely that the reduced acuity associated with infantile idiopathic congenital nystagmus will lead to extensive disability at the time the condition is identified in infancy. However, this defect is very likely to cause disability in later childhood (e.g. inability to read the blackboard in school) and adulthood (exclusion from certain professions and car driving).

Some would argue that no disability is associated with milder defects (e.g. strabismus, amblyopia, colour blindness) particularly if the defect affects only one eye. Amblyopia, as a unilateral condition, leads to significant disability only if the use of the good eye is lost, and it has been argued that the risk of this is extremely low. However, the increase in life-expectancy in recent decades has increased the significance of cataract as a visual problem of the elderly. It would be illuminating to know what proportion of first eye cataracts are in the good eye of unilateral amblyopes, leaving the patient with a relatively severe visual disability of rapid onset. More generally, longitudinal analyses of defect/disability relationships are very pertinent to the ultimate value of screening programmes on a wider scale, and, as such, deserve much more research effort than at present.

A second issue is the extent of subsequent non-visual problems as a result of a primary visual deficit. The problem is to differentiate between correlation and causality. Two areas where these issues are of current interest are: (i) in multiply handicapped visually impaired (MHVI) children; and (ii) possible visual precursors of certain learning disabilities, such as dyslexia, in otherwise normal pre-school children. Many believe that early visual defects limit motor, social and cognitive development, although there is scant evidence for these causal relationships and much evidence for clusters of correlated defects within a single individual child. Only randomized controlled studies of early intervention, with diverse outcome measures of motor, social and cognitive competence, would be able to give clear answers to these questions.

How effective are treatment regimes for the defects?

However efficient a screening programme may be in identifying strabismus, amblyopia, or their precursors, it is of very limited value unless there is some possibility of correcting the defects. There is long-standing controversy on the effectiveness of treatment for both strabismus and amblyopia.

Moseley and Fielder, in this volume, provide an account of the controversy over occlusion therapy for treatment of amblyopia. Findings of high failure rates for occlusion therapy may be caused by delay between onset of amblyopia and treatment, poor compliance with treatment, and confounding factors of other disabilities. A second major issue is the success of strabismus treatment in restoring binocularity and preventing amblyopia. It is generally believed that surgery in the first year of life for early onset strabismus provides the best outcome in terms of binocular vision. However, some recent studies suggest that even in this case the outcome in terms of stereoscopic vision is frequently poor (Atkinson *et al.* 1991*a*) and that the primary justification for early treatment (e.g. surgery, occlusion and sometimes spectacle correction) must be the reduction of amblyopia and cosmetic improvement. There is a need for controlled trials of late and early surgery with careful longitudinal outcome measures, although such studies would present considerable problems of ethical acceptability.

The trials of infant refractive screening discussed above have been linked to evaluations of refractive correction by spectacles. However, the results show some disagreement on whether such correction can successfully prevent later amblyopia and strabismus. The two studies (Ingram *et al.* 1979; 1985; Atkinson *et al.* 1984; 1987; Atkinson 1993), differed in the exact criteria and protocol for spectacle prescription and the compliance level that was achieved, and these may be critical factors in deciding effectiveness.

How cost-effective are vision screening programmes?

To date, there is very little information on comparisons between current screening and surveillance programmes in terms of outcome or costs. Many hidden costs have not been taken into account (e.g. the relative costs of training medical practitioners, ophthalmologists, orthoptists or nurses, who may be the personnel carrying out screening). There is a paucity of effectiveness measures and very limited ideas as to what constitutes disability. Until these issues are researched, proper cost-effectiveness analysis is not possible.

THE CAMBRIDGE INFANT SCREENING PROGRAMME

In this refractive screening programme, every infant living in the City of Cambridge over a 2-year period was sent an appointment to attend at a local clinic at age 6–8 months. A trained orthoptist conducted a basic orthoptic examination, and isotropic photorefraction following cycloplegia with 1% cyclopentolate. Full details of this methodology and study are given in Atkinson *et al.* (1981; 1984); Atkinson and Braddick (1983*a,b*); Howland *et al.* (1983).

All children identified at screening with an abnormal refraction were followed up at 4–6 month intervals. At 4 years of age, there were careful tests of the child's acuity and binocular vision. These tests represent the main outcome measures of the study. Children who at any stage in the screening or follow-up showed manifest strabismus, demonstrable amblyopia or ocular pathology were referred directly to the regular hospital eye clinic and follow-up information was derived from their examinations there.

The possibility of countering any effects of early hyperopia on visual development was tested in a randomized control trial of treatment by spectacle correction, to reduce the child's habitual accommodation and/or image blur. Infants identified as hyperopic at screening were assigned randomly to 'spectacles' and 'non-spectacles' groups. Spectacles were prescribed according to a defined protocol that was deliberately conservative, especially for astigmatism, to minimize the risk of over-correction (Atkinson 1993). Compliance in wearing the spectacles was closely but sympathetically monitored; around 70 per cent of those prescribed wore the correction for 50 per cent or more of waking hours.

Incidence of strabismus and refractive errors

In this study, 3166 infants were screened (74 per cent of the total population), and 9.3 per cent of these were followed up. The largest single category of refractive errors was the 4.6 per cent who were hyperopic (over +3.5 dioptres in any meridian). Astigmatism, which is common at this age (Howland *et al.* 1978; Mohindra *et al.* 1978; Atkinson and Braddick 1983*a,b*) was not treated as a separate category. However, infants with large astigmatisms were likely to meet the criterion for the hyperopic group.

The number who already showed a clear, manifest strabismus at this age was small (0.7 per cent). There was concern that our figures might omit a strabismic group who did not attend screening because they had already seen an ophthalmologist before 6 months. A sample of 100 infants was therefore investigated out of those who had not attended their appointments. Only two cases were found to have been referred to a hospital eye clinic with possible strabismus, and in neither case was this confirmed. Any bias arising from differential attendance must therefore be very small, and the true figure for manifest strabismus before 6 months in this population is almost certainly below 1 per cent.

Outcome at 4 years

It should not be assumed that an early refractive error necessarily of itself represents a visual deficit. Rather, it must be asked, how far does identification of early refractive errors predict lasting, functionally significant vision problems? There were two main outcome measures at 4 years—strabismus and monocular and binocular acuity. Acuity was tested with the Cambridge Crowding Cards, which give an equivalent to Snellen but were usable with 4-year-olds (Atkinson *et al.* 1986*a*; 1988; Anker *et al.* 1989). For acuity testing, children wore the appropriate refractive correction if they still had a refractive error, even if the child was not wearing spectacles regularly as part of the trial. The criterion of failure on this multiple-letter test was 6 out of 12 or poorer.

A total of 21 per cent (16 out of 76) of the children who had been hyperopic initially and had not worn a correction throughout infancy became strabismic, compared with 1.6 per cent (2 out of 123) of the control group (emmetropic in infancy) and 6.3 per cent (3 out of 48) of the children who had complied by wearing spectacles. The difference between the incidence of strabismus in the treated and non-treated groups was statistically significant; however, there was no significant difference between the treated hyperopic group and controls (although the incidence is still higher in the former group).

There was an analogous pattern of results for the acuity test. Here 68 per cent (47 out of 69) of the non-treated group failed, with 28.6 per cent (12 out of 42) of the treated group and 11.1 per cent (11 out of 99) of the controls failing to obtain 6/9 equivalent in one or both eyes. Many of these acuity failures were bilateral, so were not a result of conventional strabismic or anisotropic amblyopia. Meridional amblyopia from persisting astigmatism (Mitchell *et al.* 1973) appears to be a contributing but not exclusive cause of these failures (Atkinson 1993).

It appears that persisting vision problems among children who had been infant hyperopes may result from several causes. Some are truly amblyopic, unilaterally, and/or meridionally at 4 years. In other children, failure on the Crowding Cards appeared to have a cognitive component; as for some younger children, they showed difficulty in understanding the task of matching the central letter of the array. It is speculated that hyperopia may be associated with mild delays that are not specific to the visual domain. In a second screening programme, now underway in Cambridge, it is hoped that measures including cognitive, motor and linguistic as well as visual development will allow us to test this hypothesis further.

The complex set of data, briefly described here, indicate several relationships among the variables of visual development over the first years of life, although most of the causal mechanisms involved are still quite unclear:

1. A high level of hyperopia at around 6 months is a strong predictor of later visual problems, including relatively poor pre-school acuity. A likely mechanism is deprivation amblyopia caused by image blur. Infant hyperopia is also a predictor of strabismus. This relationship is often explained in terms of accommodative esotropia; however, this hypothesis leaves much to be explained.

2. Developmental visual problems of hyperopes can be alleviated by spectacle correction, suggesting that image blur and/or accommodation have a causal role. However, it is possible that hyperopia may be correlated also with more general developmental variables.

3. Refractions that are initially hyperopic and myopic tend to emmetropize over the pre-school years; children with small refractive errors show little change.

The use of cycloplegia is a practical complication (and in some places a legal or professional complication) in a vision screening programme. A close relationship between non-cycloplegic and cycloplegic videorefraction has been found in our studies (Braddick *et al.* 1988), and so our current, second infant screening programme is examining whether infant hyperopes can be detected from videorefraction when freely accommodating. Results so far confirm that a suitable non-cycloplegic criterion can identify most of the infants who have marked hyperopia under cycloplegia. The study will investigate whether these children, who typically under-accommodate, show the same visual outcome as the group identified by a cycloplegic criterion, and whether there is a relationship between delays or aberrant visual development and abnormal development motorically, cognitively and linguistically.

APPROACHES TO VISUAL ASSESSMENT

Visual assessment, as distinct from screening, has the goal of characterizing in detail the individual child's visual capabilities. Where a specific ocular condition has been diagnosed, the requirements may be quite specific, for example, measurement of acuity, visual fields, or stereoscopic function. However, such cases are a minority of those for whom visual assessment is required. In our experience, most are children with major neurological problems. Such children can show very variable performance and uneven profiles, and so extensive testing in several different visual domains may be necessary (Atkinson *et al.* 1989). For example, a dissociation has been shown between attentional visual defects and sensory loss of resolution acuity in some neurologically impaired children (Hood and Atkinson 1990). Procedures testing one aspect of visual functioning (e.g. a measure of acuity alone) may yield valuable information, however, they may fail to identify important deficits or fail to reveal significant areas of visual competence.

The need, therefore, is for batteries of tests appropriate to the range of levels of visual and cognitive function that may be encountered. Over the past 20 years, assessment techniques from various sources have been introduced into clinical practice, for example: (i) from the vision laboratory, behavioural psychophysical measures of acuity, a variety of amplitude and latency measures from visual evoked potentials; (ii) from paediatrics, tests based on developmental milestones of visual and visuo-motor behaviour; (iii) from developmental psychology, tests based on Piagetian visuo-cognitive tasks. The selection of procedures often depends on the particular professional background of those carrying out the assessment, rather than the visual problems under investigation. In many of these tests there is little indication of the relationship between the results and the level of disability in the child's everyday tasks for the infant or child. Indeed this relationship has yet to be made explicit in future research.

The range of recently developed tests of infant and child vision, which have been considered in recent reviews (e.g. Atkinson 1985; Atkinson and van Hof-van Duin 1993), will not be described here. Rather, an outline of a vision test battery protocol developed in our Unit, which draws on all the sources mentioned above, will be presented. Brief descriptions of this battery have already been published (Atkinson *et al.* 1989; Atkinson and van Hof-van Duin 1993); in this chapter some normative data are also presented.

THE ATKINSON BATTERY OF CHILD DEVELOPMENT FOR EXAMINING FUNCTIONAL VISION (ABCDEFV)

The battery has been devised in order to provide information about whether infants are reaching the goals in vision for everyday tasks appropriate for their age, and to assess the level of visual functioning in children with multiple disabilities. The battery combines ideas from current methods of assessment of infant vision (e.g. FPL, videorefraction), from established paediatric tests (Sheridan 1976; Griffiths 1970) and from developmental psychology (e.g. Piagetian search tasks). The professional groups interested in using the battery might be in paediatric neurology, paediatrics, ophthalmology, developmental clinical and educational psychology, and optometry.

The battery is being normalized for birth to 3.5 years. Here, normative data for the first year of life are reported. Initially, 139 babies were tested, within the age ranges 0–6 weeks (mean age 4.3 weeks), 8–17 weeks (mean age 13.8 weeks), 18–29 weeks (mean age 22.4 weeks) and 30–52 weeks (mean age 32.8 weeks). Each infant received the same tests on two visits within a 2-week period, to yield reliability measures. The component tests evaluated for inclusion in the battery were:

1. *Preferential looking*: a shortened staircase procedure (Atkinson *et al.* 1986*b*) is used with an automated FPL set-up, the Teller acuity cards and the Keeler acuity cards. Published Teller card norms are applied as criteria of the normal acuity range on each test.

2. *Videorefraction (without cycloplegia)*: using the Cambridge Paediatric Video-refractor (Clement Clark VPR1). To pass, infants have to change focus reliably in the appropriate direction for targets between 20 cm and 150 cm distance, from a camera position at 75 cm.

3. *Direct and consensual pupil response*: the standard orthoptic procedure is used (with small pen torch).

4. *Tracking*: a conspicuous target (e.g. a silent, shiny Christmas decoration, at least 5 cm diameter at 30 cm viewing distance), is moved slowly laterally (at 5–10°/s) from the infant's midline at eye level. The infant should be in an alert state and semi-upright position. To pass at the newborn level, the infant must track at least once in both directions out to around 15–20° laterally (up to five separated test trials were allowed). Saccadic tracking with several seconds' latency is allowed. For older ages, the criterion for passing the test is changed to success on two out of three trials by 3 months of age and two out of two trials by 6 months of age.

5. *Diffuse light reaction*: in a darkened room, the infant is placed to the side of the door, which is opened slowly and silently allowing light to enter. The response is a slow head-and-body turn towards the light (allowing two trials, and 5–10 s latency in newborns). This was repeated with the light source on the other side. The newborn should turn in both directions.

6. *Peripheral re-fixation*: with the child's attention gained on the tester 30 cm in front of the child's face, a high contrast silent toy (e.g. the Christmas decoration in 4) is moved from the peripheral field (on a level with the child's eyes) in an arc movement in towards the midline at 2–3 cm/s at a distance of 20–30 cm from the child's eyes. The angle is noted at which a saccadic refixation is made. Up to 2–3 trials were allowed on each side. The newborn passed the test if they refixate on both sides out to 15° eccentricity. This should increase to at least 45° by age 6 months.

7. *Response to smiling face*: the tester, smiling, approaches the child slowly and silently from across the room, and observes whether the child made an attentional response, e.g. smiles back. Between 6 weeks and 4–5 months post-term, children generally smile at friendly strangers; the response is not reliable in newborns and may be either positive or negative in older children.

8. *Regards hands and feet*: the parent is asked whether the child looks at or plays with his or her hands or feet at any time. A positive response is not expected until after 3 months of age.

9. *Defensive blink*: (after van Hof-van Duin and Mohn 1986). A plexiglass screen is held 5 cm from child's face and tapped with the fingers. Then the hand

is withdrawn from the screen and moved smoothly with palm forward towards the screen. A pass is scored if there is blinking on either 1/1 trials or 2/3 trials.

10. *Batting or reaching for a toy*: a silent conspicuous toy (as in 4 above) was held in the midline, 5–15 cm from the child's eyes. Any attempt to reach or bat for the toy is noted.

11. *Follows a falling toy*: the child's attention is attracted to a silent lightweight toy, which is then allowed to drop to the ground, noting any eye and head movements to follow the toy's trajectory to the ground. Pass is scored if head or eye movements follow the toy on 1/1 or 2/3 trials.

12. *Follows to 3 m distance*: the tester obtains the child's attention and then silently retreats to 3 m away, noting the distance when eye contact was lost. Up to three trials were allowed (pass 1/1 or 2/3 following to at least 3 m).

13. *Convergence*: a penlight with a toy on the end is presented at 30 cm from the child's eyes, and is brought towards the child's nose, smoothly at around 10–20 cm/s. The tester notes if both eyes converged and at what distance convergence was lost. Pass is convergence on 1/1 or 2/3 trials.

14. *Corneal reflex*: (i.e. standard Hirschberg test). The penlight is pointed midway between the child's eyes at approximately 30 cm distance. Whether the reflections in each eye were symmetrically positioned was observed.

15. *Reaches for toy*: same as 10 above for batting but, for older age groups, a reaching and grasping action is required. Which hand was used was recorded.

16. *Partially covered object*: a toy that is interesting to the child, and preferably silent, is partially covered with a dark cloth (20 × 20 cm). A child passes if they remove the cloth and retrieve the toy (1/1 or 2/3 passes).

17. *Totally covered object*: as for the partially covered toy but totally concealed.

RESULTS AND REVISION OF TEST BATTERY

In Fig. 10.1 the results for the different acuity tests with each age group are compared. There was no significant difference between the three tests of acuity at any age. In general, the means obtained were somewhat higher than the published Teller norms.

The results of the other, pass/fail tests on the four age-groups are shown in Fig. 10.2. These results have been used to select items for a revised set of age batteries. The revised batteries include only those tests meeting a criterion of 80 per cent or better pass rate in the age range concerned. For example, at 30–52 weeks there was a high failure rate for retrieving a totally covered toy and so this test has been discarded. For any test where there was a high failure rate on one out of the two test sessions, the test was retained but it was recommended that the test was carried out twice and a pass on either occasion counted.

The revised battery is divided into a set of core tests and a branching pass/fail section, as shown in Fig. 10.3. (This chart includes some tests appropriate for older age groups that have not been discussed here.) The core tests are used

Acuity by three PL tests across the four age groups

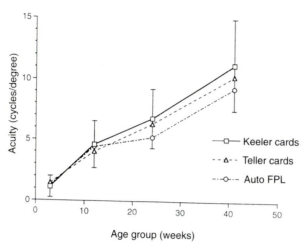

Fig. 10.1 Comparison of mean acuities on Teller cards, Keeler cards and automated forced choice preferential (FPL) looking for four age groups.

to identify general motor delay, motor asymmetries and several specific visual problems (e.g. strabismus and field deficits). They are suitable for children of any age, from birth to 3.5 years, who are able to make some head and eye movements. The tests are not time limited. (In children with very severe limitations of head and eye movement control, the results can be useful to those working with the child but do not necessarily give a specific measure of visual deficit in isolation.)

The core tests are followed by a branching sequence, in which certain tests can be omitted if immediate success is shown on a more advanced version of the same test (e.g. if a child successfully retrieves a totally covered toy it is not necessary to test for retrieval of a partially covered object). This structure allows tests at an appropriate level to be used even for a child who is far from the age norms, and whose performance is very non-uniform. Some children with neurological problems may reach the age norms in one branch but fail tests passed by a much younger normal group on another, so dissociations between different aspects of visual development can be identified. Using this revised protocol, 78 children have been assessed successfully, who had been referred for visual assessments, including many with neurological deficits.

These tests should be taken as a starting point for identifying the areas of possible visual problems. Specific follow-up tests, to delineate further the visual problems may then be carried out (e.g. measures of visual-evoked potentials for ascertaining cortical damage, measures of saccadic latencies for shifting visual attention from one target to another). Such tests involve more specialist equipment and expertise.

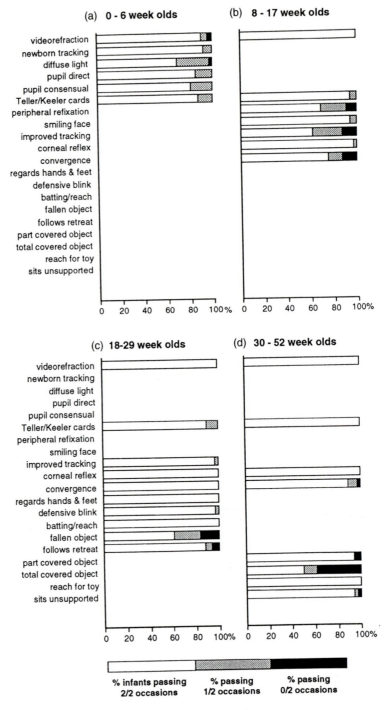

Fig. 10.2 Summary of four age groups on ABCDEFV test.

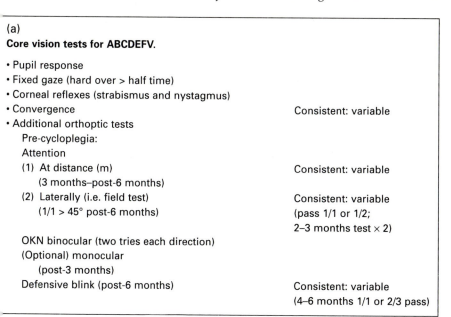

(a)
Core vision tests for ABCDEFV.

• Pupil response
• Fixed gaze (hard over > half time)
• Corneal reflexes (strabismus and nystagmus)
• Convergence   Consistent: variable
• Additional orthoptic tests
   Pre-cycloplegia:
   Attention
   (1) At distance (m)   Consistent: variable
       (3 months–post-6 months)
   (2) Laterally (i.e. field test)   Consistent: variable
       (1/1 > 45° post-6 months)   (pass 1/1 or 1/2;
                                                        2–3 months test × 2)

   OKN binocular (two tries each direction)
   (Optional) monocular
       (post-3 months)
   Defensive blink (post-6 months)   Consistent: variable
                                                        (4–6 months 1/1 or 2/3 pass)

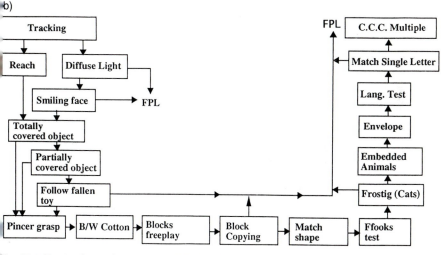

(b)

Fig. 10.3 Revised test battery for ABCDEFV. (a) Core vision tests; (b) flow-chart of events.

APPLICATION TO VLBW INFANTS

One application of this type of test battery is to infants who are at high risk of visual problems (e.g. those with a family history of genetic ophthalmological disorder, very premature infants). The battery has been used to assess visual development in a group of healthy very-low-birthweight (VLBW) infants. (Results from this study have been reported elsewhere: Atkinson *et al.* 1990; 1991*b*; Atkinson and van Hof-van Duin 1993).

The ABCDEFV battery was carried out with the VLBW group and their controls between 4–6 months post-term. The results are shown in Fig. 10.4. Overall there was a higher incidence of failures on all tests for the VLBW group compared with the controls. Children who failed two or more tests were considered to be showing some delay or defect in visual development and were followed up, although the exact nature of the failure and the specifics of the tests failed, are also important considerations.

CONCLUSIONS

In this chapter, the general questions raised by visual screening and assessment have been considered and illustrated with specific programmes underway in the Visual Development Unit. New tests and methodologies are being developed in child vision testing all the time; however, it is important to keep in mind the many unanswered scientific and policy questions in this area. These can be summarized as:

1. How effective are present vision screening and assessment procedures in identifying those who either have or are likely to have visual problems?
2. What vision problems are at present treated successfully? and when treatment fails do we understand why?
3. Should vision screening and assessment be equally available for all children, or should it be concentrated on those considered to be most at risk?
4. What is the relationship between defect or abnormality and disability, and how does this relationship change with the age of the child and with the presence of additional non-visual problems?

To answer these questions, professionals will need to co-operate and combine their knowledge and skills and to cross the boundaries between neuroscience, clinical practice, epidemiology and health economics.

ACKNOWLEDGEMENTS

This work is supported by the Medical Research Council of Great Britain. I would like to thank current members of the Visual Development Unit and in

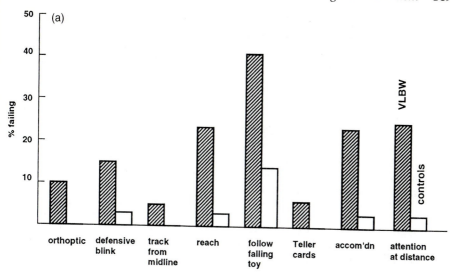

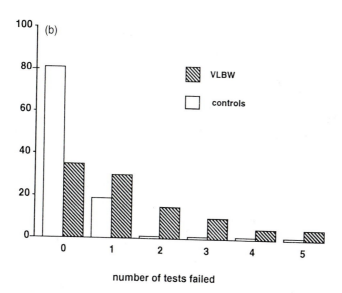

Fig. 10.4 Summary data of VLBW group on ABCDEFV.

particular Shirley Anker, Claire Hughes, Fiona Macpherson, Sara Rae and Frank Weeks for their assistance in the ABCDEFV and VLBW studies. Professor Oliver Braddick is a co-director of this research programme and has been heavily involved in the preparation of this chapter.

REFERENCES

Angi, M. R, Pucci, V., Forattini, F., and Formentin, P. A. (1992). Results of photo-refractometric screening for amblyogenic deficits in children aged 20 months. *Behavioural Brain Research*, **49**, 91–7.

Anker, S., Atkinson, J., and McIntyre, A. M. (1989). The use of the Cambridge Crowding Cards in pre-school vision screening programmes, ophthalmic clinics and assessment of children with multiple disabilities. *Ophthalmic and Physiological Optics*, **9**, 470.

Atkinson, J. (1985). Assessment of vision in infants and young children. In *The at-risk infant: psycho/socio/medical aspects,* (ed. S. Harel and N. J. Anastasiow), Paul H. Brookes Publishing, Baltimore.

Atkinson, J. (1993). Infant vision screening: prediction and prevention of strabismus and amblyopia from refractive screening in the Cambridge photorefraction programme. In *Early visual development: normal and abnormal,* (ed. K. Simons), Oxford University Press, New York.

Atkinson, J. and Braddick. O. J. (1983*a*). The use of isotropic photorefraction for vision screening in infants. *Acta Ophthalmologica*, **157** (suppl.), 36–45.

Atkinson, J. and Braddick, O. J. (1983*b*). Vision screening and photorefraction—the relation of refractive errors to strabismus and amblyopia. *Behavioural Brain Research*, **10**, 71–80.

Atkinson, J. and van Hof-van-Duin, J. (1993). Assessment of normal and abnormal vision during the first years of life. In *Management of visual impairment in childhood,* (ed. A. Fielder and M. Bax), Mac Keith Press, London.

Atkinson, J., Braddick, O. J., Ayling, L., Pimm-Smith, E., Howland, H. C., and Ingram, R. M. (1981). Isotropic photorefraction: a new method for refractive testing of infants. *Documenta Ophthalmologica Proceedings Series*, **30**, 217–23.

Atkinson, J., Braddick, O. J., Durden, K., Watson, P. G., and Atkinson, S. (1984). Screening for refractive errors in 6–9 month old infants by photorefraction. *British Journal of Ophthalmology*, **68**, 105–12.

Atkinson, J., Pimm-Smith, E., Evans, C., Harding, G., and Braddick, O. J. (1986*a*). Visual crowding in young children. *Documenta Ophthalmologica Proceedings Series*, **45**, 210–13.

Atkinson, J., Wattam-Bell, J., Pimm-Smith, E., Evans, C., and Braddick, O. J. (1986*b*). Comparison of rapid procedures in forced choice preferential looking for estimating acuity in infants and young children. *Documenta Ophthalmologica Proceedings Series*, **45**, 192–200.

Atkinson, J., Braddick, O. J., Wattam-Bell, J., Durden, K., Bobier, W., Pointer, J., and Atkinson, S. (1987). Photorefractive screening of infants and effects of refractive correction. *Investigative Ophthalmology and Visual Science*, **28** (suppl.), 399.

Atkinson, J., Anker, S., Evans, C., Hall, R., and Pimm-Smith, E. (1988). Visual acuity testing of young children with the Cambridge Crowding Cards at 3 and 6 metres. *Acta Ophthalmologica*, **66**, 505–8.

Atkinson, J., Gardner, N., Tricklebank, J., and Anker, S. (1989). Atkinson Battery of Child Development for Examining Functional Vision (ABCDEFV). *Ophthalmic and Physiological Optics*, **9**, 470.

Atkinson, J., Braddick, O. J., Anker, S., Hood, B., Wattam-Bell, J., Weeks, F., Rennie, J., and Coughtrey, J. (1990). Visual development in the VLBW infant. In *Transactions of the IVth European Conference on Developmental Psychology*, University of Stirling, p. 193.

Atkinson, J., Smith, J., Anker, S., Wattam-Bell, J., Braddick, O. J., and Moore, A. T. (1991*a*). Binocularity and amblyopia before and after early strabismus surgery. *Investigative Ophthalmology and Visual Science*, **32**, 820.

Atkinson, J., Braddick, O. J., Anker, S., Hood, B., Wattam-Bell, J., Weeks, F., Rennie, J., and Coughtrey, H. (1991*b*). Visual development in the VLBW infant. In *Transactions of the 3rd Meeting of the Child Vision Research Society*, Rotterdam.

Bax, M. C. O. and Whitmore, K. (1990). Health for all children, (book review). *Archives of Disease in Childhood*, **65**, 141–2.

Beardsell, R. (1989). Orthoptic visual screening at 3½ years by Huntingdon Health Authority. *British Orthoptics Journal*, **46**, 7–13.

Braddick, O. J. and Atkinson, J. (1984). Photorefractive techniques: application in testing infants and young children. *Transactions of the British College of Ophthalmic Opticians (Optometrists) 1st International Congress*, **2**, 26–34.

Braddick, O. J., Atkinson, J., Wattam-Bell, J., Anker, S., and Norris, V. (1988). Video-refractive screening of accommodative performance in infants. *Investigative Ophthalmology and Visual Science*, **29** (suppl.), 60.

Castanera de Molina, A., Munoz, L. G., and Castanera, A. S.. (1989). El metodo de foto-refraccion coaxial isotropica (VPR-1) en la deteccion precoz de la ambliopia. Presented at the *X Congreso de la Sociedad Espanola de Estrabologia*, Madrid.

Ehrlich, M. I., Reinecke, R. D., and Simons, K. (1983). Preschool vision screening for amblyopia and strabismus. Programs, methods, guidelines, 1983. *Survey of Ophthalmology*, **28**(3), 145–63.

Griffiths, R. (1970). *The abilities of young children: A comprehensive system of mental measurement for the first eight years of life*. Child Development Research Centre.

Hall, D. B. M (ed.) (1989). *Health for All Children (Report of the Joint Working Party on Child Health Surveillance)*, Oxford University Press.

Holland, W. W. and Stewart, S. S. (1990). *Screening in Health Care*. Nuffield Provincial Hospitals Trust, London.

Hood, B. and Atkinson, J. (1990). Sensory visual loss and cognitive deficits in the selective attentional system of normal infants and neurologically impaired children. *Developmental Medicine and Child Neurology*, **32**, 1067–77.

Howland, H. C. (1991). Advances in instrumentation for biometry of infant refractive error. *Investigative Ophthalmology and Visual Science*, **32**(4 suppl.), xii.

Howland, H. C., Atkinson, J., Braddick, O. J., and French, J. (1978). Infant astigmatism measured by photorefraction. *Science*, **202**, 331–3.

Howland, H. C., Braddick, O. J., Atkinson, J., and Howland, B. (1983). Optics of photo-refraction: orthogonal and isotropic methods. *Journal of the Optical Society of America*, **73**, 1701–8.

Hyvarinen, L. (1988). Vision and eye screening in Finland: an overview. Presented at the *Joint Meeting of the American Orthoptic Council and the American Association of Certified Orthoptists*, Dallas, Texas.

Ingram, R. M., Walker, C., Wilson, J. M., Arnold, P. E., Lucan, J., and Dally, S. (1985). A first attempt to prevent squint and amblyopia by spectacle correction of abnormal refractions from age one year. *British Journal of Ophthalmology*, **69**, 851–3.

Ingram, R. M., Traynar, M. J., Walker, C., and Wilson, J. M. (1979). Screening for refractive errors at age 1 year: a pilot study. *British Journal of Ophthalmology*, **63**, 243–50.

McClellan, A. V. (1977). Area vision screening. *British Orthoptic Journal*, **34**(26), 28–33.

Mitchell, D. E., Freeman, R. D., Millodot, M., and Haegerstrom, G. (1973). Meridional amblyopia: evidence for modification of the human visual system by early visual experience. *Vision Research*, **13**, 535–58.

Mohindra, I., Held, R., Gwiazda, J., and Brill, S. (1978). Astigmatism in infants. *Science*, **202**, 329–31.

Sheridan, M. D. (1976). *Manual for the STYCAR Vision Tests*. National Federation for Educational Research, Slough.

Somov, E. E. (1989). The videorefractometry for children of different ages on the device of Clement Clarke International Ltd (London). Presented at the *Plenary Meeting of the Leningrad Scientific Medical Society of Ophthalmologists*.

van der Lem, G. J., Verbrugge, H. P., Almind, G., Baart de la Faille, L. M. B., Loewer-Sieger, D. H., and de Ridder-Sluiter, J. G. (ed.) (1990). *Early detection of vision, hearing, and language disorders in childhood*. Final report of workshop sponsored by Commission of the European Communities, Concerted Action Committee on Health Services Research.

van Hof-van Duin, J. and Mohn, G. (1986). Visual field measurements, optokinetic nystagmus and the visual threatening response: normal and abnormal development. In: *Detection and measurement of visual impairment in preverbal children. Documenta Ophthalmologica Proceedings Series*, **45**, 305–16.

11

Photorefraction for the detection of amblyogenic defects: past and present

M. R. Angi and E. Pilotto

INTRODUCTION

Amblyopia is a developmental disorder of binocular vision resulting from an anomalous visual experience early in life. It is the primary cause of monocular vision loss in children and young adults, affecting more than 2% of the population (Shaw *et al.* 1985). Many investigators have strongly recommended the screening and correction of amblyogenic factors—such as high refraction errors, strabismus and dioptric media opacity—at the earliest feasible age (from 6 months onwards) to improve visual outcome and reduce cases of squint and the progression of myopia (Angi *et al.* 1992; Atkinson *et al.* 1984; Romano 1990; Vaegan and Taylor 1979). The major obstacle to early, mass visual-screening programmes is currently the lack of agreement on appropriate methods (Hoyt 1987). Amblyopia can be screened by subjective or objective testing. From birth, an estimation of visual acuity can be obtained from preferential direction of gaze (Fulton *et al.* 1981; Vital-Durand 1992) but this method is unsuitable for large-scale screening because it is time-consuming and relies on the subject's co-operation. Objective refractometry without cycloplegia may represent the ideal method for screening infants for amblyogenic factors because the test is fast, it requires no contact, and it can be performed by non-professional staff. Howland and Howland (1974) were the first to use a photographic technique to evaluate refractive status from a distance, using a co-axial light source. Atkinson *et al.* (1984) introduced an isotropic co-axial photorefractor for use in large-scale screening programmes. Kaakinen (1979) suggested a photorefractor with an eccentric light source. In subsequent years, the latter model of photorefractor has been used predominantly in paediatric vision screening. Various improvements have been proposed in an attempt to solve problems such as controlling image quality, accurate fixation and accommodation, to extend the range of sensitivity to refractive defects and to measure ocular deviation.

After a brief review of the technical features and clinical outcome of photorefractors described in the literature, the latest developments in automated image analysis will be discussed in this chapter.

PHOTOREFRACTION IN THE PAST

Optical principles of eccentric photorefraction

In 1979, working from the static skiascopy method (Rosengren 1937; Strampelli 1931) and the Brückner test (Brückner 1962), Kaakinen *et al.* (1987) developed a new method for screening for strabismus and ametropias using the simultaneous photographic documentation of the corneal and retinal reflex generated by a flash eccentric to the optical axis of the lens. A refractive defect coming within the instrument's sensitivity range causes a light crescent to appear in the pupil. Several ray-tracing analyses of eccentric photorefraction have been published, defining the parameters that explain the behaviour of the crescent, both in spherical ametropia (Bobier and Braddick 1985; Howland 1980; 1985) and in an astigmatic eye with an oblique axis (Wesemann *et al.* 1991). Basically, the **width** of the crescent is given by the following equation:

$$S = 2r - \frac{E + Y}{D\,d}$$

where S = light crescent width; r = subject's pupillary radius; E = distance of light source from edge of lens aperture; Y = parallax between tested eye and edge of lens aperture; d = distance between subject and camera; and D = degree of refractive error.

The **position** of the crescent in the pupil depends on the radial position of the light source around the lens: the crescent appears on the side opposite the light source in hyperopic eyes and on the same side in myopic eyes. If the values E, r, Y and d are kept constant, the width of the crescent will only depend on the refractive error D. The luminous crescent in the pupil appears at the critical value defined by the blind interval (i.e. the interval in which a refractive error does not make a crescent of light appear in the pupil) and increases according to a curve that quickly becomes asymptotic for refractive defects about 2 dioptres beyond the detection threshold. The angular tilt of the crescent is a function of the cylinder axis; the degree of ametropia in a model eye has been calculated from the size and tilt of the crescent measured in two orthogonal positions (Wesemann *et al.* 1991).

The evolution of photorefractors

The first photorefractor described by Kaakinen *et al.* in 1979 was composed of a 35 mm camera with a flash placed alongside a 100 mm f: 2.8 lens. On a test eye with a 9 mm pupil, the blind interval at 1 metre was 4.75 dioptres (+1.75 to –3); astigmatism could not be detected because the photorefraction involved only one meridian. Since then, at least 10 new prototypes of photorefractor have been described. Technical evolution has aimed to increase their sensitivity in detecting refractive defects and to improve image quality.

Reducing the blind interval and detecting astigmatism

In order to improve the method's sensitivity and permit the evaluation of astigmatism, Kaakinen *et al.* reduced the **eccentricity** of the light source and simultaneously triggered two small orthogonal flashes (Kaakinen *et al.* 1987). On the test eye with a pupil of 4 mm, the blind interval dropped to 3.50 dioptres (+1 to –2.50). To eliminate parallax error between the vertical measurement of the right and left eyes in detecting astigmatism, Angi and Baravelli (1989) proposed using a photorefractor with a single, miniaturized flash at an eccentricity of 10 mm and taking at least three photographs with the camera placed first horizontally, then vertically to the right and left. The blind interval at 1 m was 2.50 dioptres (+0.50 to –2) for the test eye with a pupil of 9 mm. Other models of Polaroid photorefractor (Hsu-Winges *et al.* 1989; Wanger and Waern 1988) produced identical blind intervals. Freedman and Preston (1992) reduced the eccentricity of the flash to 5 mm and thus obtained a blind interval of 0.5 dioptres (–0.50 to 0.0) on a test eye with a pupil of 8 mm. Schaeffel *et al.* (1987) proposed an infrared photoretinoscope that reduced the blind interval to zero with a minimum light source eccentricity of 2 mm.

Other authors reduced the blind interval by increasing the distance between the camera and the eye using a catadioptric 500 mm lens (Abramov *et al.* 1990; Day and Norcia 1986; Norcia *et al.* 1986); with these photorefractors, the blind interval was 1.50 dioptres (+0.50 to –1). However, this apparatus calls for the head to be immobilized against a chin rest and astigmatism is not detected because the camera cannot be turned through 90°, the greater distance (4.5 m) also makes it difficult to ensure the subject's fixation, especially in the case of very young children.

Expanding the range of measurable ametropia

In principle, any magnitude of refractive error can be measured with the right light source eccentricity (Hamer *et al.* 1992). In practice, the eccentricity is low (5–7 mm) in almost all photorefractors: this facilitates refractive error measurement around the blind interval but makes it impossible in high ametropias because the amount of light reflected from the posterior pole becomes too weak. In fact, the photorefraction calibration curves on the test eye reported in the literature stop at +6/–6 dioptres; behaviour of the crescent at high ametropias is not considered. Shaeffel *et al.* (1987) extended the range of measurement by using several infrared (IR) LEDs positioned at different eccentricities (2–20 mm) from the camera axis; they report a linear relationship between refractive defect and eccentricity in an artificial eye for a range of at least ±8 dioptres. Using 7 and 20 mm eccentricity of the IR LEDs in a model eye, Angi *et al.* (1993) find a progressive collapse in crescent size for a myopic error greater than 10 dioptres. These findings are borne out in clinical practice. High ametropias (above ±10 dioptres) risk giving rise to insidious false negatives, because the pupillary field appears illuminated evenly in the same way as in mild myopia of the blind interval. In fact, Norcia *et al.* (1986) found no myopic anisometropia greater than –7 dioptres while screening children whereas Angi *et al.* (1992) found a myopic anisometropia of −20 dioptres; with currently used photorefractors, there is a risk of high ametropia being overlooked in an orthotropic eye.

Controlling image quality fixation and accommodation
Using a 35 mm camera, image quality can only be verified after the film has been developed, which makes it impossible to check for any problems such as the subject's blinking, shifting and faulty fixation or focusing. This problem is evident particularly when screening premature children or the handicapped. Preslan and Zimmerman (1993) found unreadable photorefractions in 23% of a group of 182 infants: 85% of the children unsuccessfully screened were premature (<3 months corrected age). An attempt was made to overcome the fixation problem by means of a luminous and acoustic fixation target to attract the subject's attention. However, this proved inadequate because a child's fixation lasts only a matter of seconds and the observer has to be able to check the result immediately. The problem of controlling image quality has been solved in two ways: using either instantly-developed film or the video camera. Kaakinen (1981) used instant image development with a Polaroid backing in a 6 × 6 camera; Wanger and Waern (1988) and Freedman and Preston (1992) in a 35 mm camera; Hsu-Winges *et al.* (1989) used a commercial Polaroid model. Shaeffel *et al.* (1987, 1993) and Angi and Cocchiglia (1990) used an IR-sensitive video camera connected to a computer, with an image grabber that enables continuous observation of the eye's refractive status. In emmetropic eyes, binocular fixation can easily be observed on-line through the Brückner pupillary reflex: conjugacy of the IR-emitting diodes in the apparatus with the fovea causes the pupil to appear darkened in an eye that is fixating and focusing on the light source (Roe and Guyton 1984). Frames of interest can be captured at a click of the mouse and stored for subsequent analysis. By comparison with the still camera, sampling precision is higher because of the multiple choice option offered by the video and because the operator freezes an image he or she can see, whereas with a still camera the shutter hides the image that is actually recorded. In the darkness, the test performed by the IR videorefractor enables the operator to check continuously the subject's fixation. In addition, unlike the still camera's flash, the IR LEDs create no glare and therefore have no effect on the subject's visual performance.

Assessing strabismus
When reporting clinical trials with the photorefractor, Kaakinen *et al.* (1987) pointed out that microtropias with a deviation of less than 2° were not detectable from observation of the asymmetry of the corneal/retinal reflexes. Freedman and Preston (1992) confirmed that photo camera screening systems do not screen adequately for phorias or for small-angle or intermittent tropias. These drawbacks stem from problems of accuracy in the measurements and the method of collecting the diagnostic images. To estimate the angle of strabismus in photorefraction, the clinician uses the Hirschberg test and compares the

corneal reflex positions of the light source in the two eyes (Griffin and Boyer 1974). The difficulty lies in exactly estimating the reflex displacement in millimetres and in the fact that it is impossible to know the kappa angle with only one picture taken by conventional photorefractors. At high magnification, the corneal reflex appears as an oval area with blurred edges and the transition of the cornea to the sclera is gradual, making the choice of limits somewhat subjective in both cases. An error in the estimated position of the corneal reflex of 0.3 mm (caused by, for instance, a different physiological kappa angle) will give rise to 7 prism dioptres of false strabismic deviation. To overcome such problems, DeRespinis *et al.* (1989) suggest using a Hirschberg phototest taking three pictures (binocular view, RE fixating, LE fixating) so that the kappa angle can be calculated. The measurements are taken manually with callipers. By comparison with the alternate prism/cover test, the accuracy of this method is 6.58 prism dioptres. Barry *et al.* (1992) introduced a reflex camera with three horizontally aligned flashes and measured the angle of strabismus from the reflection patterns of the first and fourth Purkinje images of each light source. Measurements are made by a computer with a frame grabber after digitizing the slides with a CCD video camera. The accuracy of this method, which requires only one shot with both eyes open, is between 2 and 4.5 prism dioptres. Angi *et al.* (1993) performed the Hirschberg phototest with the IR videorefractor, introducing an IR filter to occlude the non-fixating eye. The IR occluder enables the detection and measurement of the angle of both tropias and phorias. Positioning of the markers and calculations are automatically processed by the instrument. The accuracy of this method is 3.86 prism dioptres.

The sensitivity and specificity of eccentric photorefraction

Several controlled clinical trials and screening programmes have evaluated the sensitivity and specificity of photorefraction with and without cycloplegia. The findings are summarized in Table 11.1. The lack of any standardization of failure criteria restricts the comparison between different studies; nonetheless, there is a general consensus on the validity of the method in screening for significant refractive errors (> ±3.50 dioptres).

Analysis of false-negative cases reported

At low risk of amblyopia   These are as follows:

(1) cases of mixed astigmatism (e.g. +1 sph −2.50 cyl): a significant difference between the two main axes can be overlooked if their focal planes are falling in front of and below the retina, within the blind interval of the instrument;

(2) moderate spherical hyperopia (e.g. +4.25 to +5 sph) compensated by accommodation: without cycloplegia, hyperopic eyes may appear normal if the subject accommodates on the fixation target at a distance of 1 metre and is orthotropic;

Table 11.1 Accuracy of photorefraction in the detection of amblyogenic defects.

Reference	Photorefractor model	Distance (m)	Mean age (range)	No. of cases	Cycloplegic refraction	Limits of inclusion in the 'at risk' group (D = dioptres; PD = prism dioptres)	Sensitivity (%)	Specificity (%)	Positive prediction value (%)	Pre-screening probability (%)
Morgan and Johnson (1987)	35 mm camera catadioptric	4.5	(3 months–8 years)	63	No	>+2.50 D meridional hyperopia ≥2.00 D anisometropia ≥2.00 D astigmatism strabismus: any	91	74	84	60
Hamer et al. (1992)	35 mm camera catadioptric	4.5	3 years (8 weeks–4.3 years)	92	No / Yes	>+2.25 D meridional hyperopia / >+2.75 D meridional hyperopia	83 / 83	72 / 73	31 / 32	13
Hsu-Winges et al. (1989)	Polaroid SE camera	1	7 months (2–18 months)	187	No	≥+3.50 D sphere 2.50 D astigmatism ≥1.50 D anisometropia	83	63	43	22
Kennedy and Sheps (1989) Kennedy and Sheps (1989)	35 mm camera catadioptric Otago	3.1 0.5	6 years (2–6 years) 6 years (2–6 years)	236 236	No Yes No Yes	>±3.00 D sphere >±2.00 D astigmatism " "	85 90 94 95	87 83 94 88	82 79 92 85	42 42
Angi et al. (1992)	35 mm camera	1	19 months (18–20 months)	795	No	>+2.50 D meridional hyperopia <−2.50 D meridional myopia >2.00 D anisometropia strabismus > 5 PD	80	95	45	4
Angi et al. (1993)	IR video-refractometer	1 1	3 years (3–4 years)	198	No	>+2.50 D meridional hyperopia <−2.50 D meridional myopia >2.00 D anisometropia strabismus > 5 PD	82	97	65	5.5
Freedman and Preston (1992)	Eyecor	1	7 years (5 months–23 years)	202	No	>+3 D sphere at 2–6 years <−1.00 D sphere >1.50 D astigmatism >1.50 D anisometropia strabismus: any	87	89	93	63
Preslan and Zimmerman (1993)	35 mm camera catadioptric	4.5	28 weeks gestational age (0–13 months)	181	No	≥+4 D sphere ≤−2 D sphere ≥2 anisometropia strabismus > 5 PD	77	90	65	18

3) borderline low myopia (e.g. 2.25 dioptres);
4) variable, small-angle accommodative esophoria/tropia.

Amblyopia was excluded clinically in most of these children, despite the presence of a refractive error above the risk threshold (Angi *et al.* 1992). Overall, this group represented most of the false negatives found while screening selected groups of children (Freedman and Preston 1992; Hamer *et al.* 1992; Hsu-Winges *et al.* 1989).

At high risk of amblyopia These are as follows:

1) high myopic/hyperopic defects (greater than ± 10 dioptres) simulating a low error within the blind interval;
2) microtropia or small-angle esotropia;
3) anisometropia >2 dioptres masked by insufficient mydriasis;
4) refractive errors above the threshold and visible in the photograph but missed by human error of interpretation.

Amblyopia was clinically confirmed in all these children: in mass screening, they represented 0.4% of the population examined (Angi *et al.* 1992).

PHOTOREFRACTION IN THE PRESENT

Since 1987, all children born in the Cittadella area to the north of Padova (Veneto Health Unit No. 19) have been invited to undergo non-cycloplegic photorefractive screening at the age of 18 months. From between 795 and 860 children a year (mean attendance: 82% of the cohort) have been screened by an orthoptist and a nurse in the past 6 years. The sensitivity and specificity of the method in screening for amblyogenic defects was found to coincide with the results of other studies (Table 11.2). After 2 years of mass screening with a 35 mm camera-based photorefractor, the VRB binocular videorefractor (Angi and Cocchiglia 1990) was developed to satisfy the need to check image quality immediately in order to reduce the number of fixation errors and false positives. Specific software was developed to reduce the number of false negatives.

Videorefractor hardware

The apparatus has been described in detail elsewhere (Angi *et al.* 1993). Briefly, it comprises a CCD TV camera with maximum sensitivity in the near infrared band (720 nm). The lens is set for a focal distance of 1 m. A battery of infrared LEDs is installed outside the lens to illuminate the subject's eyes from the meridians 90°, 0° and 180°. The operator can select their eccentricity from the edge of the camera aperture (7 mm and 20 mm). A 386/33 MHz computer with 4MB RAM, equipped with a camera digitizing board image-grabber with a monochrome, 262,144 pixels per square inch CCD sensor, processes the images from the TV camera and displays them on a screen. The apparatus provides a continuous sequence (30 frames/s) of the subject's fixation and accommodative performance. In order to better emphasize variations in pupillary light crescents caused by accommodation, the operator can view images on the screen in equalized form (i.e. by selecting only three threshold levels on the grey scale). A fixation target is provided by a matrix of diodes, which reflects non-repetitive moving patterns in the centre of the lens.

Videorefractor software

The refraction programme

Test method   The test is performed in dim light at a distance of 102 ± 5 cm. Once the subject's eyes are in the right focus (sharp corneal reflex) and position, the operator induces fixation by turning on the fixation target. Using a mouse, the operator can then select a suitable frame: three images are obtained automatically in 60 ms, lighting the eyes from the 90°, 0°, and 180° meridians. The images are displayed on the screen for immediate verification and are discarded if they are found unsuitable. The diagnostic images can be stored and printed with other clinical results.

Algorithms for the automated measurement of refraction   Owing to the scattered reflections of light in the human eye, it is difficult to define the edges of the pupillary light crescent because the pupillary irradiation distribution profiles tend to have the form of a smooth ramp rather than a steep cliff shape (Hodgkinson *et al.* 1991). An experimental calibration has been suggested to convert the crescent shape into refractive error (Schaeffel *et al.* 1993). Meridional refractive errors were measured in seven emmetropic subjects (mean age 24.6 years, range 19–35 years), simulating refractive errors from 0 to ±7 dioptres in 1 dioptre steps. Lenses of different powers were placed in a trial frame in front of one eye occluded by a Hoya R72 IR filter to prevent accommodation, while the contralateral eye was covered. Plotting the refractive defect vs. the dimension of the light crescent gave rise to an excessively high variability. The refractive defect was estimated more reliably by the light crescent dimensions, the pupil size and the integral of pupillary irradiation. An error signal was displayed on the screen when the reliability index for the image quality was below the threshold of 90%. The reliability index was altered by pupil size below 5 mm in diameter, by the poor focusing of images, when the crescent intensity saturated the CCD sensor, or when the crescent collapsed in ametropias > ±4 dioptres.

Validation of the refraction programme   Retrospectively, 75 consecutive clinical cases were used, and these were recorded at the Preventive Ophthalmology Unit of the Padua University Eye Clinic. There were 40 males and 35 females; (mean age 4.5 years, range 3–14 years, median 6) with refractive errors ranging from +9 to –12 dioptres. Overall, a total of 284 meridians were examined. Cases of strabismus or opacity of ocular media were excluded. Each patient provided:

(1) videorefractor pupillary images of fixating eyes obtained with 7 mm eccentricity, without cycloplegia;
(2) manifest and cycloplegic refraction values (Cyclopentolate 10% × 2 after 40′) evaluated with the Topcon 3000 autorefractor;
(3) visual acuity: an eye was considered amblyopic below the visual acuity of 0.5 with the best correction.

The prevalence of amblyogenic defects in this group was 30%. The recorded pupillary images displayed by VRB were scored by an observer who was unaware of the results of the final clinical examination. The observer subjectively measured pupil diameter and crescent size on the screen, then classified the meridional defect either as **safe** (0 to +2.50; –1.50 to –4), or **at risk** (> +2.50 or < –4), comparing the picture with a set of standard images with known refractive errors. The VRB objectively measured the meridional refractive error, expressed in dioptres, indicating its reliability index.

The strabismus programme

Principles   The Hirschberg test gives an estimate of strabismic angle by comparing the positions of the corneal images of a light held in front of the subject. The photographic estimation of the amount of corneal reflex displacement has been suggested to evaluate ocular deviation as an alternative to using the prism/alternated cover test (DeRespinis *et al.* 1989). Values from 19.5 to 25 prism dioptres per millimetre of corneal reflex displacement had been indicated as the factor of conversion from reflex displacement to strabismic angle (Paliaga 1992; Wick and London 1980).

Test method   The method has been described in detail elsewhere (Angi *et al.* 1993). Briefly, the subject is seated in front of the VRB at a distance of 1 m, in a dim environment to induce natural mydriasis. Three images are captured while the subject's gaze is fixing on the VRB target:

(1) binocular viewing (primary deviation);
(2) left eye fixing with right eye occluded by an IR transmitting filter (secondary deviation RE);
(3) right eye fixing with left eye occluded (secondary deviation LE).

The images are then processed by the VRB, which automatically identifies the positions of the corneal reflex and pupillary border in each image and thus calculates the angle of horizontal and vertical tropia and the secondary deviation under the occluder.

Calibration   Equally-spaced targets induce a progressive underestimation of the simulated angle of strabismus (Brodie 1987). To solve this problem, we corrected the distance of the fixation targets according to the following formula:

$$D = \text{arc tan} \left(\frac{1}{102} \right) d$$

where D = distance of fixation target; d = equally-spaced distance of target; and 102 = distance between camera and eye (in cm). This enables a calculation of the intersection of the extended line of gaze with the tangent at the circumferential arc subtended by a simulated angle of strabismus expressed in prism dioptres. A strabismus of 10, 20, 30, 40, 50, and 60 prism dioptres at 102 cm was obtained with a fixation target placed at a distance of 10, 20.2, 30.9, 42.2, 54.4, and 68 cm. The VRB programme was validated using the Hirschberg phototest (DeRespinis *et al.* 1989) as a gold standard. Nine emmetropic and orthophoric volunteers with a mean corneal curvature radius between 7.5 and 8 mm were photographed from a distance of 102 cm while fixing on a series of 12 targets (six temporal and six nasal). The conversion factor used was 21 prism dioptres/mm (DeRespinis *et al.* 1989). Repeatability was assessed comparing the measurements obtained by two observers, and by one observer on two different days, in the same subject.

RESULTS

The refraction programme

The VRB correctly revealed the *presence* and the *sign* of refractive errors from +9 to –12 dioptres (eccentricity $E = 7$ mm; mean pupillary diameter 7.3 mm ± 0.45 SD; blind interval +0.00 to –1.50 dioptres). Naturally, spherical hyperopic errors in eyes without cycloplegia were underestimated by VRB because of accommodation. Astigmatism was detected in combination with spherical errors < ±5 dioptres. In all cases presenting simple spherical and/or astigmatic errors orthogonal to the VRB light sources, the defect was estimated to within a difference of ±3 dioptres around the blind interval. A progressive underestimation of the defect was observed in the refractive errors above +3.50/–5 dioptres, when the pixel brightness saturated the CCD sensor or the crescent began to collapse (Fig. 11.1). All 11 cases of refractive error >7 dioptres were revealed correctly by the VRB when the reliability index was taken in account (Fig. 11.2).

The accuracy of the automated and subjective interpretation is reported in Table 11.2.

Error analysis produced the following results:

(1) *False negatives*: both the VRB and the observer failed to identify three eyes with mixed astigmatism >2.50 dioptres and nine eyes with > +2.50 dioptres sphere because of insufficient scotopic mydriasis and/or accommodation. The observer classified four eyes with ametropias > ±8 dioptres as 'safe'.

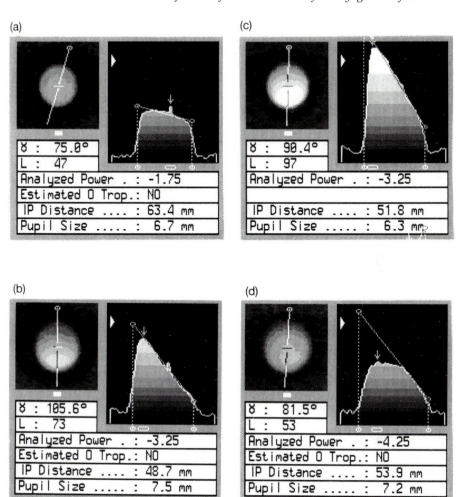

Fig. 11.1 Equalized two-dimensional videorefractor images of myopic human eyes: (a) –1.75 dioptres—the crescent intensity distribution profile has the shape of a truncated cone with slightly tilted top; the estimated error is correct; (b) –3.25 dioptres —the truncated cone has a straight, tilted top with sharp edges, the estimated error is correct; (c) –6.50 dioptres—the upper edge of the cone saturates the CCD sensor: therefore, the refractive error is underestimated (–3.25 dioptres); (d) –10.25 dioptres— the truncated cone is dome-shaped with smooth edges (collapse); the refractive error is underestimated (–4.25 dioptres).

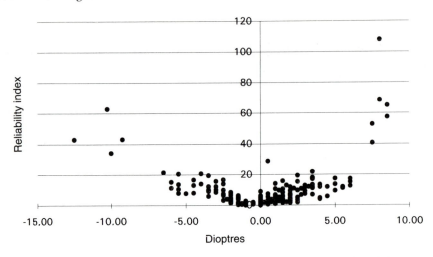

Fig. 11.2 Distribution of refractive errors plotted *vs* the reliability index of the crescent in the pupillary area. High ametropias (> ±7 dioptres) are easily detected.

Table 11.2 Accuracy of automated and subjective interpretation of refractive errors.

	Sensitivity	Specificity	PPV
VRB	85%	94%	86%
Observer	81%	87%	73%

VRB = IR videorefractor; PPV = positive prediction value.

(2) *False positives*: the VRB and the observer both overestimated the defect respectively in 12 and 25 borderline hyperopic eyes. Overall, the VRB correctly identified more eyes at risk than the observer.

The strabismus programme

In simulated squint, the VRB automated measurement of horizontal corneal reflex displacement showed a significant, constant underestimation by comparison with the photographic Hirschberg test. However, when a conversion factor of 23 prism dioptres/mm was used in the VRB, the difference became insignificant and the correlation between the simulated and measured angles was excellent (esotropia $r = 0.986$; exotropia $r = 0.984$) up to ±60 prism dioptres (Fig. 11.3).

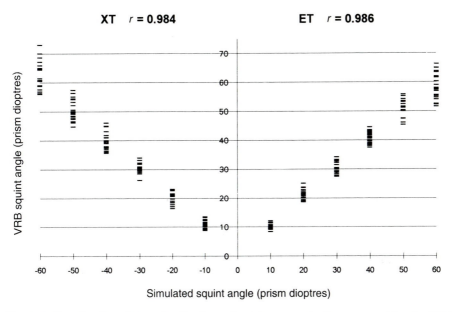

Fig. 11.3 Simulated squint angles (horizontal axis) automatically measured by the VRB (vertical axis) in 9 normal subjects. *r*, correlation coefficient calculated by multiple regression; XT, exodeviations; ET, esodeviations.

Repeatability was assessed with the ANOVA test for repeated measurements. Data obtained with the VRB by two observers and by the same observer on two different days were similar ($p = 0.76$ and 0.96 respectively) in 40 prism dioptres simulated exotropia, less concordant in 40 prism dioptres simulated esotropia ($p = 0.09$ and 0.12). Data obtained with a 35 mm camera, however, gave a significant variation in repeated measurements of esotropia on the same subject (40 prism dioptres simulated exotropia with $p = 0.75$ and 0.87; 40 prism dioptres simulated esotropia with $p = 0.05$ and 0.07).

DISCUSSION

In this study software programmes have been developed for automatic off-line analysis of the images generated with an IR eccentric videorefractor in human eyes without cycloplegia. In the evaluation of refractive amblyogenic errors and strabismus, this method proved qualitatively more accurate than results obtained by subjectively scoring the images. Alternatively, the quantitative assessment of refractive errors needs major improvements, which perhaps are beyond the reach of the photorefractive method. In fact, the amount of refractive error was correctly measured within ±3 dioptres around the blind interval, then a progressive underestimation was detected. However, by including in this evaluation the reliability index based on the crescent's saturation/collapse evaluation, all high ametropic errors were identified correctly. Crescent shape, tilt of crescent top and the integral of pupillary irradiation distribution are the keys for distinguishing between low and high ametropia. This distinction proves very difficult if it is based on two-dimensional analogue images.

In our opinion, automated videorefraction represents a major step forward in the search for an appropriate method for visual screening of infants for three reasons.

1. The on-line evaluation of images has solved two problems involved in all other photorefraction techniques (i.e. exact control of fixation and continuous evaluation of accommodative response during the test).

2. The quantitative estimation of refractive error in the two eyes, and the 'error' message indicating the presence of ametropia above the range measured by the instrument make the test more suitable for handling by non-professional staff. It is impossible to quantify high refractive errors on the basis of the crescent's width. The crescent does not have a clear margin because the retina acts as an angularly diffuse partial reflector in photorefraction (Hodgkinson et al. 1991). The quantitative assessment of meridional refractive defects in eccentric photoretinoscopy has been obtained over a range of ±5 dioptres by comparing the crescent width detected at different light source eccentricities (Bobier and Braddick 1985; Schaeffel et al. 1987). We suggest a further extension of the measurable range by means of the nulling technique (i.e. neutralizing the refractive error with spherical lenses until it falls within the linear measurement interval).

3. Automatic measurement of the binocular horizontal and vertical angle of tropia and phoria decreases the time and increases the accuracy of the method by comparison with the prism/alternate cover test, making it feasible in a screening setting. Inter-observer reliability of the masked interpretation of squint angles was excellent. On plotting the VRB estimates of squint angle against the simulated value, it was found that the most appropriate nominal conversion factor of reflex displacement was 23 prism dioptres/mm; the difference from the 21 prism dioptres/mm used in the phototest may depend on the different flash wavelength and IR LED sources, which generate different depths of Purkinje's reflections in the anterior chamber.

CONCLUSION

In conclusion, the automated analysis of videorefraction images is a powerful new method for screening for amblyogenic factors in infants or uncooperative patients. New software developments provide reliable data on ocular deviation and a qualitative evaluation of the eye's refractive error. Since relationship between refractive error and light crescent width is markedly non-linear, its quantitative estimates above +5/−6 dioptres must be preceded by at least partial neutralization. Mass clinical trials are needed to clarify whether automated videorefractometry can be considered as a suitable technique to lower the age of amblyopia detection.

ACKNOWLEDGEMENTS

The authors wish to thank the engineers A. Cocchiglia and G. Meneghini from Fortune Optical srl, Padova (Italy) for providing technical support in the development of VRB software programs.

REFERENCES

Abramov, I., Hainline, L., and Duckman, R. H. (1990). Screening infant vision with paraxial photorefraction. *Optometry and Vision Science*, **67**, 538–45.

Angi, M. R. and Baravelli, S. (1989). La fotorefrazione statica non cicloplegica. I: descrizione dell'apparato e del metodo. *Bollettino di Oculistica*, **68**, 133–43.

Angi, M. R. and Cocchiglia, A. (1990). The binocular infrared videorefractometer: an instrument for the screening of amblyogenic factors and the dynamic study of accommodation in children. *Bollettino di Oculistica*, **69** (suppl. 4), 305–20.

Angi, M. R., Pucci, V., Forattini, F., and Formentin, P. A. (1992). Results of photo-refractometric screening for amblyogenic defects in children aged 20 months. *Behavioural Brain Research*, **49**, 91–7.

Angi, M. R., Bergamo, L., and Bisantis, C. (1993). The binocular videorefractoscope for visual screening in infancy. *German Journal of Ophthalmology*, **2**, 182–8.

Atkinson, J., Braddick, O. J., and Durden, K. (1984). Screening for refractive errors in 6–9-month-old infants by photorefraction. *British Journal of Ophthalmology*, **68**, 105–12.

Barry, J. C., Effert, R., and Kaupp, A. (1992). Objective measurement of small angles of strabismus in infants and children with photographic reflection pattern evaluation. *Ophthalmology*, **99**, 320–9.

Bobier, W. R. and Braddick, O. J. (1985). Eccentric photorefraction: optical analysis and empirical measures. *American Journal of Optometry and Physiological Optics*, **62**, 614–20.

Brodie, S. E. (1987). Photographic calibration of the Hirschberg test. *Investigative Ophthalmology and Visual Science*, **28**, 736–42.

Brückner, R. (1962). Exacte Strabismusdiagnostik bei 1/2-3 jährigen Kindern mit einem einfachen Verfahren, dem 'Durchleuchtungstest'. *Ophthalmologica*, **144**, 184–98.

Day, S. H. and Norcia, A. M. (1986). Photographic detection of amblyogenic factors. *Ophthalmology*, **93**, 25–8.

DeRespinis, P. A., Naidu, E., and Brodie, S. E. (1989). Calibration of Hirschberg test photographs under clinical conditions. *Ophthalmology*, **96**, 944–9.

Freedman, H. L. and Preston, K. L. (1992). Polaroid photoscreening for amblyogenic factors. *Ophthalmology*, **99**, 1785–95.

Fulton, A. B., Manning, K. A., and Dobson, V. (1981). A behavioral method for efficient screening of visual acuity in young infants. *Investigative Ophthalmology and Visual Science*, **17**, 1151–7.

Griffin, J. R. and Boyer, F. M. (1974). Strabismus measurement with the Hirschberg test. *Optometry Weekly*, **65**, 863–6.

Hamer, R. D., Norcia, A. M., Day, S. H., Haegerstrom-Portnoy, G., Lewis, D., Hsu-Winges, C. (1992). Comparison of on- and off-axis photorefraction with cycloplegic retinoscopy in infants. *Journal of Pediatric Ophthalmology and Strabismus*, **29**, 232–9.

Hodgkinson, U., Chong, K. M., and Molteno, A. C. (1991). Characterization of the fundal reflectance of infants. *Optometry and Vision Science*, **68**, 513–21.

Howland, H. C. and Howland, B. (1974). Photorefraction: a technique for study of refractive state at a distance. *Journal of the Optical Society of America*, **64**, 240–9.

Howland, H. C. (1980). The optics of static photographic skiascopy. *Acta Ophthalmologica*, **58**, 221–7.

Howland, H. C. (1985). Optics of photoretinoscopy: results from ray tracing. *American Journal of Optometry and Physiological Optics*, **62**, 621–5.

Hoyt, C. S. (1987). Photorefraction. A technique for pre-school visual screening. *Archives of Ophthalmology*, **105**, 1497–8.

Hsu-Winges, C., Hamer, R., Norcia, A. M., Weserman, H., and Chan, E. (1989). Polaroid photorefractive screening of infants. *Journal of Pediatric Ophthalmology and Strabismus*, **26**, 254–60.

Kaakinen, K. A. (1979). A simple method for screening of children with strabismus, anisometropia or ametropia by simultaneous photography of the corneal and the fundus reflexes. *Acta Ophthalmologica*, **57**, 161–71.

Kaakinen, K. A. (1981). Simultaneous two flash static photoskiascopy. *Acta Ophthalmologica*, **59**, 378–86.

Kaakinen, K. A., Kaseva, H. O., and Teir, H. H. (1987). Two-flash photorefraction in screening of amblyogenic refractive errors. *Ophthalmology*, **94**, 1036–42.

Kennedy, R. A. and Sheps, S. B. (1989). A comparison of photoscreening techniques for amblyogenic factors in children. *Canadian Journal of Ophthalmology*, **24**, 259–64.

Morgan, K. S. and Johnson, W. D. (1987). Clinical evaluation of a commercial photorefractor. *Archives of Ophthalmology*, **105**, 1528–31.

Norcia, A. M., Zadnik, K., and Day, S. H. (1986). Photorefraction with a catadioptric lens. *Acta Ophthalmologica*, **64**, 379–85.

Paliaga, G. P. (1992). Linear strabismometric methods. *Binocular Vision*, **7**, 139–54.

Preslan, M. W. and Zimmerman, E. (1993). Photorefraction screening in premature infants. *Ophthalmology*, **100**, 762–8.

Roe, L. D. and Guyton, D. L. (1984). The light that leaks: Brückner and the red reflex. *Survey of Ophthalmology*, **28**, 665–70.

Romano, P. E. (1990). Advances in vision and eye screening: screening at 6 months of age. *Pediatrician*, **17**, 134–41.

Rosengren, B. (1937). A method of skiascopy with the electric ophthalmoscope. *Acta Ophthalmologica*, **15**, 501–6.

Shaeffel, F., Farkas, L., and Howland, H. C. (1987). Infrared photoretinoscope. *Applied Optics*, **26**, 1505–9.

Shaeffel, F., Wilhelm, H., and Zrenner, E. (1993). Inter-individual variability in the dynamics of natural accommodation in humans: relation to age and refractive errors. *Journal of Physiology (London)*, **461**, 301–20.

Shaw, D. E., Fielder, A. R., Minshull, C. *et al.* (1985). Amblyopia—factors influencing age of presentation. *Lancet*, **i**, 207–9.

Strampelli, B. (1931). Pratiche applicazioni dell'oftalmoscopio del May. Esame oftalmoscopico a luce lineare. Metodo rapido di schiascopia. *Atti Società Italiana di Oftalmologia*, **7**, 739–50.

Vaegan, W. and Taylor, D. (1979). Critical period for deprivation amblyopia in children. *Transactions of the Ophthalmological Society of the United Kingdom*, **99**, 432–9.

Vital-Durand, F. (1992). Acuity card procedures and the linearity of grating resolution development during the first year of human infants. *Behavioural Brain Research*, **49**, 99–106.

Wanger, P. and Waern, G. (1988). Instant photographic refractometry in children. *Acta Opthalmologica*, **66**, 165–9.

Wick, B. and London, R. (1980). The Hirschberg test: analysis from birth to age 5. *Journal of the American Optometry Association*, **51**, 1009–10.

Wesemann, W., Norcia, A. M., and Allen, D. (1991). Theory of eccentric photo-refraction (photoretinoscopy): astigmatic eyes. *Journal of the Optical Society of America*, **8**, 2038–47.

12

The Rotterdam C-chart: visual acuity and interocular acuity differences in very low birth weight and/or very prematurely born children at the age of 5 years

J. van Hof-van Duin and
J. W. R. Pott

INTRODUCTION

It is generally accepted that children born very prematurely or with a very low birth weight (VLBW; <1500 g) are at risk for visual impairment, at least during the first few years after birth. Whether visual impairment such as low visual acuity is only a sign of delayed development, or is irreversible, is still questionable (van Hof-van Duin et al. 1989). Visual acuity development continues until puberty (Slataper 1950; Frisen and Frisen 1981; Hohmann and Haase 1982; De Vries-Khoe and Spekreijse 1982; Kothe and Regan 1990; Pott and van Hof-van Duin 1992), which possibly allows a catching up in this lag in development.

The purpose of our study was to determine whether VLBW and/or very prematurely born children are at risk for permanent impairment of visual acuity by comparison of acuity values obtained in 5-year-old children who are at risk for an impaired visual development because of a very low birth weight and/or a very short gestational duration, to those of healthy control 5-year-olds.

Landolt-C acuity was measured using a new C-chart (the Rotterdam C-chart) on which according to the recommendations of the Committee on Vision (1980), optotypes on successive lines decreased in 1/3-octave (0.1 log) steps and on which crowding was comparable over the entire chart (Pott and van Hof-van Duin 1992). In this earlier study, we demonstrated that with the Rotterdam C-chart acuity estimates of both 5-year-old control children and adults show a normal distribution and no ceiling effect. Therefore, the Rotterdam C-chart seemed suitable for acuity assessment in young and visually impaired children.

SUBJECTS

Landolt-C acuity was tested in 450 5-year-old children who were born after less than 32 weeks of gestation and/or whose birth weights had been less than 1500 g; their mean age, corrected for prematurity, was 5.06 ± 0.23 years. These children represented a geographical subpopulation of the 'Project On Preterm and Small for gestational age infants in the Netherlands 1983' (POPS), a National study, started in Leiden in 1983 (Verloove-Vanhorick and Verwey 1987). Informed consent was obtained from the parents, who were present during testing. Children were screened for eye misalignment. Refractive state was examined by means of isotropic photorefraction without cycloplegia (Atkinson and Braddick 1982; Howland *et al.* 1983; Howland *et al.* 1987; Braddick *et al.* 1988). They wore their own correction if prescribed.

METHODS

The Rotterdam C-chart

The Rotterdam C-chart (Pott and van Hof-van Duin 1992) consisted of black Landolt Cs on a white background, arranged in 16 horizontal rows. The orientation of the Cs was either horizontal or vertical, with a random distribution of the four directions over the chart. The number of optotypes on each line varied from five on the upper row to 11 optotypes on the lower 6 rows. Optotypes on successive rows decreased in 1/3 octave (0.1 log) steps (that is a decrease in optotype height by a factor of two on every third row). Comparable crowding was maintained over the chart by keeping inter-letter and inter-line distances relatively constant. The inter-letter distance on each row was 0.25 octaves smaller than the horizontal diameter of each optotype. Inter-line distances were 0.26 octaves smaller than the optotype height on the preceding line. For acuity measurements at 6 m the size of the chart was 95 cm wide by 110 cm. For acuity measurements at 40 cm this chart was reduced to 6.3 cm by 7.3 cm (a reduction of 15:1). Charts were printed on photographical paper. The contrast of the optotypes was 88%.

Acuity assessment

Binocular and monocular acuity was assessed at 6 m and 40 cm, with the children wearing their own correction if prescribed. For the 6 m assessment, the luminance of the chart was 100 cd/m^2. Subjects were seated at 6 m distance, with a helper seated beside the child, to encourage the child during testing. One of the parents was seated nearby. The examiner was positioned beside the chart and pointed at the optotypes, using a black pointer. The children were asked to indicate the position of the gap in the Landolt C by pointing with a finger or with the hand in the relevant direction. If the children preferred, they could use a black cardboard 'C' to mimick the direction of the indicated optotype. This was practised with large optotypes until the examiner felt confident that the child understood the procedure. Starting with lines with large optotypes, the examiner pointed out five optotypes on each row in a random order. When a child made a mistake, the examiner would go back to the previous line and present two or three of the larger optotypes to keep the child's attention, and then resume testing the line with the smaller optotypes. Acuity threshold was determined by the line with the smallest optotypes on which the child could still make four correct responses out of five.

For testing near acuity, the luminance of the chart was 450 cd/m². The child was seated at a distance of 40 cm with the head supported by a headrest. Only one examiner was needed. The procedure was similar as for distant acuity assessment. Monocular testing was achieved by means of occluding glasses.

To calculate mean acuities, variances and comparison of group means, acuity estimates were converted into the logarithm of the minimal angle of resolution (logMAR) (Westheimer 1979; Holladay and Prager 1991). Results were compared with norm values obtained in 180 5-year-old control children (Pott and van Hof-van Duin 1992). Visual acuity values below the 2.5% lower limits of the normal distribution were considered abnormal.

RESULTS

Binocular acuity could be assessed in 433 children at 6 m distance and in 431 children at 40 cm. Monocular acuity assessment at these distances was possible in 421 and 428 children. Failure in 24 children in one or more conditions was caused by monocular ROP with retina detachment in one child, psychomotor retardation in 10 and lack of co-operation in 13 children. The mean testing time for binocular and monocular acuity assessment at 6 m was 5.25 min (SD ± 2.5 min) and at 40 cm 4.67 min (SD ± 0.92 min).

Mean Landolt-C acuities and variabilities assessed at the various testing conditions are given in Table 12.1, together with norm values as obtained in 5-year-old control children and control adults in an earlier study (Pott and van Hof-van Duin 1992). Binocular acuities of all subjects, children and adults, were both at 6 m and at 40 cm significantly better than monocular acuities (paired *t*-test, $p < 0.001$). At 5 years of age, mean acuities in children were significantly lower than mean acuities in adults. As indicated in Table 12.1, binocular and monocular C acuities obtained in at-risk children were found to be significantly lower than in control children (*t*-test, $p < 0.001$), except for binocular near acuity. Near acuity was significantly better than far acuity in at-risk children, for both binocular and monocular assessments (paired *t*-test, $p < 0.01$). These results contradict those of 5-year-old controls; their binocular acuity assessed at 6 m was significantly better than at 40 cm (paired *t*-test, $p < 0.05$), whereas their

Table 12.1 Mean C acuity at (a) 6 m and (b) 40 cm.

Age group	n	VLBW/Preterms 5-year-olds (n = 450)	Controls 5-year-olds (n = 180)	Controls Adults (n = 25)
		min.arc ± octave	min.arc ± octave	min.arc ± octave
(a) 6 m				
OU	433	1.69* ± 0.39	1.50 ± 0.31	0.82 ± 0.27
OD	422	1.91* ± 0.47	1.63 ± 0.34	0.93 ± 0.27
OS	421	1.92* ± 0.49	1.64 ± 0.34	0.91 ± 0.31
(b) 40 cm				
OU	431	1.62 ± 0.41	1.55 ± 0.31	0.69 ± 0.31
OD	422	1.83* ± 0.51	1.64 ± 0.37	0.75 ± 0.31
OS	421	1.82* ± 0.51	1.64 ± 0.36	0.77 ± 0.31

* $p < 0.001$ (t-test).

monocular acuity was not significantly different at the two distances (paired *t*-test, $p > 0.1$).

The frequency distribution of acuity estimates as obtained with the Rotterdam C-chart in at-risk (black columns) and control (stippled columns) children at the various test conditions is shown in Fig. 12.1. The 2.5% lower limit of the normal distribution ($p_{2.5}$) was found between 2.5 and 3.1 min.arc for all test conditions. Compared with the acuity distribution of control children, acuity estimates in at-risk children were shifted into the direction of lower acuities. In Table 12.2, the number of at-risk children with acuity values below 2.5 min. arc is given, together with the frequency of impaired acuity for each test condition. In some at-risk children more than one acuity value appeared impaired. The coincidence of more than one visual impairment in the same patient is indicated in Table 12.3 (incidences of other visual impairments are taken from Pott, 1992). Bold digits indicate the total number out of 450 children tested with a certain impairment; on horizontal and vertical lines the coincidences with other impairments are given in regular digits. As can be seen in Table 12.3, binocular C acuity values at 6 m were below the $p_{2.5}$ (worse than 2.5 min.arc) in 21 and at 40 cm in 14 children; binocular C acuity values at 6 m *or* at 40 cm were impaired in **21** − 8 + **14** = 27 at-risk children (6.2%), monocular acuity was impaired in 101 children (23.9%).

Acuity values obtained in at-risk children were subdivided into three groups according to birth weights (<1500 g *vs.* ≥1500 g) and gestational duration (<32 *vs.* ≥32 weeks). Results are presented in Table 12.4. No significant differences (σ^2-test, corrected according to Yates) were found between C acuity estimates obtained in VLBW children born after a short (n = 147) or a long gestational

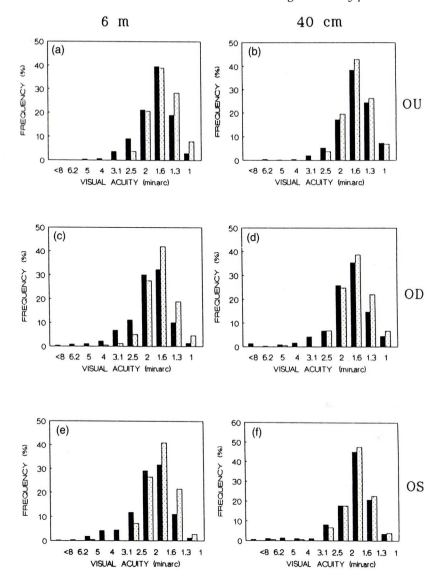

Fig. 12.1 Distribution of binocular (OU) and monocular (OD, right eye; OS, left eye) acuity estimates as obtained with the Rotterdam C-chart in 5-year-old VLBW/very preterm (black columns) and control (stippled columns) children at testing distances of 6 m and 40 cm. (a) binocular 6 m; (b) binocular 40 cm; (c) right eye 6 m; (d) right eye 40 cm; (e) left eye 6 m; (f) left eye 40 cm.

period ($n = 217$), or in very prematurely born children but with a birth weight of ≥ 1500 g ($n = 86$).

Interocular acuity differences are shown in Fig. 12.2, with differences between left eye and right eye presented in 1/3 octave (0.1 log) steps. Whereas

Table 12.2 Mean Rotterdam C acuity, number and incidence of individual acuity impairments (>2.5 min.arc) in 450 VLBW/preterm children tested at 5 years of age.

	6 m			40 cm		
	min.arc ± octave	Below normal		min.arc ± octave	Below normal	
		n	%		n	%
OU	1.69 ± 0.39	21/43	4.8	1.62 ± 0.41	14/431	3.2
OD	1.91 ± 0.47	51/422	12.1	1.83 ± 0.51	37/428	8.6
OS	1.92 ± 0.49	50/421	11.9	1.82 ± 0.51	42/428	9.8

Table 12.3 Occurrence of combinations of visual impairments in 450 at-risk 5-year-olds.

	RC 6 m		RC 40 cm		Strabismus	Binocular debth	OKN	
	Binocular	Monocular	Binocular	Monocular			Binocular	Monocular
RC 6 m								
Binocular	**21**							
Monocular	21*	**92**						
RC 40 cm								
Binocular	8*	14*	**14**					
Monocular	14*	57*	12*	**66**				
Strabismus	9*	38*	6*	33*	**65**			
Binocular.depth	11*	47*	9*	43*	58*	**83**		
OKN								
Binocular	5	11	3	10	12	16*	**49**	
Monocular	8	35*	7	30*	35*	44*	41*	**107**

* $p < 0.01$ (χ^2-test).

interocular acuity differences in 95.6% and 97.8% of the control children (stippled columns) were not more than 0.1 log step for far and near acuity respectively, 12.8% of the at-risk children (black columns) had an interocular acuity difference of 2/3 octave or more at testing at 6 m and 9.3% for near acuity testing.

Strabismus was present in 65 at-risk children (14.4%) (Pott 1992). As to the outcome of isotropic photorefraction without cycloplegia, the distribution of photorefractive values in at-risk children was similar to that of controls; however, the incidence of myopia of ≥ –1.5 dioptres was significantly higher in at-risk 5-year-olds (6.3%) than in control children (2.1%) (Pott 1992).

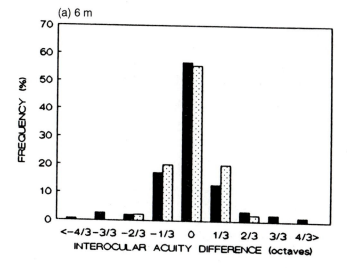

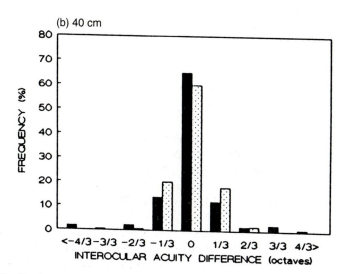

Fig. 12.2 Distribution of monocular acuity differences as obtained with the Rotterdam C-chart in 5-year-old VLBW/very pre-term (black columns) and control (stippled columns) children at testing distances of 6 m (a) and 40 cm (b). Results are presented in 1/3 octave (0.1 log) steps. An interocular acuity difference of one line on the C chart equals a difference of 1/3 octave. Acuity differences between left and right eye are presented: 0 indicates no interocular difference; a positive difference means better acuity for the right eye; a negative difference better acuity for the left eye.

Table 12.4 Visual impairments in 5-year-old at-risk children, divided according to birth weight and gestation.[a]

Visual impairments	Birth weight <1500 g Gestation ≥32 weeks (n = 147)		Birth weight <1500 g Gestation <32 weeks (n = 217)		Birth weight ≥1500 g Gestation <32 weeks (n = 86)	
	n	(%)	n	(%)	n	(%)
Visual acuity Landolt Cs						
6 m						
Binocular	9	(6.4%)	11	(5.3%)	1	(1.2%)
Monocular	27	(19.1%)	49	(23.6%)	16	(19.3%)
40 cm						
Binocular	5	(3.5%)	9	(4.3%)	–	
Monocular	19	(13.6%)	34	(16.5%)	13	(15.9%)
Strabismus	20	(13.6%)	34	(15.7%)	11	(12.8%)
Binocular depth perception	26	(17.7%)	44	(20.3%)	13	(15.1%)

[a] Chi square corrected according to Yates not significant.

DISCUSSION

Success rates for binocular and monocular acuity assessment in the at-risk children ranged between 94% and 96%. This means that as in control 5-year-olds (Pott and van Hof-van Duin 1992), the Rotterdam C-chart can be recommended for visual acuity assessment in 5-year-old children who have suffered from perinatal complications and who are at risk for later visual impairments.

Mean C acuity assessed by means of the Rotterdam C-chart was found to be significantly lower in 5-year-old at-risk children than in controls, except for binocular near acuity (see Table 12.1). This applied both to children born with a birth weight of less than 1500 g and those born after a gestational period of less than 32 weeks duration (see Table 12.4). Binocular C acuity was found impaired in 6.2% of the at-risk children, whereas in 23.9% monocular C acuity was below normal.

In contrast to results obtained in controls, near acuity of at-risk children was significantly better than far acuity, at both binocular and monocular assessments. A possible explanation for the relatively good mean near acuities obtained in at-risk children might be found in the frequency distribution of the acuity values. As can be seen in Fig. 12.1, the shape of the distributions of acuity values obtained in at-risk children at 40 cm distance is different in comparison to those of controls, with more acuities shifted to the left and more values of

Table 12.5 Low acuity estimates in at-risk children compared with ophthalmological impairments.

	6 m			40 cm		
	Binocular	OD	OS	Binocular	OD	OS
Number and incidence with impaired acuity	21 (4.8%)	51 (12.1%)	50 (11.9%)	14 (3.2%)	37 (8.6%)	42 (9.8%)
Possibly ophthalmological	9 (2.1%)	34 (8.1%)	33 (7.8%)	6 (1.4%)	23 (5.4%)	22 (5.1%)
Strabismus		8	10		7	10
Refractive error	5	21	14	3	9	6
Strabismus + refractive error	2	3	5		4	3
Other	2	2	4	3	3	3
Non-ophthalmological	12 (2.8%)	17 (4.0%)	17 (4.0%)	8 (1.9%)	14 (3.2%)	20 (4.7%)

$\geq$2.5 min.arc. However, the incidence of better acuities (1 and 1.3 min.arc) is remarkably high, possibly resulting in relatively high mean acuities. In turn, the relatively high incidence of better acuity values measured at 40 cm, might be caused by an increased incidence of myopia in the at-risk group (6.3% compared with 2.2% in controls).

A further comment on the results shown in Fig. 12.1 concerns the 2.5% lower limit of the normal distribution ($p_{2.5}$), found between 2.5 and 3.1 min.arc for all test conditions. As can be seen in this figure, none of the binocular control values (stippled columns) were below 2.5 min.arc, and in only 4% of the children a binocular acuity of 2.5 min.arc was measured. Since acuities were measured binocularly and monocularly, the $p_{2.5}$ and not the p_5 was chosen as the lower limit of the normal distribution. As a consequence, the number of at-risk children with impaired binocular acuity, as given in Table 12.2, based on values higher than 2.5 min.arc, is probably an underestimate of the incidence of binocular acuity impairments.

At-risk children often had more than one visual deficit, as demonstrated in Table 12.3 (incidences of other visual impairments are taken from Pott 1992). This means that acuity deficits in some of the children could be related to ophthalmological impairments. Table 12.5 indicates whether low acuity estimates, assessed in at-risk children, could possibly be explained by ophthalmological impairments. Refractive errors in this table are based on results obtained with isotropic photorefraction without cycloplegia, and do not include children with correcting glasses prescribed by an ophthalmologist.

IMPAIRED C-ACUITY

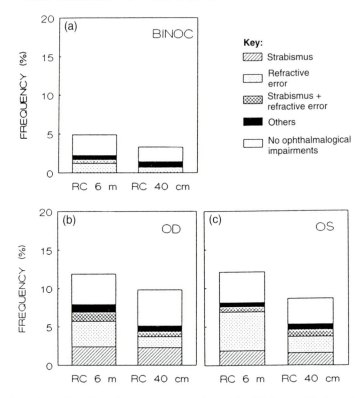

Fig. 12.3 Bar chart showing the percentage of at-risk children with impaired visual acuity as assessed with the Rotterdam C-chart (RC) at 6 m and at 40 cm distance (a) binoc, binocular; (b) OD, right eye; (c) OS, left eye. Subdivisions in each bar indicate percentages of deficits possibly related to ophthalmological impairments.

Corrected refractive errors were not considered to cause low vision. In addition, a binocular acuity impairment was considered neither to be caused by a monocular refractive error nor strabismus. 'Strabismus' in Table 12.5 refers to children with an impaired monocular acuity and the presence of continuous convergent strabismus. Abnormalities such as serious retinopathy of prematurity ($n = 2$), cataract ($n = 2$), spontaneous nystagmus ($n = 2$), and cornea dystrophia ($n = 1$) are indicated as 'other' in Table 12.5, Fig. 12.3 and Fig. 12.4. In Fig. 12.3 the incidence of ophthalmological abnormalities, possibly related to impaired binocular or monocular C acuity is illustrated. As can be seen, acuity deficits could not be related to ophthalmological abnormalities in 30–50% of the at-risk children. These results provide evidence that VLBW and/or very prematurely born children are at risk for permanently impaired visual acuity of both ophthalmological and cerebral origin.

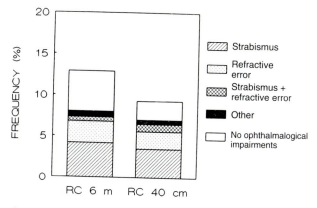

Fig. 12.4 Bar chart showing the percentage of at-risk children with an interocular difference of >1/3 octave, as assessed with the Rotterdam C-chart (RC) at 6 m and at 40 cm distance. Subdivisions in each bar indicate percentages of deficits possibly related to ophthalmological impairments.

Interocular difference appeared impaired (more than 1/3 octave) in 14.3% of the at-risk children. Compairson of interocular acuity differences in at-risk and control children (shown in Fig. 12.2), indicated an acuity difference between left and right eye of ≥2/3 octave in respectively 12.8 *vs.* 4.4% at 6 m testing distance and 9.8 *vs.* 2.2% at 40 cm distance. A difference of 0.2 log steps (or two rows on the Rotterdam C-chart) or more is an indication of a monocular acuity deficit (Pott and van Hof-van Duin 1992). An interocular difference of 1/3 octave was more often present in control than in at-risk children (40 *vs.* 30%). In both groups about 55–65% of the children had no interocular acuity differences. As illustrated in Fig. 12.4, interocular acuity differences of ≥2/3 octave assessed at 6 m testing distance, could be related to ophthalmological abnormalities in 21 out of 55 at-risk children. At 40 cm testing distance this was possible in 30 out of 40 at-risk children.

The present study has given evidence that the Rotterdam C-chart is suitable for acuity assessment in young children at risk for visual impairments. At 5 years of age, 101 out of 422 tested at-risk children (23.9%) had one or more acuity deficits. In 49 of these children the presence of a visual acuity deficit was unknown until testing in our department, despite the fact that these children were known to be at-risk for impaired development, owing to a birth weight of less than 1500 g and/or a gestational period of <32 weeks. In the at-risk children, impaired acuity could be related to ophthalmological abnormalities in 26 cases and is probably a cerebral visual impairment in at least 23 children. Our results suggest that VLBW and/or very prematurely born children are at risk for permanent acuity impairment, both of ophthalmological and of cerebral origin.

ACKNOWLEDGEMENTS

We gratefully acknowledge the co-operation of our colleagues who started the Project On Preterm and Small for gestational age infants, in particular Dr S. P. Verloove-Vanhorick and Dr A. M. Schreuder, Department of Paediatrics, Division of Perinatology, Leiden University. We would like to thank Mrs C. Reus-van Haeren for her help in testing the children and for administrative support, and B. L. F. Weijer for technical assistance. We also would like to thank all the children and their parents.

This work was supported by Praeventiefonds #28-1544, The Hague, The Netherlands.

REFERENCES

Atkinson, J., and Braddick, O. (1982). The use of isotropic photorefraction for vision screening in infants. *Acta Ophthalmologica*, **157** (suppl.), 36–45.

Braddick, O., Atkinson, J., Wattam-Bell, J., Anker, S., and Norris, V. (1988). Video-refractive screening of accommodative performance in infants. *Investigative Ophthalmology and Visual Science*, **suppl. 29**, 60.

Committee on Vision (1980). Recommended standard procedures for the clinical measurement and specification of visual acuity. *Advances in Ophthalmology*, **41**, 103–48.

De Vries-Khoe, L. H. and Spekreijse H. (1982). Maturation of luminance and pattern EPs in man. *Documenta Ophthalmologica, Proceedings Series*, **31**, 461–75.

Frisen, L. and Frisen, M. (1981). How good is normal visual acuity? *Graefes Archive of Clinical and Experimental Ophthalmology*, **215**, 149–57.

Hohmann, A. and Haase, W. (1982). Development of visual line acuity in humans. *Ophthalmological Research*, **14**, 107–12.

Holladay, J. T. and Prager, T. C. (1991). Mean visual acuity. *American Journal of Ophthalmology*, **111**, 372–4.

Howland, H. C., Braddick, O., Atkinson, J., and Howland, B. (1983). Optics of photorefraction: orthogonal and isotropic methods. *Journal of the Optical Society of America*, **73**, 1701–8.

Howland, H. C., Dobson, V., and Sayles, N. (1987). Accommodation in infants as measured by photrefraction. *Vision Research*, **27**, 2141–52.

Kothe, A. C. and Regan, D. (1990). The component of gaze selection/control in the development of visual acuity in children. *Optometry and Visual Science*, **67**, 770–8.

Pott, J. W. R. (1992). Visuele functies bij 5-jarige kinderen in relatie tot een zeer laag geboortegewicht en/of een zeer korte zwangerschapsduur. Published Thesis Erasmus University Rotterdam, University Press, Rotterdam, pp. 1–184.

Pott, J. W. R. and van Hof-van Duin, J. (1992). The Rotterdam C chart: norm values for visual acuity and interocular differences in 5-year-old children. *Behavioural Brain Research*, **49**, 141–7.

Slataper, F. J. (1950). Age norms of refraction and vision. *Archives of Ophthalmology*, **43**, 466–81.

van Hof-van Duin, J., Evenhuis-Leunen, A., Mohn, G., Baerts, W., and Fetter, W. P. F. (1989). Effects of very low birth weight (VLBW) on visual development during the first year after term. *Early Human Development*, **20**, 255–66.

Verloove-Vanhorick, S. P. and Verwey, R. A. (1987). Project on preterm and small for gestational age infants in the Netherlands 1983. Published Thesis, Rijksuniversiteit Leiden, 'S Gravenhage: J. H. Pasman B. V.

Westheimer, G. (1979). Scaling of visual acuity measurements. *Archives of Ophthalmology*, **97**, 327 –30.

13

Acuity cards and the search for risk factors in infant visual development

*François Vital-Durand, Louis Ayzac,
and Gabriel Pinzaru*

INTRODUCTION

It is widely accepted that the major steps of visual development occur during the first 18 months of life. Resolution, measured with acuity cards, improves steadily from birth where it is close to 1 cycle per degree (20/600) to near 15 cycles/degree (20/40) toward the end of the first year (Teller *et al.* 1986; Dobson *et al.* 1987; van Hof-van Duin and Mohn 1986; Sebris *et al.* 1987; Vital-Durand 1992). Accommodation is present when needed so that it does not limit resolution (Braddick *et al.* 1979; Howland *et al.* 1987; Hainline *et al.* 1992). The hyperopic refractive error of 1–2 dioptres often seen in most children may be an artefact of the method used for the measure (Howland 1993; Thorn *et al.* 1996 (this volume)). Binocularity and stereopsis appear at about 4 months of age (Birch *et al.* 1985). Chromatic sensitivity allows detection of reasonable colour contrasts by 3 months of age, if not earlier (Brown and Teller 1989; Morrone *et al.* 1990; Knoblauch and Vital-Durand 1994; Dale *et al.* 1993; Burr *et al.*, Chapter 5, this volume). Finally, velocity and accuracy of saccadic eye movements and gain of pursuit have reached adult performance levels by 5 months of age (Hainline *et al.* 1984; Harris *et al.* 1993; Wattam-Bell, Chapter 6, this volume).

Knowledge of these developmental trends, as well as data obtained from animal experiments, focuses attention on the sensitivity and plasticity of this early period. It is not surprising that amblyopia is most likely to occur at this stage as a consequence of any imbalance between the two eyes. In most cases, amblyopia does not precede refractive imbalance or the onset of strabismus but follows a short time afterwards.

Clinical techniques available have proven their reliability in assessing resolution, normal eye alignment and refractive errors. It is also clear that amblyopia can be prevented easily in almost every case if the treatment is initiated before 1 year of age (Vital-Durand and Patin 1991). Most strabismus can be avoided with early detection and when optical correction is prescribed before 1 year of age (Atkinson 1993).

There remain three questions to be answered to clarify the increasing request for early detection of strabismus (Essman and Essman 1992):

(1) Should the whole population be screened and, if not, which part of it should be, and according to which risk factors?
(2) At what age should the screening be performed to get an optimal response and to allow maximum compliance and efficiency of the therapeutic means used, usually occlusion and optical correction?
(3) How do acuity cards stand in the battery of tests to be used in a screening procedure as well as in the follow-up of screened children.

These questions can be addressed by analysing the data from a large population of infants assessed by various personnel with various techniques (Bishop 1991). A photographic technique was used by Effert *et al.* (1991) to detect strabismus. Da Silva *et al.* (1991) and Schmidt (1991) have compared several tests including acuity cards in order to determine the most efficient technique. Photorefraction and videorefraction are being more widely investigated (Atkinson *et al.* 1984; Angi *et al.* 1992; Freedman and Preston 1992; Preslan and Zimmerman 1993; Angi and Pilotto, Chapter 11, this volume). Introduction of Teller Acuity Cards (TAC) has been a strong incentive to promote early detection of visual defects by allowing estimation of resolution at any age as well as in infants afflicted by visual deficits.

Specifically, this chapter investigates the sensitivity and specificity of TAC in clinical practice, when considered as a single test in a standard battery of tests. Few studies have described a general population of infants in terms of visual capacity. The present study is based on data gathered over 4 years from a large population of infants. However, it should be stressed that this population cannot be considered as representative of the general population.

POPULATION AND METHODS

Infants were referred either to the hospital by general practitioners, paediatricians, medical workers, or they came spontaneously for any reason (walk-ins). As a consequence, there may be an unmeasurable bias in this study population. A population of 2413 infants aged 4–15 months (120–457 days) is considered. Fig. 13.1 shows the age distribution at which individual assessments were performed. Since the authors recommend that infants should be assessed between 7 and 10 months the distribution is inflated over this age range.

There were 1633 (67.7%) referrals and 766 (31.7%) walk-ins. There were 1168 girls (48.4%) and 1245 boys from a wide geographical area, although the largest number of individuals lived in the vicinity of the city of Lyon. Some subjects have been examined more than once, amounting to a total of 5238 eyes tested.

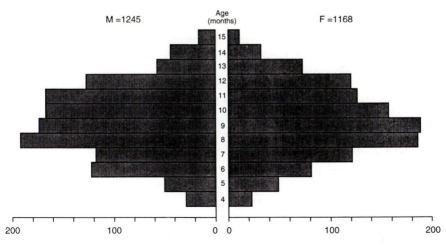

Fig. 13.1 Age distribution at which individual assessments were performed. M, male; F, female.

Clinical assessment

All children were assessed by a single group of trained examiners. For each subject, a record was taken of family and personal history. Binocular and monocular resolution were measured with Teller Acuity Cards using a rapid preferential looking procedure as described by Vital-Durand (1992). In short, the low-frequency gratings were presented only once if the response was immediate and clear. When higher frequencies were reached, the threshold was determined as the highest spatial frequency for which a clear gaze orientation was obtained four times in a row, including two consecutive presentations on the same side. Grating frequencies are separated by one-half octave intervals. Binocular acuity was measured first, then each monocular acuity using an adhesive patch.

Orthoptic assessment included the cover/uncover test, diagnostic spectacles (equipped with a small bi-nasal translucent sector to check independent fixation of each eye), assessment of eye movements, pupillary and stereoscopic responses (Lang test). Direct retinoscopy was performed under cycloplegic (tropicamide) with non-strabismic infants below 18 months. Squinting subjects were refracted after 4 days of 0.30% atropine instillation. In a population of 54 infants (128 eyes, 256 comparisons), data obtained with the two drugs were compared. The ocular fundus was examined by an ophthalmologist.

Children positively screened for any defect or doubtful response were re-examined 2–3 months later. Children with pathologies were prescribed an appropriate treatment, usually based on optical correction and patching, and re-examined subsequently by the same team.

Procedure to measure test validity

The population was divided into four categories: pathological cases (PC) and non-pathological cases (NC), positive results (PR) and negative results (NR). The test distinguishes:

(1) positive cases who may be pathological or true positive (TP) and non-pathological cases or false positive (FP);
(2) negative cases who may be pathological cases or false negative (FN) and non-pathological or true negative cases (TN).

The following definitions are given:

- The sensitivity of the test is defined as $\dfrac{TP}{PC}$

- The specificity of the test is defined as $\dfrac{TN}{NC}$

- The predictive value of positive results is defined as $\dfrac{TP}{PR}$

- The predictive value of negative results is defined as $\dfrac{TN}{NR}$

- The global validity of the test is defined as $\dfrac{TP + TN}{\text{Total number of cases}}$.

Any test undertaken falls between two extremes:

(1) more sensitive but less specific with a high proportion of false positives. Such a test is useful for detection of all pathologic cases. The pathologic condition is checked with a more specific test.
(2) more specific but less sensitive with a high proportion of false negatives. Such a test is useful to confirm the existence of a pathology with a high reliability.

Our population was divided into four groups according to the following criteria:

- Group 1: Normals
  - full-term
  - no abnormality was diagnosed
  - no tropia, no phoria/tropia, no esophoria
  - no refractive error ≤0 dioptres on any axis (myopia), or >2.5 dioptres on any axis (hyperopia)
  - no refractive error difference <–1 or >1.5 dioptres between axes (astigmatism)
  - normal ocular fundus.

- Group 2: Hyperopes
  - same except refractive error difference >2.5 dioptres on any axis.
- Group 3: Myopes
  - same except refractive error difference ≤0 dioptres on any axis.
- Group 4: Astigmats
  - same except refractive error difference <−1 or >1.5 dioptres between two axes.

According to these definitions 927 infants were found to be normal. Table 13.1 shows the distribution of refractive error, strabismus and amblyopia. Some cases showed more than one symptom.

The Epi-Info program was used to process the data, and the odds ratio (OR) was used to quantify the strength of the association between a factor and the occurrence of a pathology. The higher the odds ratio, the greater the strength. The population was divided into cases exposed and non-exposed to the risk factor on one side and into pathological and non-pathological cases on the other.

RESULTS

Resolution

All responses were included, even from poorly co-operative infants. No attempt was made to rate the quality of co-operation. Few instances of lack of

Table 13.1 Incidence of refractive errors and strabismic pathology in the population. In this table each refractive error is considered independently of any other pathology.

	Infants		Eyes	
	n	%	*n*	%
Total	2413		5238	
Normals	927	38.4	1946	37.2
Hyperopes				
≥2.0	386	16.01	757	14.45
≥2.5	254	10.53	480	9.16
≥3.0	168	6.96	314	5.99
Myopes				
≤−2	56	2.33	101	1.93
Strabismics	300	12.4	–	–
Amblyopes				
1/2 octave	262	10.84	–	–
1 octave	129	5.36	–	–

responses were recorded. These, when they occurred, were usually from infants older than 12 months of age. Compliance was 95.9% for binocular testing and 87.43% for monocular testing in the whole population. Missing data usually originated from strabismic or brain-damaged patients who did not tolerate monocular occlusion.

Mean geometric resolution from 927 normals developed fairly linearly between 4 months and 16 months of age (Fig. 13.2). A difference of one third of an octave was observed between binocular and monocular acuity. The large interval of ±1 standard deviation (SD) reflects the variability of the individual scores.

Comparison of resolutions obtained from myopic, hyperopic and astigmatic subjects with normal subjects showed slightly lower values that do not differ significantly from the normal subjects because of the large confidence interval (Fig. 13.3). This means that TAC are useful to signal the possibility of poor vision and evaluate acuity differences between the two eyes, but cannot be considered as a reliable tool to sort out bilateral refractive errors.

Validity of TAC

Sensitivity and specificity tests, as described in the methodology have been used to characterize the validity of TAC in relation to age and refractive errors. These two factors are dependent upon the definition of amblyopia. If we assume that amblyopia should be defined as a difference of two units between the values obtained from the two eyes (one octave), then the test is not very sensitive but highly specific (Table 13.2(a)). If we choose one half octave interval as a sign of amblyopia, then the test is fairly sensitive but moderately specific (Table 13.2(b)).

Refraction

Most children were refracted using tropicamide cycloplegia, except the squinting subjects who were refracted under 30% atropine. To compare the two cycloplegic drugs, the data from a population of 128 eyes that were refracted under the two conditions at short intervals were analysed. Comparison of refractive errors shows a positive correlation of 0.95 with a slight tendency toward higher refractive errors under atropine (Fig. 13.4). Only 5.8% of the measures differed by more than 2 dioptres. Table 13.1 shows the proportion of spherical refractive errors. Some subjects may have a cylindrical error or an anisometropia in addition to their spherical error.

Stereoscopy

The Lang test was found unreliable at early ages. From 7 months of age onward the Lang test was positive on at least two pictures in an increasing percentage of normal subjects. It becomes fairly reliable in a clinical situation after 9 months (Fig. 13.5).

Binocular resolution

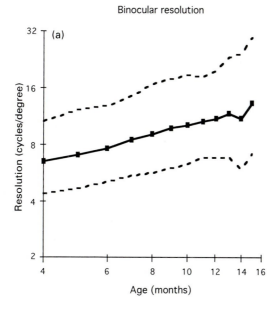

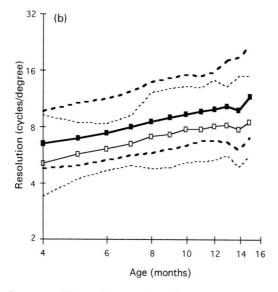

Fig. 13.2 (a) Development of binocular visual resolution in normal eyes. (b) Comparison with monocular resolution. Thick line, binocular resolution; thin line, monocular resolution. Dotted lines indicate S.D.

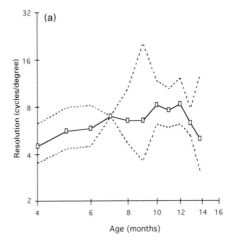

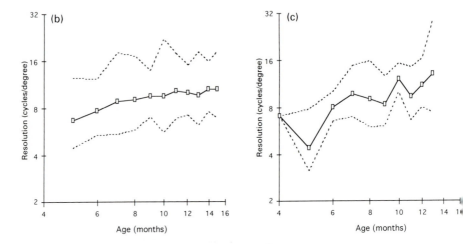

Fig. 13.3 Development of resolution in infants with refractive error: (a) hyperopia; (b) myopia; (c) astigmatism.

Risk factors

Personal and family risk factors of strabismus have been tested in the population of strabismic infants. The data are given in Table 13.3 for each category of putative risk. It shows that the following factors of personal history increase the risk of having a strabismus and hence of developing amblyopia: prematurity, birthweight <2500 g, cerebral pathology and squint reported by the parents or medical agents. This latter point will be discussed specifically later.

Table 13.2 Validity of Teller acuity cards.

	Sensitivity	Specificity	Positive predictive values	Negative predictive values	Global validity
(a) 1 octave					
All subjects	10.90%	96.36%	68.66%	59.67%	60.27%
4	16.67%	86.21%	60.00%	45.45%	47.69%
5	24.27%	86.29%	59.52%	57.84%	58.15%
6	14.61%	97.80%	86.49%	54.28%	56.95%
7	4.69%	98.61%	68.18%	61.97%	62.14%
8	11.42%	95.44%	63.79%	60.52%	60.76%
9	11.42%	95.44%	63.79%	60.52%	60.76%
10	7.45%	97.96%	70.37%	61.94%	62.29%
11	5.88%	98.21%	66.67%	63.22%	63.33%
12	5.88%	97.46%	60.00%	61.52%	61.46%
13	26.62%	91.88%	74.00%	59.04%	61.54%
14	16.87%	89.16%	60.87%	51.75%	53.01%
15	24.00%	100.00%	100.00%	42.42%	51.28%
(b) 1/2 octave					
All subjects	56.46%	56.41%	48.64%	63.93%	56.43%
4	63.89%	39.66%	56.79%	46.94%	53.08%
5	41.75%	71.77%	55.13%	59.73%	58.15%
6	56.62%	59.47%	57.41%	58.70%	58.07%
7	30.94%	83.13%	53.80%	65.47%	62.86%
8	76.85%	41.87%	48.16%	72.01%	56.31%
9	76.85%	41.87%	48.16%	72.01%	56.31%
10	58.43%	48.72%	42.57%	64.31%	52.55%
11	57.14%	58.16%	45.33%	69.09%	57.78%
12	50.98%	57.14%	43.51%	64.29%	54.72%
13	89.93%	6.88%	45.62%	44.00%	45.48%
14	84.34%	9.64%	48.28%	38.10%	46.99%
15	92.00%	14.29%	65.71%	50.00%	64.10%

Surprisingly, it is clear that the family pathologies have a protective effect for the child, possibly through a selection artefact (see discussion). This protective effect means that in this population, infants are less prone to develop the pathology if the parents are affected by the pathology. Family history and heredity show a strong protective effect in the cases of strabismus, amblyopia, hyperopia, myopia, astigmatism and other ophthalmological pathologies. This fact shall be discussed using arguments derived from the analysis of the population studied.

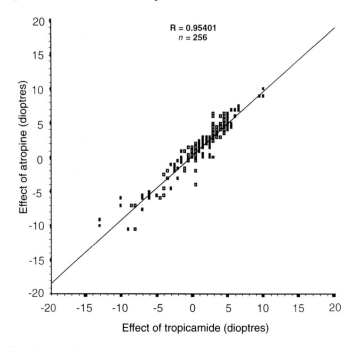

Fig. 13.4 Correlation of atropine and tropicamide cycloplegia.

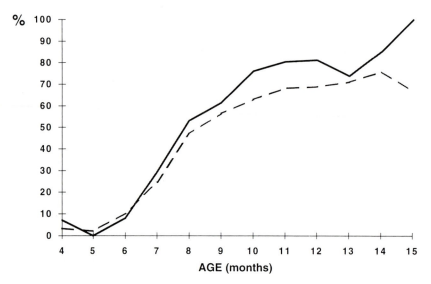

Fig. 13.5 Percentage of positive responses to Lang test as a function of age. Solid line, all normal subjects (*n* = 861). Dotted line, all non-strabismic non-amblyopic subjects (*n* = 1733).

Table 13.3 Risk factors for strabismus. When the OR is high the population concerned is highly exposed to the risk. When the OR is low the population is barely exposed to the risk. When the OR is negative it means that the population is 'protected' against the risk.[a, b]

Risk factors	OR	Confidence interval (95%)	Effect
Personal history			
Pathological childbirth	1.18	0.84–1.66	–
Prematurity	1.53	1.12–2.08	F
Birthweight <2500 g	1.45	1.02–2.05	F
Cerebral pathologies	4.68	2.96–7.39	F
Cross eyes reported	2.96	2.28–3.85	F
Other ophthalmological pathologies	1.24	0.68–2.23	–
Family history			
Strabismus	0.7	0.53–0.91	P
Amblyopia	0.53	0.38–0.73	P
Hyperopia	0.72	0.5–1.05	–
Myopia	0.55	0.42–0.71	P
Astigmatism	0.7	0.5–0.97	P
Other ophthalmological pathologies	0.41	0.17–0.93	P
Strabismic cases/normals		300/2113	

[a] P = protective; F = favouring.
[b] For instance, an infant born from blind parents is 'protected' since the hypothesis is that his or her parents are very likely to have him or her examined, whereas an infant born normally from normal parents is at relatively high risk since it is hypothesized that his or her parents will not have their child examined because they are not anxious about visual defects.

DISCUSSION

Subjects

The age distribution of our population is biased by the recommendation that the optimal age for the test should range from 7–10 months. At this age, a pathology that would not be accompanied by obvious signs is detected easily. In addition, infants comply more easily with our testing procedures, and therapeutic means are more readily accepted and effective. As a consequence, the age classes studied are unequal, all of them are larger than needed, however, to yield a good estimation of acuity values in a population of normal subjects. The same cannot be said about the proportion of pathological cases because we have no control of the recruitment of a clinical population. However, it is likely that the possible bias bears more on the proportion of pathological cases than on the nature of the pathology.

One can only hypothesize about the bias present in our population. It could well be that parents are more prone to have their children examined if they are affected by a pathology, even if they detect no sign of it. Families with no ophthalmological pathology are probably less attentive to information about eye defect and may form a small contingent of our consulting population. The opposite may be postulated for families including pathological members.

Acuity

When considering the data presented in Fig. 13.2 showing the development of resolution in normals, it is clear that these children fall within the limits of normal infants' resolution as described by many (Heersema and van Hof-van Duin 1990). In addition, the data presented largely confirm previous studies whose populations were not any more controlled as samples of the general population. This limit is inherent to most clinical studies and stresses the need for the study of a representative sample. Although the data are reasonably comparable, it is clear that normative data are still needed because procedures vary greatly across clinical settings (Lewis *et al.* 1993).

Resolution increases very regularly throughout the first year of life (Vital-Durand 1992). This could simply reflect the dynamic of cone packing in the fovea (Yuodelis and Hendrickson 1986). There is no obvious explanation for the fact that some authors have observed a pause in the development of resolution between 6 months and about 1 year of age (McDonald *et al.* 1986). This could be caused by the behavioural conditions of the testing. It could also originate from the fact that the intervals between the gratings of the acuity cards are constant (one-half octave), while the slope of the psychometric function varies with age. Obviously such a limitation applies also to this study.

Finally, the scale coarseness enlarges the range of the confidence intervals, thus increasing the overlap of the confidence interval for normals and pathological subjects (Bailey *et al.* 1991; Arditi and Cagenello 1993). This limitation could be controlled with the use of acuity cards printed with spatial frequencies separated by a smaller interval (Heersema and van Hof-van Duin 1990).

Precision of a measure is determined by the interval between the units of the instrument. In order to be certain of a difference between two measures, the acuity values recorded should differ by more than one unit. As TAC are separated by half-octave intervals, a difference of acuity between the two eyes can only be ascertained if the figures differ by one octave or more. This limitation can be avoided by altering the distance of presentation of the cards, an awkward manoeuvre. Practically, a difference of a half octave between the two eyes was not classified as an amblyopia, except when it was strongly supported by the results of other tests.

Refraction

There is no clear agreement among authors concerning the refractive state of infants (Howland 1993; see Thorn *et al.*, Chapter 8, this volume). Two large-scale studies concur with some degree of hyperopia during the first year in normal children (Dobson *et al.* 1981; Atkinson *et al.* 1984), although it has been hypothesized that it could be an artefact resulting from a weaker sensitivity of infants to cycloplegic drugs (Mutti *et al.* 1994). It should be noted that refractive errors measured with two different drugs, tropicamide and atropine, were very similar in our study (Fig. 13.4). However, it appears that some individuals show a striking difference, up to 4.5 dioptres in one case. As a consequence, it should be recommended that atropine cycloplegia is used when an optical correction is to be prescribed, but see Thorn *et al.*, Chapter 8, this volume.

Risk factors

When addressing the question of which infants should be screened for visual risks, it is clear that a series of personal risk factors can be isolated. The infants concerned are referred for visual assessment, apparently because the parents and the medical personnel are aware of a possible pathology. However, it appears that family history of visual pathology has a strong protective effect. One clear evidence is the high proportion of infants referred for a squint, which subsequently appeared to be a normal epicanthus. Our study was not designed to show if there was an increased proportion of such 'false' referrals among parents squinting or with pathology.

It can be hypothesized that the parents concerned are very prone to have their children assessed and introduce a major bias in our population. As a consequence, the category of infant at high risk of not being referred for visual assessment comprises infants with no apparent risk. In that population, the incidence of a visual pathology is low but the probability that it is identified is also very low. The logical consequence is that all infants would benefit from a screening. It remains to be determined which battery of tests is the most efficient to detect the highest proportion of true positive cases.

An increasing number of medical centres use acuity cards (Chandna *et al.* 1988; Speeg-Shatz *et al.* 1991; Fielder *et al.* 1992; Schenk-Rootlieb *et al.* 1992) although some have questioned their value as a screening test (Katz and Sireteanu 1990). However, the question as to which is the best, fastest and most inexpensive procedure to detect the most pathological infants in a screening programme is still open. An alternative method using videorefraction, which would yield data on refraction, strabismus and ocular opacities is currently being tested by several groups.

CONCLUSIONS

In this study it has been shown that acuity cards stand as a unique test to measure visual resolution but contain some flaws because they are not sensitive and specific enough to screen large populations. Known risk factors do not allow a proper detection of infants at risk of developing amblyopia. To help determine the best way to alleviate visual deficiencies in early infancy, more data on the refractive condition of this age group and determination of the most reliable test that can be applied to large populations at a cost acceptable to society are required for the future.

REFERENCES

Angi, M. R., Pucci, V., Forattini, F., and Formentin, P. A. (1992). Results of photo-refractometric screening for amblyogenic defects in children aged 20 months. *Behavioural Brain Research*, **49**, 91–7.

Arditi, A. and Cagenello, R. (1993). On the statistical reliability of Letter Chart visual acuity measurements. *Investigative Ophthalmology and Visual Science*, **34**, 120–9.

Atkinson, J., Braddick, O. J., Durden, K., Watson, P. G., and Atkinson, S. (1984). Screening for refractive errors in 6–9-month-old infants by photorefraction. *British Journal of Ophthalmology*, **68**, 105–12.

Atkinson, J. (1993). Infant vision screening: prediction and prevention of strabismus and amblyopia from refractive screening in the Cambridge Photorefraction Program. In *Early visual development, normal and abnormal*, (ed. K. Simmons), pp. 335–48. Oxford University Press, New York.

Bailey, I. L., Bullimore, M. A., Raasch, T. W., and Taylor, H. R. (1991). Clinical grading and the effects of scaling. *Investigative Ophthalmology and Visual Science*, **32**, 422–32.

Birch, E. E., Shimojo, S., and Held, R. (1985). Preferential-looking assessment of fusion and stereopsis in infants aged 1–6 months. *Investigative Ophthalmology and Visual Science*, **26**, 366–70.

Bishop, A. M. (1991). Vision screening of children: a review of methods and personnel involved within the UK. *Ophthalmic and Physiological Optics*, **11**, 3–9.

Braddick, O., Atkinson, J., French, J., and Howland, H. C. (1979). A photorefractive study of infant accommodation. *Vision Research*, **19**, 1319–30.

Brown, A. M. and Teller, D. Y. (1989). Chromatic opponency in 3-month-old human infants. *Vision Research*, **29**, 37–45.

Chandna, A., Pearson, C. M., and Doran, R. M. L. (1988). Preferential looking in clinical practice: a year's experience. *Eye*, **2**, 488–95.

Dale, A., Banks, M., and Norcia, A. M. (1993). Does chromatic sensitivity develop more slowly than luminance sensitivity? *Vision Research*, **33**, 2553–62.

Da Silva, O. A., Henriques, J., Pinto, F., and Neves, C. (1991). Rastreio visual em crianças. *Acta Medica Portuguesa*, **4**, 183–7.

Dobson, V., Fulton, A. B., Manning, K., Salem, D., and Petersen, R. A. (1981). Cycloplegic refractions of premature infants. *American Journal of Ophthalmology*, **91**, 490–5.

Dobson, V., Schwartz, T. Z., Sandstrom, D. J., and Michel, L. (1987). Binocular visual acuity of neonates: the acuity card procedure. *Developmental Medicine and Child Neurology*, **29**, 199–206.

Effert, R., Barry, J. C., Dahm, M., and Kaupp, A. (1991). Eine neue photographische Methode zur Messung von Schielwinkeln bei Sauglingen und kleinen Kindern. *Klinisches Monatsblatt Augenheilkunde*, **198**, 284–9.

Essman, S. W. and Essman, T. F. (1992). Screening for pediatric eye disease. *American Family Physician*, **46**, 1243–52.

Fielder, A. R., Dobson, V., Moseley, M. J., and Mayer, D. L. (1992). Preferential looking—clinical lessons. *Ophthalmic Paediatrics and Genetics*, **13**, 101–10.

Freedman, H. L. and Preston, K. L. (1992). Polaroid photoscreening for amblyogenic factors. An improved methodology. *Ophthalmology*, **99**, 1785–95.

Hainline, L., Turkel, J., Abramov, I., Lemerise, E., and Harris, C. M. (1984). Characteristics of saccades in human infants. *Vision Research*, **24**, 1771–80.

Hainline, L., Riddell, P., Grose-Fifer, J., and Abramov, I. (1992). Development of accommodation and convergence in infancy. *Behavioural Brain Research*, **49**, 33–50.

Harris, C. M., Jacobs, M., Shawkat, F., and Taylor, D. (1993). The development of saccadic accuracy in the first seven months. *Clinical Vision Science*, **8**, 85–96.

Heersema, D. J. and van Hof-van Duin, J. (1990). Age norms for visual acuity in toddlers using the acuity card procedure. *Clinical Vision Science*, **5**, 167–74.

Howland, H. C., Dobson, V., and Sayles, N. (1987). Accommodation in infants as measured by photorefraction. *Vision Research*, **27**, 2141–52.

Howland, H. C. (1993). Early refractive development. In *Early visual development, normal and abnormal*, (ed. K. Simmons), pp. 5–13. Oxford University Press, New York.

Katz, B. and Sireteanu, R. (1990). The Teller acuity card test: a useful method for the clinical routine? *Clinical Vision Science*, **5**, 307–23.

Knoblauch, K. and Vital-Durand, F. (1994). Développement de la sensibilité aux couleurs. *Bulletins des Sociétés d'Ophtalmologie de France*, **2** (XCIV), 217–21.

Lewis, T. L., Reed, M. J., Maurer, D., Wyngaarden, P. A., and Brent, H. (1993). An evaluation of acuity card procedures. *Clinical Vision Science*, **8**, 591–602.

McDonald, M. A., Sebris, S. L., Mohn, G., Teller, D. Y., and Dobson, V. (1986). Monocular acuity in normal infants: the acuity card procedure. *American Journal of Optometry and Physiological Optics*, **63**, 127–34.

Morrone, M. C., Burr, D. C., and Fiorentini, A. (1990). Development of contrast sensitivity and acuity of the infant colour system. *Proceedings of the Royal Society, (Series B)*, **242**, 134–9.

Mutti, D. O., Zadnick, K., Egashira, S., Kish, L., Twelker, J. D., and Adams, A. J. (1994). The effect of cycloplegia on measurement of the ocular components. *Investigative Ophthalmology and Visual Science*, **35**, 515–27.

Presland, M. W. and Zimmerman, E. (1993). Photorefraction screening in premature infants. *Ophthalmology*, **100**, 762–8.

Schenk-Rootlieb, A. J., van Nieuwenhuizen, O., van Zoggel, J., van der Graaf, Y., and Willemse, J. (1992). Grating-acuity in children. Normal values of visual acuity in children up to 13 years as assessed by the acuity card procedure. *Ophthalmic Paediatrics and Genetics*, **13**, 155–63.

Schmidt, P. P. (1991). Effectiveness of vision-screening in pre-school populations with preferential looking cards used for assessment of visual acuity. *Optometry and Vision Science*, **68**, 210–19.

Sebris, S. L., Dobson, V., McDonald, M. A., and Teller, Y. (1987). Acuity cards for visual acuity assessment of infants and children in clinical settings. *Clinical Vision Science*, **2**, 45–58.

Speeg-Schatz, C., Lobstein-Henry, Y., and Flament, J. (1991). Intérêt des cartons de Teller dans l'évaluation de l'acuité visuelle du jeune enfant. *Journal Français d'Ophtalmologie*, **14**, 583–6.

Teller, D. Y., McDonald, M. A., Preston, K., Sebris, S. L., and Dobson, V. (1986). Assessment of visual acuity in infants and children: the acuity card procedure. *Developmental Medicine and Child Neurology*, **28**, 779–89.

van Hof-van Duin, J. and Mohn, G. (1986). The development of visual acuity in normal fullterm and preterm infants. *Vision Research*, **26**, 909–16.

Vital-Durand, F. and Patin, C. (1991). La méthode du regard préférentiel dans une étude longitudinale de 150 enfants de 2 mois à 6 ans. *Revue ONO*, **9**, 10–11.

Vital-Durand, F. (1992). Acuity card procedures and the linearity of grating resolution development during the first year of human infants. *Behavioural Brain Research*, **49**, 99–106.

Yuodelis, C. and Hendrickson, A. E. (1986). A qualitative and quantitative analysis of the human fovea during development. *Vision Research*, **26**, 847–56.

Part III
Oculomotor and binocular processes

Vision is not simply a process of passive reception. There is an intimate reciprocal relationship between the delicate processes of oculomotor control that determine how images fall on the two retinae, and the analysis of those images, which provides the input to the control processes.

The relation between eye movement and visual processing is of particular importance in development for several reasons. First, oculomotor behaviour, through measures of fixation, tracking, and optokinetic responses, has always provided one of the main routes for understanding the visual processing capacities of the infant. The methodologies based on children's eye movements are the subject of Buquet and Charlier's Chapter 18. Second, the mechanisms for shifting gaze are themselves not simple but require several components to be smoothly co-ordinated. For example, the movement of eye and head, with their different dynamics, have to be controlled together if we are to pursue or fixate an object. How such co-ordination can be established is a classic developmental problem on which Carchon and Bloch provide evidence in Chapter 16.

The strongest example of the developmental interrelation between visual and oculomotor processes is in binocular vision. The binocular analysis of disparity, whose development around the fourth month is discussed by Held and his co-workers in Chapter 17, can only operate if the two eyes are well enough aligned to bring image points within a limited range of disparities. Conversely, maintaining accurate eye alignment is usually presumed to require a controlling signal based on the analysis of binocular disparity. To understand how this two-way relationship becomes established, the kind of information provided by Hainline and Riddell in Chapter 15 is needed, which examines in detail how well infants align their eyes and converge them at different target distances, before and around the time that sensory binocularity becomes established.

The association of binocular and oculomotor function can be extended to other functions. The mechanism of convergence is coupled closely to that of accommodation, and accommodative changes in focus determine image quality which is one of the determinants of fine stereopsis. It is this web of associations that is developmentally disrupted in children with strabismus, and its complexity is responsible for the fact that after a century of clinical and scientific study, our understanding of strabismus is very incomplete. Chapter 18, by Schmidt and colleagues, examines one element of this linkage, the relation between defocus and steroacuity, in the context of comparing stereo and resolution measures as means for detecting children with impaired resolution and/or binocular disorders.

Finally, oculomotor function is important because it provides a route to analyse the developmental relationships between different visual pathways. Subcortical centres are known to be involved in the control of visual fixation and of optokinetic responses. In Chapter 14, Braddick, Atkinson and Hood re-examine hypotheses about these pathways in relation to the cortical areas that underlie the analysis of pattern and motion. The investigation of children with known cerebral damage provides new evidence about this relationship.

14

Striate cortex, extrastriate cortex, and colliculus: some new approaches

Oliver Braddick, Janette Atkinson, and Bruce Hood

INTRODUCTION

It has been widely accepted, since Bronson (1974) first suggested it, that many aspects of visual development over the first months of life can be understood in terms of visual function becoming increasingly dominated by cortical processes. More recent formulations have developed this idea in terms of cortical processes modulating continuing visual functions of subcortical structures (Atkinson 1984; Braddick and Atkinson 1988) and of differential development of distinct visual cortical streams and areas (Atkinson 1992).

One important source of evidence for visual cortical development is the development of capabilities that require the specific kinds of stimulus selectivity found in cortical neurons. These include selectivity for orientation, for directional motion selectivity, and binocular disparity. The work of ourselves and others in these areas has been quite extensively reviewed (Atkinson 1992; Braddick 1993; Braddick *et al.* 1989; Birch 1993). This chapter, therefore, will concentrate on three other lines of evidence; from the control of shifts in visual attention, from optokinetic responses in children with localized brain damage, and from sensitivity to 'second-order' stimuli that are presumed to require relatively elaborate cortical processing. These new kinds of evidence are consistent with the broad idea of increasing cortical dominance in the early months but also make clear that the developmental relationships between cortical and subcortical processing, and between cortical areas, are complex ones.

CONTROL OF SHIFTS IN VISUAL ATTENTION

The ability of infants to shift attention from one visual target to another is an area where cortical and subcortical processes interact particularly closely. The superior colliculus contains cells in the superficial layers, which respond to visual stimuli, and cells in deeper levels, which are involved in the initiation of saccadic eye movements; thus it is likely that reflexive orienting of the head and eyes to a sudden visual event can be accomplished with entirely subcortical circuitry. According to the hypothesis that subcortical visual function is dominant in newborns, it is these pathways that determine the newborn's fixation preferences.

However, normal visual environments contain many potential targets so subjects are rarely orienting to the only stimulus in the field of view, or even to the most prepotent in terms of variables such as contrast. Further many saccades are not exogenous (i.e. triggered by an external event) but endogenous (i.e. the result of some internal process selecting a new target). Thus most saccades must involve analysis of multiple stimuli, and processes to determine which requires the further analysis that is possible in foveal fixation.

These analyses and processes must depend on cortical structures. Several pathways are known, which link cortical visual areas to the frontal eye fields and directly or indirectly to the superior colliculi (Schiller *et al.* 1979; Schiller 1985). These pathways, some of which are excitatory and others inhibitory, provide possible routes by which cortical processes can modulate a subcortical reflex loop between visual stimulation and an orienting response. Modulation is required in at least two ways; to inhibit fixation shifts to irrelevant peripheral events and clamp fixation on a target, which requires continuing processing and to disengage from the current target of fixation when cortical processes determine that an exogenous or endogenous shift is required.

Such modulatory effects can be examined in infants by comparing shifts of fixation to the onset of a peripheral target when the current fixation target disappears (non-competition) or remains visible (competition). Several studies have found that the continuing presence of a central target restricted the area over which a stimulus could elicit a foveating saccade (Harris and MacFarlane 1974; Aslin and Salapatek 1975; Finlay and Ivinski 1984).

'Competition' effects have been extensively investigated in our laboratory (Atkinson and Braddick 1985; Atkinson *et al.* 1988; 1992; Hood and Atkinson 1991). Using the display of Fig. 14.1, the effect appears considerably stronger in 1-month-old than in 3-month-old infants and has generally been found to decrease with age. Switching attention would, of course, be expected to improve with age because of the infants' increasing sensitivity for detecting peripheral targets. Our work attempted to dissociate changes of sensitivity from the ability to disengage, by setting the contrast of the peripheral target for different age groups to levels that produced the same performance in the non-competition situation. The increase in latency to fixate the peripheral target with competition from a persisting central target was much greater in 1-month-olds than in 3-month-olds (Atkinson *et al.* 1992).

Further conditions used in our studies have also shown that 1-month-olds also have latency increased more than 3-month-olds when two peripheral targets (one on each side of fixation) appear simultaneously. Again, the younger group show a difficulty in operating an attention-switching mechanism, in this case in selecting one of two peripheral targets and inhibiting the effect of the other (Atkinson *et al.* 1992).

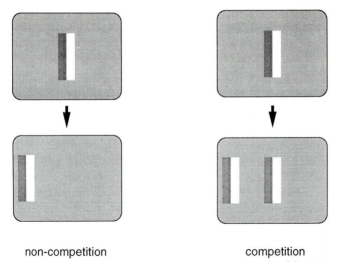

non-competition   competition

Fig. 14.1 Display sequences used to examine competition effects in the fixation shift experiments of Atkinson *et al.* (1992). The initial central target either disappears ('non-competition', left) or remains visible ('competition', right) at the onset of the peripheral target, which may appear at either side. Central and peripheral targets both underwent contrast reversal six times per second. The inner edge of the peripheral target lies 23° from the midline. (Subsequent testing, e.g. that reported in Braddick *et al.* (1992) used an alternating schematic face display instead of the dark/light strip as a central target.)

Our suggestion from all these studies of competition was that the additional mechanism necessary to operate disengagement was cortical rather than sub-cortical, and argued, by analogy, for this system to involve the superior collic-ulus and parietal lobes (Atkinson and Braddick 1985; Atkinson *et al.* 1988; 1992; Hood and Atkinson 1991). Johnson (1990) took this idea one stage further in arguing that changes in the ability to disengage were related to the matura-tional sequence of various cortical layers. Direct evidence on the neural systems underlying these effects comes from our recent study of two infants who underwent complete hemispherectomies at 5 and 8 months of age to relieve intractable focal epilepsy (Braddick *et al.* 1992). These infants provided a rare opportunity to investigate the activity of the subcortical pathway in isolation from cortical influence, allowing a direct test of the subcortical contribution to infants' visual orienting, as well as the role of cortical mechanisms in the com-petition effect. Removal of one cerebral hemisphere obliterates the cortical rep-resentation of the contralateral visual field. However, as the surgery involves the removal of tissue from above the level of the thalamus, it leaves the retino-collicular pathways intact.

In post-operative testing, both children were visually alert with a full range of eye movements. As might be expected from the loss of visual processing by one hemisphere, they completely ignored toys presented in the half-field contralateral to the damage, although they promptly reached for the same toys in the ipsilateral 'good' half-field. Tested in the non-competition condition of the fixation-shift procedure described above, both infants oriented to the peripheral target in either half field, at levels strongly above chance. Thus orienting responses are clearly possible to targets that have no cortical representation and are presumably mediated by subcortical structures such as the superior colliculus acting without cortical control, as has been hypothesized for normal newborns. However, one child was also tested in the competition condition. In this case, saccadic responses to targets appearing in the 'bad' half-field were greatly reduced. This finding supports the idea that, when fixation is switched between targets that are present together, cortical mechanisms are required to modulate subcortical mechanisms of fixation control.

One child's orienting response was also tested using each eye separately. With the right eye (contralateral to the removed left hemisphere), she could respond above chance to both the left and right half fields. However, with the left eye, she only made saccades to targets in the left half field. This result suggests that in the absence of cortex, no uncrossed pathway, transmitting information from the left eye to the damaged left side of the brain, is capable of eliciting saccadic eye movements. It resembles findings that, with monocular viewing, infants younger than 2 months are much more likely to orient to a visual target presented in their temporal visual field compared with their nasal visual field (Lewis *et al.* 1985; Lewis and Maurer 1992). It has been argued that such asymmetries between nasal and temporal visual fields reflect a strong preponderance of crossed fibres in the retino-collicular projection (Hubel *et al.* 1975; Pollack and Hickey 1979) although there are contrasting anatomical reports that the uncrossed (i.e. nasal field) projection to the primate superior colliculus is substantial (Schiller 1984; Cowey, personal communication).

The effects of competition between fixation targets will depend on their relative timing. Even in adults, the presence of a foveal stimulus overlapping in time with the onset of a peripheral target can be shown to have an inhibitory effect on saccades (Fischer 1986). Conversely, a temporal gap between the offset of a central stimulus and the onset of a peripheral target can substantially shorten saccadic latencies (Saslow 1967). The disappearance of the fixation target during the gap is thought to produce an automatic disengagement of attention, thereby by-passing one of the processes that contribute to the latency (Posner and Petersen 1990; Fischer 1986). This disengagement is believed to depend on extra-striate processes, while the initiation of a fast saccade depends on the retino-collicular pathway. Thus if subcortical mechanisms are mature before cortical ones in normal development, relatively short latencies in the 'gap' paradigm would be expected from the earliest age, and latencies in the 'overlap' case should become shorter with age as cortical disengage mechanisms develop. Studies by Hood (1991; Hood and Atkinson 1991; 1993) on infants aged 6 weeks to 6 months support these predictions: saccadic latencies overall reduced with age, but this reduction was significantly greater in 'overlap' than in 'gap' conditions. The important period for this change occurred between 6 weeks and 3 months.

Rapid temporal sequences of targets can produce more complex effects. In adults, a prior target to which subjects briefly switch attention even without an overt orienting response can either facilitate or inhibit a subsequent response to the same location, depending on the time interval (Posner and Cohen 1980). The inhibitory effect ('inhibition of return' or IOR), in particular, has been argued to depend heavily on collicular mechanisms, on the basis of naso-temporal asymmetries (Rafal *et al.* 1989; Rafal *et al.* 1991) and on the interference with IOR from collicular damage in progressive supranuclear palsy (Posner *et al.* 1985). Unlike adults, infants cannot be told that they should not orient to the first target; however, the competition effect can be exploited to prevent them doing so to a brief target. Hood (1993; Hood and Atkinson 1990; 1991), using this technique, found evidence both for facilitation and IOR at different intervals in 6-month-olds but found neither effect in 3-month-olds. Johnson and Tucker (1993), using slightly different stimuli, found IOR in 4-month-olds but not in 2-month-olds. These results suggest that the interactions leading to IOR and facilitation do not arise from those cortical contributions to visual behaviour that first become prominent between birth and 3 months. They also suggest that, if indeed collicular processes underlie these phenomena, the level of collicular function present from birth is not adequate for them. (However, the effects may depend on the detailed stimulus characteristics and a recent report suggests that IOR effects may be demonstrated even in newborns (Valenza *et al.* 1994).) Overall, the most striking developmental change in attentional control is the enhanced ability to disengage from one target and engage with another that is simultaneously present. This probably reflects the modulation of a subcortical fixation reflex by emerging cortical processes. However, effects such as IOR show more subtle modulations of control that emerge later, and may reflect improving integration of the network linking striate and extra-striate cortical areas (including parietal and frontal eye fields) to the superior colliculus, which is believed to be responsible for the control of fixation in the mature system (Schiller 1985).

OPTOKINETIC RESPONSES

Shifts of fixation are not the only eye movements for which cortical–subcortical relations must be considered. Optokinetic nystagmus (OKN) consists of a repetitive pattern of slow eye movements, interspersed with saccade-like return movements in the reverse direction. It is elicited by uniform movement of pattern in a large part of the visual field. Responses of this kind are very pervasive across species, and so are often thought of as a very basic visual reflex that must be mediated by phylogenetically ancient structures in the visual system.

With binocular viewing, OKN can be elicited in infants from birth onwards, to patterns moving either to the left or right. However, infants up to about 3 months show a strong asymmetry of OKN in *monocular* viewing; the response to temporal-to-nasal (T→N) stimulus movement is brisk, while that to nasal-to-temporal (N→T) movement is absent or weak (Atkinson 1979). In cat, the T→N response is known to be driven by a crossed pathway direct to the nucleus of the optic tract (NOT) while the N→T response depends on a route via ipsilateral visual cortex (Hoffmann and Schoppmann 1975). The response asymmetry in young infants has generally been taken to indicate that the subcortical pathway through the NOT is functional from birth, while the cortical pathway matures later.

However, observations of the hemispherectomized infants, whose fixation responses have already been discussed, mean that this conclusion must, at least, be questioned. In each of these children, there was an asymmetry in binocular as well as monocular viewing: normal OKN could only be driven for the direction of pattern movement towards the side of the intact hemisphere (Braddick *et al.* 1992). Following the removal of a cerebral hemisphere, the subcortical pathway from the eye contralateral to the damage, direct to the NOT on the opposite side, ought still to be intact. The failure of binocular OKN in one direction suggests that, in these children, the response in the T→N direction as well as N→T one depends on a cortical pathway that has been abolished by hemispherectomy.

Asymmetries of binocular OKN do not require cerebral damage as extreme as hemidecortication. We and others (van Hof-van Duin and Mohn 1983) have found qualitatively similar asymmetries in several children known to have lateralized brain damage (Table 14.1), and we have also seen asymmetries in children where the localization of damage had not been determined (Table 14.2) but where there has been some asymmetry of motor control and often asymmetry of visual fields.

Developmentally, there are several alternative interpretations of binocular asymmetry of OKN. The first possibility is that, at all ages from birth, T→N OKN requires cortical control. The initial asymmetry would then represent an asymmetry of cortical development in the processing of the two directions, rather than a subcortical property. Such an asymmetry has been proposed by Norcia *et al.* (1991) to account for unbalanced contributions of the two directions to visual-evoked potentials generated by oscillatory grating motions. (However, it is possible that this unbalance may reflect an asymmetrical optokinetic response elicited by the oscillating grating, rather than being a direct result of an asymmetry in motion processing). If there *is* a cortical mechanism sensitive to motion direction from birth, this needs to be reconciled with the evidence that direction-based discriminations do not seem to be possible before 6–8 weeks (Wattam-Bell 1992; 1993; Braddick 1993).

A second alternative is that OKN in newborns is controlled by a subcortical route but that this function is taken over by cortex for both directions sometime after 3 months of age. To explain the hemispherectomy results, one would need

Table 14.1 OKN in children with lateral focal lesions.

Name	Age	Lesion from images	Field deficit	Better binocular OKN towards:		
				Symmetrical	'Bad side'[a]	'Good side'
FD	20 months	Right occipito-temporal posterior infarct (meningitis)	L		+	
JO	9 months	Left occipito-parietal haemorrhage and infarct	R	+		
SP	2.5 years	Left infarct of entire hemisphere (and right fronto-parietal region)	R		+	
AW	12 months	Right glioma	L		+	
LW	21 months	Left contusion (and minor right contusion)	R			+

[a] 'Bad side' = side of body on which motor/field deficit is manifest, i.e. contralateral to brain damage.

to suppose that the subcortical mechanism functionally drops out even if the cortex cannot take over the function on one side. The gross developmental abnormality of one hemisphere means that this failure could have occurred before the hemisphere was removed.

The third possibility is that T→N function remains mediated by the NOT but that the development of this route depends on cortical control. In these patients the input, or absence of input, from abnormal cortex may have affected the development of the NOT (Cowey and Stoerig 1993).

Whichever turns out to be the correct interpretation, it is clear that OKN in either direction cannot be considered as a subcortical function without reference to the cortex. There seems to be increasing role of cortical pathways from cats to non-human primates to humans (Hoffmann 1989; Harris *et al.* 1993), which needs to be taken into account in understanding human development.

FIRST- AND SECOND-ORDER PROCESSING

Recently, the concept of 'first-order' and 'second-order' processes has come to play an important part in the analysis of cortical function. Can this distinction help us to analyse the development of visual cortical processing?

Table 14.2 OKN in children with cerebral palsy.

Name	Age	Motor deficit	Field deficit	Better binocular OKN towards:				
				Symmetrical	'Bad' side[b]	'Good' side	'Left' side	'Right' side
(a) Children with motor asymmetry								
JTC	4 years	L	Left		+			
IL	3.5 years	R	Symmetrical		+			
LEA	4 years	L	Symmetrical		+			
EA	10.5 years	R	Symmetrical			+		
US	5 years	L	Symmetrical		+			
BAM	7.5 years	L	Left		+			
DW	7.5 years	L	Symmetrical		+			
BP	7.0 years	R	Symmetrical	+				
(b) Cerebral palsy without motor asymmetry								
RH	2 years		Symmetrical					+
JT	3.5 years		Symmetrical				+	
SS	17 years		Symmetrical					+
DJ	5 years		Left				+[a]	
MM	2.5 years		?					+
CD	4 years		Right					+[a]
AM	1.5 years		Right					+[a]
KB	7.0 years		Left				+[a]	
MS	13.5 years		Symmetrical	+				
KF	2.5 years		Symmetrical				+	

[a] Direction is towards better hemisphere (as found for hemispherectomy cases).

[b] 'Bad' side, 'Left side', etc. refer to side on which motor/field deficit is manifest, i.e. contralateral to presumed brain damage.

'First order' refers to early stages of visual processing that, it has been widely proposed, are effectively sets of linear filters, signalling how well the local pattern of light and dark matches particular spatial (or spatio-temporal) profiles. The operation of simple-cell receptive fields in cat and monkey has been described in this way (Movshon *et al.* 1978; de Valois and de Valois 1988). However, there are many visual features that are readily perceived but which cannot be registered by linear filters. For example, two textured regions can have the same average luminance and so the boundary between them does not generate a signal from any linear filter. Yet, if the textures differ enough in contrast, grain size or orientation, a conspicuous boundary is perceived immediately. If the boundary (but not the texture elements themselves) moves then the sense of a moving object is compelling, although linear analysis would not reveal any spatio-temporal energy component with this velocity (Chubb and Sperling 1988). 'Second-order' refers to stationary or moving features created in this way (Cavanagh and Mather 1989). The idea behind this term is that linear operators acting directly on the luminance pattern can serve the detection of 'first-order' shapes or movements but that, to detect second-order shape or movement, an additional stage is required. This additional processing must include non-linear operations if it is to be sensitive to spatial boundaries and regions defined by differences of texture or contrast without mean luminance differences.

It is tempting to propose that if area V1 contains simple cells that are linear in many respects and so respond to first-order stimuli, then sensitivity to second-order stimuli is a result of subsequent operations carried out in higher cortical visual areas (Wilson *et al.* 1992). Indeed, striking responses to edges (von der Heydt and Peterhans 1989) and motion (Albright 1992) defined by non-luminance stimuli have been reported in macaque areas V2 and MT respectively. However, the fact that responses can be demonstrated in 'higher' cortical areas does not prove they are absent in V1. There is, in fact, evidence of sensitivity to second order stimuli in neurones recorded in V1 of cat (Zhou and Baker 1993) and monkey (Grosof *et al.* 1993), and human evoked potentials related to second-order stimuli have also been interpreted as arising from V1 (Lamme *et al.* 1993). Of course, given the extensive descending connections to V1 from other cortical areas (Zeki and Shipp 1988; Felleman and van Essen 1991) effects could well be detected in V1 responses that arose from non-linear operations in extra-striate cortical areas. In any case, sensitivity to these stimuli requires a more elaborate form of cortical processing than linear filtering.

How does sensitivity to second-order properties arise in the course of infants' visual cortical development? This question has been examined by us, both for static texture segmentation, and for motion of regions defined by dynamic second-order properties.

INFANTS' ABILITY TO SEGMENT ORIENTED TEXTURES

Our experiments on texture segmentation (Atkinson and Braddick 1992) examined whether 8–12-week-old and 14–18-week-old infants could detect, within a field of oriented oblique-line segments, a target region where the texture orientation differed from that of the surround by 90° (Fig. 14.2). From evoked potential and behavioural measures, infants before 8 weeks are sensitive to the difference between opposite oblique orientations (Braddick 1993). The experiment was intended to test whether this established sensitivity could be used by a second-order system to detect a region boundary that is defined by orientation difference. Detection was assessed by forced-choice preferential looking, and compared with a target that could be detected by its luminance contrast within the same kind of texture field. Both age groups showed significant preference for the side containing the contrast-defined target, but only the older group demonstrated significant preference for the orientation-defined target. Some similar experiments have been reported by Sireteanu and Rieth. In their first experiments (Sireteanu and Rieth 1992), they found no preferential fixation of an orientation-defined texture patch until infants were 9–12 months old, with negative results for 0–3- and 3–6-month-old groups. However, the texture was presented in apertures only 15° arc across within a dark surround, giving a rather small area of both background texture and target, and also rather prominent luminance contours at the edge of the apertures, which may have reduced the salience of the texture boundaries for the infants. More recently (Rieth and Sireteanu 1994a), they have repeated these experiments with a display in which (as in our study) the texture patch appears within a larger region of background texture, which extends uninterrupted into both half fields. With this display, they have found statistically significant preferential looking in 3–4- and 5-month-old groups. Thus when these conditions are used, which appear more nearly optimal for infants' detection of texture-defined objects, the results from Sireteanu's laboratory and ours are much more consistent.

Rieth and Sireteanu (1994b) have also examined infants' texture segmentation with a habituation recovery technique. They found a discrimination of a region containing opposite oblique texture, from a uniform texture field, in 5–6-month infants but not in younger groups. (However, this experiment used the small apertures that yielded poorer discrimination in their preferential looking experiment, so it is possible that younger infants would show habituation recovery with a more optimal configuration.) While this discrimination could possibly have been based on texture discrimination without segmentation, the view that the infants perceived a texture-defined form is strongly supported by the fact that, habituated to a texture-defined square shape, they showed a significant preference for a luminance-defined diamond over a luminance-defined square.

A related stimulus has been examined by Freedland and Dannemillar (1990). They habituated infants to 'herringbone' patterns in which alternating bands

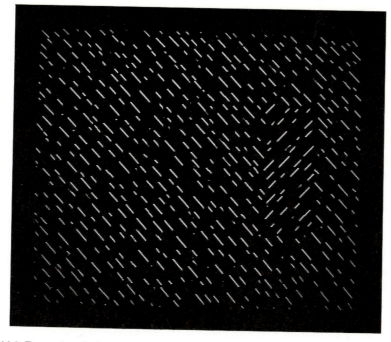

Fig. 14.2 Example of the displays used for preferential-looking testing of texture segmentation by Atkinson and Braddick (1992).

contained gratings oriented at 45° and 135°. 12-week-old infants (the only age group tested) showed shorter looking time to a luminance grating with the same orientation as these bands (e.g. vertical) than to the orthogonal orientation. These infants, therefore, also must have registered a second-order, texture-defined, form.

Taken together, our results and those from Sireteanu's and Dannemillar's laboratories imply that regions defined by orientation differences can form visual objects that elicit fixation and discrimination in infants over 12 weeks but not in younger infants. The neural basis for extracting form based on oriented texture differences is still quite speculative. Horizontal connections between orientation columns in V1, non-linear transformations between V1 and extrastriate visual areas, and descending pathways from extrastriate areas, are all possibilities that have been suggested. As developmental neuroanatomical evidence becomes available (e.g. Burkhalter *et al.* 1993) the developmental course of behaviourally demonstrated discriminations may help to decide between these hypotheses of neural organization.

SECOND-ORDER MOTION PROCESSING BY INFANTS

Our motion experiments have made it possible to compare directly infants' sensitivity to first- and second-order motion (Atkinson *et al.* 1993) by constructing test stimuli that are very similar except in the way that they carry motion information. These stimuli were dot patterns in which dynamic visual noise was present in alternate strips (Fig. 14.3). If the interleaved strips contain static dots, shifting the boundaries between noise and static regions generates second-order motion. If the boundaries of the noise regions are stationary but dots move coherently within the interleaved windows, this provides first-order motion. For preferential-looking testing, either of these displays is paired with a non-directional pattern in which stationary boundaries separate strips of static dots and dynamic visual noise. This control pattern has spatial properties that are similar to the other patterns but contains no consistent first- or second-order motion.

Two age groups were tested, 8–12-week-olds and 16–20-week-olds (Fig. 14.4). As would be expected from other experiments (Wattam-Bell 1992) both age groups showed a significant preference for patterns containing first-order motion over the control patterns. They also showed a significant preference for the second-order motion patterns. Overall, the preference was stronger for first- than for second-order motion but this difference did not change significantly with age. Thus it appears that infants in both age groups are sensitive to the presence of second-order motion. This is not quite so effective a motion stimulus for infants (or, probably, for adults) as first-order motion but our study provides no evidence for any differential development of sensitivity to the two kinds of motion.

Our younger group was close to the age at which preferential looking tests first show any evidence of directional sensitivity (Wattam-Bell 1992; 1993). Our results, therefore, leave little scope for first-order motion sensitivity to develop before second-order sensitivity. (It should be noted, though, that our test did not strictly require any directional discrimination. Thus it is conceivable that a truly directional test would allow the development of the two kinds of sensitivity to be dissociated.)

If infants become able to detect first- and second-order motion at the same age, what are the implications for development of cortical motion systems? Adult psychophysical experiments (Pantle 1992; Derrington *et al.* 1993; Ledgeway and Smith 1993) make it unlikely that first- and second-order motion processing are handled by the same primary motion-detecting system. However, it is possible that for both first- and second-order motion, the capabilities demonstrated in infants require the functional development of extrastriate systems such as V5/MT; the need for this development might be responsible for the relatively late emergence of directional selectivity in infancy.

Second-order motion and texture segmentation have been discussed as two examples of second-order processes. The developmental contrast between

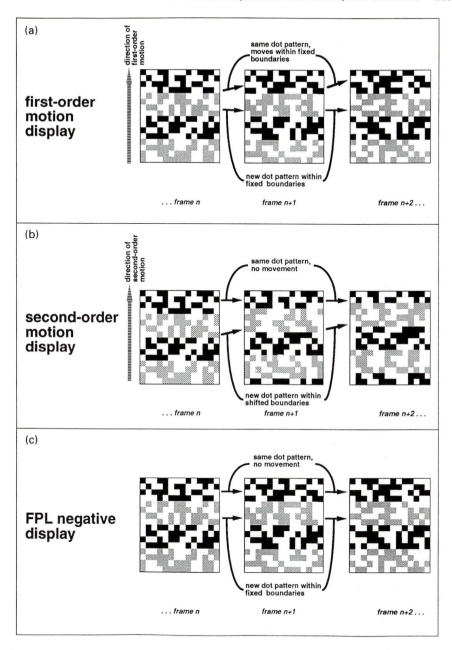

Fig. 14.3 Sequences of dot patterns used to produce first-order motion (top), and second-order motion (middle). In each trial, either of these displays on one side of the screen was paired with a control display (bottom) on the other side of the screen. Like the first- and second-order motion displays, the control display is visibly divided into horizontal bands with different dynamic properties but in this case there is no consistent motion either of the dot patterns or of the bands. These diagrams are not intended to depict correctly the relative dimensions of the pixels and the bands. The frame rate was 50 Hz.

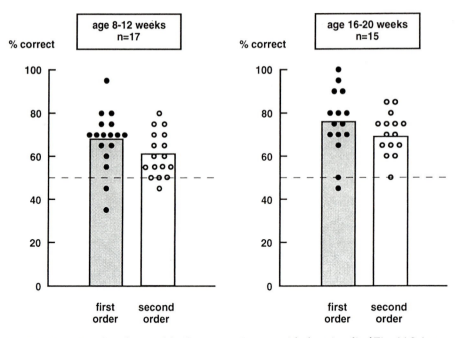

Fig. 14.4 Results of preferential-looking experiments with the stimuli of Fig. 14.3, in two age groups. Each point indicates the percentage correct over 20 trials for a single infant; bars indicate the mean results for the age group. Two-way analysis of variance (age × motion type) showed that, overall, performance improved from the younger to the older group ($p < 0.02$) and was better for the first-order than for second-order stimuli ($p < 0.05$). However, there was no significant interaction between age and motion type.

them is striking: second-order and first-order motion sensitivity appear to emerge together, whereas segmentation of oriented textures occurs much later than basic orientation discrimination. One can speculate on the comparative functional roles of motion and texture properties in development. Second-order processing involves using these properties to define boundaries, regions, and objects. It has often been emphasized that common motion is very important in defining the coherence of a visual object and its separation from background and other objects, and there is evidence that, at least by 4 months, infants are using motion as a means of organizing object perception (Kellman and Spelke 1983). Texture differences can also serve to organize the visual field into regions. However, it can be argued that this organization is associated mostly with surface properties, which may be less important to young infants who have had little opportunity to explore the nature of surfaces and their differences. Of course, there are several differences between the experimental paradigms used so far to explore texture and motion. The range and comparability of these studies needs to be extended, to understand the functional role of texture and motion vision in infancy, and the developing neural organization of the cortical systems that serve these functions.

CONCLUSIONS

It remains true that the story of visual development over the first months of life is, to a large degree, the story of developing cortical function. This development is not restricted to the kinds of stimulus selectivity found in V1 neurones. Advances in neurobiology in recent years have made our views of visual cortical function considerably richer and more complex. The idea that there is a multiplicity of cortical areas that are linked in distinct functional streams has already been used to interpret the differential course of development of pattern, motion and disparity processing (Atkinson 1992). It has also become clear that there are multiple pathways (in both directions) between cortical and subcortical visual structures, and also a wealth of 'descending' pathways between cortical visual areas. The aspects of visual function discussed in this chapter—control of attention, optokinetic responses, and second-order processing—are all likely to involve one or both of these kinds of pathway. Increasing knowledge of the functions of these pathways will help to understand development, and the sequences and dissociations of normal and abnormal development will help to understand how mature function and structure are related.

ACKNOWLEDGEMENTS

This work is supported by a programme grant from the Medical Research Council. We would like to thank John Wattam-Bell and all the staff of the Visual Development Unit in Cambridge and London for their collaboration and help.

REFERENCES

Albright, T. (1992). Form-cue invariant motion processing in primate visual cortex. *Science*, **255**, 1141–3.

Aslin, R. N. and Salapatek, P. (1975). Saccadic localization of targets by the very young infant. *Perception and Psychophysics*, **17**, 293–302.

Atkinson, J. (1979). Development of optokinetic nystagmus in the human infant and monkey infant: an analogue to development in kittens. In *Developmental neurobiology of vision*, (ed. R. D. Freeman), NATO Advanced Study Institute Series. Plenum Press, New York.

Atkinson, J. (1984). Human visual development over the first six months of life. A review and a hypothesis. *Human Neurobiology*, **3**, 61–74.

Atkinson, J. (1992). Early visual development: differential functioning of parvocellular and magnocellular pathways. *Eye* , **6**, 129–35.

Atkinson, J. and Braddick, O. J. (1985). Early development of the control of visual attention. *Perception*, **14**, A25.

Atkinson, J. and Braddick, O. (1992). Visual segmentation of oriented textures by infants. *Behavioural Brain Research*, **49**, 123–31.

Atkinson, J., Hood, B., Braddick, O. J., and Wattam-Bell, J. (1988). Infants' control of fixation shifts with single and competing targets: mechanisms of shifting attention. *Perception*, **17**, 367.

Atkinson, J., Hood, B., Wattam-Bell, J., and Braddick, O. J. (1992). Changes in infants' ability to switch attention in the first three months of life. *Perception*, **21**, 643–53.

Atkinson, J., Braddick, O. J., and Wattam-Bell, J. (1993). Infant cortical mechanisms controlling OKN, saccadic shifts, and motion processing. *Investigative Ophthalmology and Visual Science*, **34**, 1357.

Birch, E. E. (1993). Stereopsis in infants and its developmental relation to visual acuity. In *Early visual development: normal and abnormal*, (ed. K. Simons), Oxford University Press, New York.

Braddick, O. (1993). Orientation- and motion-selective mechanisms in infants. In *Early visual development: normal and abnormal*, (ed. K. Simons), Oxford University Press, New York.

Braddick, O. J. and Atkinson, J. (1988). Sensory selectivity, attentional control, and cross-channel integration in early development. In *Perceptual development in infancy: the Minnesota symposia on child psychology*, **20**. Lawrence Erlbaum, Hillsdale NJ.

Braddick, O. J., Atkinson, J., and Wattam-Bell, J. (1989). Development of visual cortical selectivity: binocularity, orientation, and direction of motion. In *Neurobiology of early infant behaviour*, (ed. C. von Euler), Wenner-Gren Symposium Series, Macmillan, London.

Braddick, O., Atkinson, J., Hood, B., Harkness, W., Jackson, G., and Vargha-Khadem, F. (1992). Possible blindsight in babies lacking one cerebral hemisphere. *Nature*, **360**, 461–3.

Bronson, G. W. (1974). The postnatal growth of visual capacity. *Child Development*, **45**, 873–90.

Burkhalter, A., Bernardo, K. L., and Charles, V. (1993). Development of local circuits in human visual cortex. *Journal of Neuroscience*, **13**, 1916–31.

Cavanagh, P. and Mather, G. (1989). Motion: the long and the short of it. *Spatial Vision*, **4**, 103–29.

Chubb, C. and Sperling, G. (1988). Drift-balanced random stimuli: a general basis for studying non-Fourier motion perception. *Journal of the Optical Society of America A*, **5**, 1986–2007.

Cowey, A. and Stoerig, P. (1993). Insights into blindsight? *Current Biology*, **3**, 236–8.

de Valois, R. L. and de Valois, K. K. (1988). *Spatial Vision*. Oxford University Press.

Derrington, A. M., Badcock, D. R., and Henning, G. B. (1993). Discriminating the direction of second-order motion at short stimulus durations. *Vision Research*, **33**, 1785–94.

Felleman, D. J. and van Essen, D. C. (1991). Distributed hierarchical processing in the primate cerebral cortex. *Cerebral Cortex*, **1**, 1–47.

Finlay, D. C. and Ivinski, A. (1984). Cardiac and visual responses to moving stimuli presented either successively or simultaneously to the central and peripheral visual fields in four-month-old infants. *Developmental Psychology*, **20**, 29–36.

Fischer, B. (1986). The role of attention in the preparation of visually guided eye movements in monkey and man. *Psychological Research*, **48**, 251–7.

Freedland, R. L. and Dannemiller, J. L. (1990). Evidence for a non-linear pattern vision process in 12-week-old human infants. *Investigative Ophthalmology and Visual Science*, **3** (suppl.), 7.

Grosof, D., Shapley, R. M., and Hawken, M. J. (1993). Macaque V1 neurones can signal 'illusory' contours. *Nature*, **365**, 550–52.

Harris, L. R., Lewis, T. L., and Maurer, D. (1993). Brainstem and cortical contributions to the generation of horizontal eye movements in humans. *Visual Neuroscience*, **10**, 247–59.

Harris, P. L., and MacFarlane, A. (1974). The growth of the effective visual field from birth to seven weeks. *Journal of Experimental Child Psychology*, **18**, 340–84.

Hoffmann, K.-P. (1989). Control of the optokinetic reflex by the nucleus of the optic tract in primates. *Progress in Brain Research*, **80**, 173–82.

Hoffmann, K.-P., and Schoppmann, A. (1975). Retinal input to the direction-selective cells of the nucleus tractus opticus of the cat. *Brain Research*, **99**, 359–66.

Hood, B. (1991). Development of Selective Visual Attention. Unpublished PhD thesis, University of Cambridge.

Hood, B. (1993). Inhibition of return produced by covert shifts of attention in 6-month-old infants. *Infant Behaviour and Development*, **16**, 255–64

Hood, B. and Atkinson, J. (1990). Inhibition of return in infants. *Perception*, **19**, 369.

Hood, B. and Atkinson, J. (1991). Shifting covert attention in infancy. *Investigative Ophthalmology and Visual Science*, **32** (suppl.), 965.

Hood, B. and Atkinson, J. (1993). Disengaging visual attention in the infant and adult. *Infant Behaviour and Development*, **16**, 405–22.

Hubel, D. H., LeVay, S., and Wiesel, T. N. (1975). Mode of termination of retinotectal fibres in macaque monkey: an autoradiographic study. *Brain Research*, **96**, 25–40.

Johnson, M. H. (1990). Cortical maturation and the development of visual attention in early infancy. *Journal of Cognitive Neuroscience*, **2**, 81–95.

Johnson, M. H. and Tucker, L. A. (1993). The ontogeny of covert visual attention: facilitatory and inhibitory effects. Paper presented at the Society for Research in Child Development, New Orleans.

Kellman, P. J. and Spelke, E. S. (1983). Perception of partly occluded objects in infancy. *Cognitive Psychology*, **15**, 483–524.

Lamme, V. A. F., van Dijk, B. W., and Spekreijse, H. (1993). Contour from motion processing occurs in primary visual cortex. *Nature*, **363**, 541–3.

Ledgeway, T. and Smith, A. T. (1993). Separate mechanisms for the detection of first- and second-order motion in human vision. *Investigative Ophthalmology and Visual Science*, **34** (suppl.), 1363.

Lewis, T. L., Maurer, D., and Blackburn, K. (1985). The development of the young infants' ability to detect stimuli in the nasal visual field. *Vision Research*, **25**, 943–50.

Lewis, T. L. and Maurer, D. (1992). The development of the temporal and nasal visual fields during infancy. *Vision Research*, **32**, 903–11.

Movshon, J. A., Thompson, I. D., and Tolhurst, D. J. (1978). Spatial summation in receptive fields of simple cells in the cat's striate cortex. *Journal of Physiology*, **283**, 53–77.

Norcia, A. M., Garcia, H., Humphry, R., Holmes, A., and Orel-Bixler, D. (1991). Anomalous motion VEPs in infants and in infantile esotropia. *Investigative Ophthalmology and Visual Science*, **32**, 436–9.

Pantle, A. (1992). Immobility of some 2nd-order stimuli in human peripheral vision. *Journal of the Optical Society of America A*, **9**, 863–7.

Pollack, J. G. and Hickey, T. L. (1979). The distribution of retino-collicular axon terminals in rhesus monkey. *Journal of Comparative Neurology*, **185**, 587–602.

Posner, M. I. and Cohen, Y. (1980). Orienting of attention. *Quarterly Journal of Experimental Psychology*, **32**, 3–25.

Posner, M. I. and Petersen, S. E. (1990). The attention system of the human brain. *Annual Review of Neuroscience*, **13**, 25–42.

Posner, M. I., Rafal, R. D., Choate, L. S., and Vaughan, J. (1985). Inhibition of return neural basis and function. *Cognitive Neuropsychology*, **2**, 211–28.

Rafal, R., Calabresi, P., Brennan, C., and Sciolto, T. (1989). Saccade preparation inhibits reorienting to recently attended locations. *Journal of Experimental Psychology: Human Perception and Performance*, **15**, 673–85.

Rafal, R., Henik, A., and Smith, J. (1991). Extrageniculate contribution to reflex visual orienting in normal humans: a temporal hemifield advantage. *Journal of Cognitive Neuroscience*, **3**, 322–8.

Rieth, C. and Sireteanu, R. (1994a). Texture segmentation and 'pop-out' in infants and children: a study with the forced-choice preferential looking method. *Spatial Vision*, **8** 173–91.

Rieth, C. and Sireteanu, R. (1994b). Texture segmentation and visual search based on orientation contrast: an infant study with the familiarization-novelty preference method. *Infant Behavior and Development*, **17**, 359–70.

Saslow, M. G. (1967). Effects of components of displacement-step stimuli upon latency of saccadic eye movements. *Journal of the Optical Society of America*, **57**, 1024–29.

Schiller, P. H. (1984). The superior colliculus and visual function. In *Handbook of physiology, The nervous system III, Sensory processes Part 1*, (ed. I. Darian-Smith) pp. 457–505. American Physiological Society, Bethesda, MD.

Schiller, P. H. (1985). A model for the generation of visually guided saccadic eye movements. In *Models of the visual cortex*, (ed. D. Rose and V. G. Dobson), John Wiley & Sons, Chichester.

Schiller, P. H., Malpeli, J. G., and Schein, S. J. (1979). Composition of geniculostriate input to superior colliculus of the rhesus monkey. *Journal of Neurophysiology*, **42** 1124–33.

Sireteanu, R. and Rieth, C. (1992). Texture segmentation in infants and children *Behavioural Brain Research*, **49**, 133–9.

Valenza, E., Simion, F., and Umilta, C. (1994). Inhibition of return in newborn infants *Infant Behavior and Development*, **17**, 293–302.

van Hof-van Duin, J. and Mohn, G. (1983). Optokinetic and spontaneous nystagmus in children with neurological disorders. *Behavioural Brain Research*, **10**, 163–75.

von der Heydt, R. and Peterhans, E. (1989). Mechanisms of contour perception in monkey visual cortex. *Journal of Neuroscience*, **9**, 1731–48.

Wattam-Bell, J. (1992). The development of maximum displacement limits for discrimination of motion direction in infancy. *Vision Research*, **32**, 621–30.

Wattam-Bell, J. (1993). One-month-olds fail in a motion discrimination task. *Investigative Ophthalmology and Visual Science*, **34** (suppl.), 1356.

Wilson, H. R., Ferrera, V., and Yo, C. (1992). A psychophysically motivated model for two-dimensional motion perception. *Visual Neuroscience*, **9**, 79–97.

Zeki, S. and Shipp, S. (1988). The functional logic of cortical connections. *Nature*, **335** 311–17.

Zhou, Y.-X. and Baker, C. L. (1993). A processing stream in mammalian visual cortex neurons for non-Fourier responses. *Science*, **261**, 98–101.

15

Eye alignment and convergence in young infants

Louise Hainline and Patricia M. Riddell

INTRODUCTION

The presence of a fovea, a region with higher spatial resolution than the rest of the retina, coincides in vertebrate evolution with the emergence of several visual characteristics. Migration of the eyes from a lateral position to the front of the head produced significant overlap of the visual fields of the two eyes, allowing the emergence of binocular visual interactions. Sensory fusion and stereopsis allow a finely tuned perception of depth that emerges through the action of disparity detectors, cortical cells that compare the simultaneous inputs from the two eyes. In addition to sensory abilities, specialized movements of the eyes such as smooth pursuit evolved to position the fovea to point at objects that move across the visual field. Convergence aligns the eyes to view objects at different distances. The result, in a mature organism, is a cortical system that represents the world in a three-dimensional binocular sensory-motor map. This allows interaction with the vestibular system to give stable, high-resolution, spatially correct vision, despite movements of the eye in the head, of the head on the body, and of the body through the world.

Many of these functions are working poorly, if at all, in the young human. Numerous accounts of infant vision attest to the degree of visual development from birth throughout the first year of life. The vision of young infants, with their immature foveae (Abramov *et al.* 1982; Yuodelis and Hendrickson 1986), reduced spatial acuity (Dobson and Teller 1978), immature smooth pursuit (Hainline 1993), absent stereopsis (Birch 1993) and other inadequacies bears little similarity to the exquisitely tuned visual system of the adult. Yet, despite its immaturity, the infant visual system is the substrate from which the mature system emerges. Paying too much attention to the sensory and motor deficiencies of young humans may cause us to lose sight of the functional abilities that allow them to relate effectively to their visual world and serve as a scaffolding for what follows (Hainline and Abramov 1992). Little is still known about how the various factors influencing visual development interact. The animal data, and the less systematic clinical data from humans who experience visually disabling conditions, tell us that early experience plays a deterministic role

(Teller and Movshon 1986). Yet, we are still far from understanding how early visual functioning ultimately leads to the adult's exquisite visual abilities.

Perhaps our lack of progress stems from failing to credit the complexity of the process. Piaget, among others, characterized infancy as a period of **sensori-motor** development (Piaget 1952). If interactions matter, consideration of single factors (sensory or motor separately) will never yield a satisfactory explanation. Examples of how infants learn to co-ordinate movements of their bodies with visual, tactual, and vestibular inputs are easy to find in descriptions of infant mouthing, reaching, grasping, standing, and walking. Curiously, 'looking' has seldom been studied.

The central topic of this chapter is an aspect of visual/motor development, specifically the development of binocular eye alignment in vergence (change in alignment of the visual axes of the two eyes to look at objects at different distances). Given the recognition of the importance of sensory–motor interactions during early development (Thelan 1989), it is perhaps surprising to find how little attention has been given to this factor in visual development. To see well we need both adequate sensory systems and reasonable oculomotor control.

DEVELOPMENT OF STRABISMUS AS AN EXAMPLE OF SENSORIMOTOR DEVELOPMENT

Many approaches have sought an answer to which modality 'comes first', the sensory or the motor. It has been common to assume that either the motor or sensory system is primary in vision and is thus required for development of the other. This perspective is seen, for instance, in descriptions of the development of visual problems such as strabismus. An example is found in the classic dispute between Worth and Chavasse over the origins of what has been termed 'essential infantile esotropia', a consistent in-turning of one eye with an onset before 6 months of age (von Noorden 1984; 1988*a;b*). Worth (1903) believed that infantile esotropia was a sensory disorder with a secondary motor consequence caused by a lack of sensory fusion (the percept of a single image after combination of images from corresponding retinal locations in the two eyes). One practical clinical consequence of this position was that early interventions to straighten the eyes were considered unhelpful, because the lack of sensory fusion was regarded as the essential deficit. Chavasse (1939) on the other hand regarded motor factors as primary, suggesting that binocular sensory fusion was a learned consequence of appropriate motor alignment. Motor alignment was believed to be dependent on minimizing retinal image disparity by fusional vergence movements. By this account, correction of squint might have the beneficial effect of allowing the system to 'learn' sensory fusion, so long as the intervention took place early enough.

The Worth/Chavasse controversy, while stated rather quaintly with respect to current knowledge and terminology, at least discusses the issue of the interaction between sensory and motor factors in vision. Most basic science research on visual development largely ignores this developmental issue. There is a substantial literature on animals suggesting that sensory function is adversely affected by deliberate early misalignment of the eyes. Surgically or prismatically induced squints in infant monkeys, as brief as 1 week's duration, decimate the number of neurones in primary visual cortex that normally receive inputs from both eyes (Crawford and von Noorden 1979; 1980). This effect is apparently irreversible even if the eyes are then realigned and the monkey receives normal binocular inputs for several years. Strabismus is not reported to occur when monkeys experience monocular deprivation or induced anisometropia early in life, although cortical binocular cells and stereopsis are clearly abnormal. In monkey, then, it has been argued that defective cortical binocular development is a consequence, not a cause, of ocular misalignment, an observation that would favour Worth's position (von Noorden 1988a). However, in much of this research, the squints that have been imposed are much larger than those that occur in typical cases of early human strabismus. The extreme forms of intervention may have interfered with recovery ordinarily allowed by normal sensory–motor feedback.

DEVELOPMENT OF BINOCULAR VISUAL FUNCTIONS IN INFANTS

Other data support the idea that strabismic human infants may not be exactly like infant monkeys made strabismic artificially. Normally, stereopsis has a sudden onset between 3 and 5 months of age (Birch *et al.* 1982), after which it improves rapidly, developing from a threshold of more than a degree of disparity to better than one minute of arc, within a matter of a few weeks (Birch 1993). Stereopsis actually represents a hierarchy of abilities (Tyler 1990), with early, coarse stereopsis more dependent on peripheral fusional mechanisms than the later fine stereopsis, which requires fusion by cells in the fovea, and is sensitive to very fine retinal disparities. The stereopsis that has been reported for infants is probably gross stereopsis. Stager and Birch (1986) report that some stereopsis is measurable in at least some 3–4 month-old infants with early onset esotropia when their ocular alignment is corrected with prisms; stereopsis is rarely shown by older strabismic infants when prism-corrected. This finding would thus seem to support innate or early central fusional mechanisms of Chavasse.

There is ample evidence that the fovea is less mature than the periphery in young infants. Abramov and our group (Abramov *et al.* 1982), and Hendrickson and hers (Yuodelis and Hendrickson 1986) have published anatomical evidence of grossly immature foveal structures, in contrast to the relative structural maturity of the periphery. This is substantiated by analyses of cone densities across the retina at different stages of monkey visual system development (Packer *et al.* 1990). Banks and Bennett (1988) and Wilson (1988) have described the functional consequences of this primary immaturity in spatial and colour vision. Clearly, acuity and contrast sensitivity for higher spatial frequencies undergo considerable development during early infancy. Behavioural work in the monkey has shown that, by contrast, acuity in peripheral regions of the retina and contrast sensitivity at lower spatial frequencies undergo less development and may attain adult levels sooner (Kiorpes and Kiper 1991). If infant vision is adaptive, the functions necessary for normal development may be more under the control of regions outside the immature fovea. It is sensible then, to shift the focus of attention from the inadequacies of infant foveal vision to the adaptive visual developments served by a more mature peripheral region.

There is evidence, for example, that sensory binocularity develops in stages with early development relying more on peripheral than foveal factors. Skarf and colleagues (Eizenman *et al.* 1989; Katz *et al.* 1991; Skarf *et al.* 1992), Baitch and Srebro (1990), and Braddick *et al.* (1983) have reported detection of cortical binocular responses in the visual-evoked potential that predate stereopsis in infant development; cortical responses to dichoptically presented correlograms depend on the existence of cells responsive to binocular inputs but not the disparity sensitive cells required for stereopsis.

Held (1985; 1988; 1993) proposed a model of the development of sensory binocularity to explain the sudden emergence and quick improvement of stereopsis. He speculates that this sudden appearance marks the emergence of cortical dominance columns labelled by eye of origin in layer IV of primary visual cortex. Ocular dominance columns are slabs of cortical cells that respond preferentially to input from one or the other eye. Eye-of-origin information is required to be able to sort out crossed and uncrossed disparities, signalling whether an object is behind or in front of the current plane of convergence. Existing evidence suggests that cortical dominance columns are only partially segregated by 4 months and only become adult-like in humans at 6 months of age (Hickey and Peduzzi 1987). In monkey, before segregation of the ocular dominance columns, visual afferents from both eyes overlap in their projection to layer IV, and even sometimes synapse on the same cells (LeVay *et al.* 1980). Owing to their common synapses, eye-of-origin information is unavailable or only partially available for subsequent processing, as would be required to detect the direction of disparity between the two eye's retinal images. Held proposes that, before the emergence of cortical disparity detectors with eye-of-origin coding, infants have neither sensory fusion nor stereopsis. He argues that sensory fusion, which he and his colleagues equate with the presence of retinal rivalry (a percept marked by a competition between the two eyes' inputs rather than fusion), emerges at about the same time as stereopsis (Shimojo *et al.* 1986). Earlier, infants are described as combining the two retinal inputs by non-selectively superimposing the two images.

Of interest here is how the infant attains the ocular alignment necessary for the appearance of these new cortical structures. Experimental work suggests that in order for disparity detectors to emerge, they must receive visual input from the two eyes with enough spatial correlation to allow some moderate level of disparity detection. If the eyes are misaligned or even poorly matched in spatial resolution, full stereopsis does not emerge. Yet, much of the data on infants' eye alignment in the months preceding measurable stereopsis leaves the impression of a system grossly mis-coordinated and apparently inadequate for the task at hand. The poor spatial resolution that has been reported for young infants has also been seen as relevant to ocular alignment; for example, von Noorden (1988b) has said that to develop stable ocular alignment requires a 'high-quality sensory input'. These are not the usual sort of terms found to describe infant vision.

DEVELOPMENT OF OCULAR ALIGNMENT AND VERGENCE

There has been long-standing interest in how well young infants align their eyes. Maurer (1975) and Wickelgren (1967) reported consistent bilateral exo-tropia for newborns, based on the quantitative scoring of the position of a corneal reflection relative to pupil centre in photographs. However, Slater and Findlay (1972) showed that the apparent exotropia was caused by a larger angle lambda (the angle between the eye's visual and optic axis) for infants than adults, so that infants were actually converging appropriately. Angle lambda reduces with age because, as the eyeball grows longer, the angle between the fovea and the optic axis reduces in proportion. These studies suggested a reasonable level of alignment to act as a platform for the binocular sensory developments described above.

A recent group of studies on early visual alignment in infants, based on stand-ard but subjective clinical evaluation, reports a different picture entirely. These studies describe a very high proportion of young infants with poor ocular alignment, with a large proportion of true exotropia reported. Nixon *et al.* (1985) observed orthotropia in 48.6% of 1219 normal newborns, exotropia in 32.7% (10.7% constant and 22% intermittent), and intermittent esotropia or esotropia combined with exotropia in 3.2%. Some 15.4% were not able to be classified because of problems with alertness. Orthotropia increased to more than 97% by 6 months. Observations were subjective, using the experimenter's face as a target. Ocular alignment was judged with an observational Hirschberg test (a measure of eye rotation based on change in position of a corneal reflec-tion of an object as the eye rotates).

Subsequently, Sondhi *et al.* (1988) and Archer *et al.* (1989) examined a large sample of 3972 infants using a modified Hirschberg test (using the experi-menter's face instead of a pen light as the source for a corneal reflection) with unsystematic repeat tests up to age 10 months. They reported an even higher incidence of moderate exodeviations in newborns (66.5%). Esodeviations accounted for less than 1% with only 29.9% orthotropic at birth, and 2.6% showing swings between eso- and exotropia. The exact proportion of constant versus intermittent exotropias alone was not reported but, overall, 54.4% of *all* deviations observed were constant and 15.7% were intermittent.

The angular equivalent of 'moderate' was not specified in these papers; however, from the description of the anatomical markers that were used, we estimate that this was classified as a misalignment of 30–60° (50–100 prism dioptres). Archer (1993) argues that the exotropia was not accounted for by the infants' larger angle lambda (because the exodeviations were larger than expected for lambda). He also claims that the experimenter could judge which was the fixating eye and which the deviating eye. He proposed that the lack of orthotropia in young infants results from vergence control that is largely 'open-loop' (i.e. not under control of visual feedback). He also proposes that stable orthotropia requires a tighter coupling of the sensory limb of vergence to motor vergence resulting in a transition to closed-loop vergence at some unspecified age (but at least by 6 months). Archer *et al.* (1989) observe, on the basis of these data, that even normal infants have 'a generally "anomalous" binocular sensory experience during the first few months of life'. This seems to be a poor context for the emergence of mature binocular functions in the normal case.

Methodological problems with these studies reduce their impact on our thinking about early visual development. From the scant procedural descriptions, it is difficult to understand important details such as testing distance and the validity of the subjective measurements. It is difficult, for instance, to discern how precisely the infant was positioned in front of the experimenter; at close distances, positioning the infant slightly off-axis can lead to large errors in estimating gaze, particularly if one eye is observed at a time. Typically, the studies use neither monocular presentation nor a cover test, both of which are important to establish the individual infant's angle lambda and which is the fixating eye. Nor do the authors estimate how much error would result from the infant fixating the extremes of a spatially extended target (the experimenter's face); when young infants' scan faces, they are reported to fixate often on the margins of the face (Hainline 1978; Haith *et al.* 1977), which means that the face is much less effective than a small target such as a penlight for such estimates.

Neonates' fleeting attention and often poor fixations must have an an impact on the experimenter's ability to make on-the-spot judgements about small changes in position of reflections on the cornea (in the order of millimetres). However, considerations about minimum resolution may be less relevant than the issue of why such extreme eye turns are being reported routinely.

At odds with this view of alignment insufficiency in early infancy are some interesting data collected by Horwood (1993). Horwood recruited orthoptist mothers to observe the status of their infants' eyes on a daily basis and to record the nature and durations of any deviations seen. The orthoptist parents were requested to complete questionnaires about their children's ocular behaviours (e.g. fixation, following, vergence, prism response, cover test etc.) between birth and 3.5 years. The results were consistently different from those reported earlier. The greatest proportion of deviations reported for 75 infants observed up to 6 months and 60 observed for 1 year or longer was for esodeviations, with exodeviations uncommon. Most babies (88.2%) showed some periods of mis-alignment at some time in the first 6 months, although most lasted only a few seconds and often were related to the infant's attentional state. At 1 week, convergent deviations represented 80.4%, divergent deviations 4.4% and variable deviations 15.2%. By 3 months, although the absolute frequency was declining, the proportion of deviations was 92% convergent when observed. The majority displayed unilateral esodeviations, more like strabismus, than bilateral deviations, which might be considered inappropriate vergence. There was steady improvement in alignment over the first 2 months but only a few infants were reported never to deviate at all.

Horwood suggests that the difference between her results and the earlier reports of high incidences of exotropia may be caused by the effects of attention and motivation on infants' ocular behaviours. She posits that a mother's face is more attractive as a stimulus than a strange experimenter's and, therefore, infants are motivated to overcome their normally divergent position. Also, since the esodeviations reported were extremely brief, mothers with their infants all day would be more likely to observe them than experimenters interacting with the infant for a few minutes. Clearly, Horwood's data imply that, while ocular motor alignment may show brief lapses (possibly related to attention), young infants have straight eyes for a much larger percentage of time than earlier work suggested. Her results are strikingly different from those of Archer and his colleagues, not in the least because she saw almost no exotropia, and certainly nothing the size of the misalignments that group had reported as typical.

There are fewer data on convergence (changes in eye alignment with target distance) but these are also somewhat contradictory. Slater and Findlay (1975) reported that newborns did alter their convergence symmetrically and appropriately for targets presented at 50 cm (2 dioptres) and 25 cm (4 dioptres), although they did not converge even more for a target at 12.5 cm (8 dioptres). It is possible that the failure to respond to extremely close targets is related to the natural hyperopia that has been reported during the newborn period; hyperopes have difficulty focusing at close target distances, and so infants may not have been eager to fixate the 12.5 cm target, although it is not clear that the connections between accommodation and convergence that occur in adults are actually functioning this early in life. The authors have presented data showing that, on average, even 1-month-old infants converge appropriately on static targets presented at distances from 25–200 cm, although there was also noted a lack of manifest convergence/accommodation links in the first few months (Hainline *et al.* 1992).

Vergence to static targets may develop at a different rate than that to moving targets. Ling (1942) judged infant convergence qualitatively from movie films as infants viewed a target moving in the midline, and reported poor convergence for near targets until 3 months of age. Aslin (1977) reported that 1-month-old infants responded with convergence in the appropriate direction for a moving fixation target, but appeared to underconverge for nearer targets

(12–50 cm) until about 3 months. They also failed to adjust their convergence when a wedge prism was placed in front of one eye until 6 months of age. This was used as evidence to suggest that younger infants do not respond to visual signals of disparity, although the response was measured only observationally and in a limited observation window. If infants made small movements or had long latencies, these responses might have been missed. Certainly, these results are at variance with the data on younger infants' ability to converge appropriately on static targets.

Relatively little attention is paid to the role of oculomotor factors in the Held model of the neural developments required for the emergence of stereopsis. Data are presented that vergence *per se* cannot account for the appearance of stereopsis (Birch *et al*. 1983) but the account predicts that dynamic vergence may be limited by sensory development. In one version of the model, Held (1988) proposes that rudimentary vergence may be controlled by a process that optimizes neural excitation of layer IV cells by registration of the inputs of the two eyes. So long as there is a richly textured visual field, deviations from correct registration may lead to a reduction in total excitation, and thus with some trial-and-error tuning, convergence on stationary or slowly moving targets may be possible.

Held predicts, and later his group provided some preliminary evidence to support the view, that infants will converge poorly on targets moving rapidly in depth or that jump from one position in depth to another, and that vergence should improve markedly when stereopsis begins. A more recent study by this group (Thorn *et al*. 1994) supports the notion that dynamic vergence may show different properties than static vergence. Infants were found to have poor control of tracking vergence eye movements to a target approaching the infant before the emergence of stereopsis but they had good steady state convergence at 1 dioptre (D; dioptres represent the reciprocal of the target distance in metres). Unfortunately, vergence control was measured only qualitatively, and speed of the target was not varied. Thus it is not known whether infants would have converged better with slower velocities or provision for the longer latencies that are typically observed in infants' oculomotor responses (Krinsky *et al*. 1990).

Feedback from eye movements may play more than a passive role in registering the inputs to cortical neurones. Oculomotor proprioception is important during this period, at least for kittens. Surgical interruption of oculomotor proprioception causes deficits in visually guided behaviour but only if performed in kittens, not in adult cats (Hein and Diamond 1983). Oculomotor proprioception was also found necessary for the development of normal segregation of cortical ocular dominance columns in kittens (Trotter *et al*. 1987; Graves *et al*. 1987); because of differences in the oculomotor systems, equivalent primate experiments are almost impossible to perform (Vital-Durand, personal communication). Still, proper oculomotor inputs are critical for normal binocular development and, while not sufficient, may be necessary for the various developments that have been described.

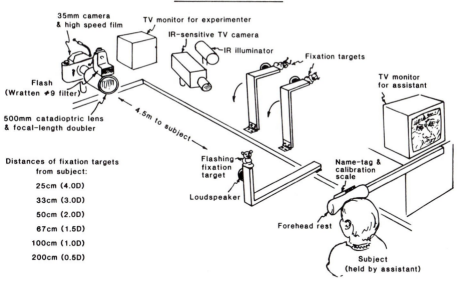

Fig. 15.1 Diagram of photorefraction equipment used to test infants. Internally lit dolls are placed at one of five distances (0.5–4 dioptres). Photographs are taken at each target distance when infants are attending to the targets.

The intent of the present chapter is to present some new analyses of the status of ocular alignment in young, normal infants. These data are relevant to the issue of how infants normally co-ordinate sensory and motor functions early in life. In part, we are trying to clarify the very confused picture now found in the literature on young infants' eye alignment and convergence. Although our data address normal development, they are still of clinical relevance, since a clear understanding of normal vergence and alignment development is essential for any clinical interpretations.

METHOD

The convergence data described here were collected using a paraxial photorefraction system that we have reported previously (Abramov *et al*. 1990) (Fig. 15.1). Briefly, the system used a 35 mm camera and a catadioptric tele-photo lens to measure accommodation and eye alignment for both eyes sim-ultaneously as the infants look at a series of small, internally lit dolls at one of five distances (25–200 cm). The infant is held briefly against a headrest to achieve correct viewing distance and right/left positioning. The targets are presented one at a time, with some short interval occurring naturally before a picture is taken. Convergence or eye alignment is measured for targets in a series of fixed locations, not for targets moving in depth, and so may be looking at the earliest forms of convergence (see earlier discussion). The demands to accommodation represented by these targets range from 0.25–4 dioptres. Required convergence angles will depend on inter-pupillary distance (IPD). For an adult with a 63 mm IPD, convergence demand ranges from 14.4° (at 4 dioptres) to 1.8° (at 0.5 dioptres). For an infant, with a smaller 40 mm IPD, the range is from 9.2° at 4 dioptres to 1.1° at 0.5 dioptres.

Infrared television cameras give feedback about positioning and allow us to monitor when the infant is attending to the targets. A flash photograph is taken for each target, using high-speed black-and-white film. The films are measured manually on a specially constructed photomicroscope that images various parts of the photo at different magnifications for measurement on a video screen; for most of the measurements, each eye's image is magnified approximately 15 times to yield high precision for changes in eye position. Measurements include interpupillary distance, pupil diameter, the size of the crescent of light reflected back from the retina by misaccommodation with respect to the plane of the camera, and the position of the corneal reflection of the camera's flash within the pupil.

From these primary measurements, we can calculate plane of accommodation and angle of convergence, the Hirschberg ratio, and angle lambda. With good adult data, these procedures can detect changes in vergence of about 1°. With infants, however, there are several factors that limit our ability to interpret a difference in convergence between the two eyes as a true error of convergence, since there are other reasons for small misalignments. Our photorefractor has a marker to show where the head should be positioned to be centred in front of the target and the camera. In the past, we were not so careful as now to achieve the best possible centring of the infant's head. It is not always easy to position squirmy or floppy infants exactly, but we also did not realize how much infants would compensate for our positioning errors with their eyes. The angular result of off-centre head position varies with target distance and IPD. For example, if the 4 dioptre target were directly in front of one eye (instead of the target being centred), for a 40 mm IPD, the convergence for the individual eyes could differ by as much as 4.5°. This might look like a tropia but it would be a correct response. At 0.5 dioptres, in contrast, the error is less than a degree.

Another source of ambiguity in interpreting misalignments arises from the fact that an extended target was used, since infants will not reliably attend to a point source. Our targets are smaller than a human face but the width of the closest target is about 6°. If on one trial, the infant was looking at one side of a target, while in the next, was fixating the other, the individual eye's convergence angles could look different because of version, not vergence. Taken together, it is difficult to discriminate true misalignments from differences in position with respect to the target or fixation point on the target for alignment differences less than about 5–6°. To put this into perspective, experimental (Reinecke *et al.* 1991) and clinical experience suggest that, using a Hirschberg test observationally in the best circumstances, one is likely to be unable to discriminate a movement of the corneal reflection of less than 1 mm. By our measurement, this is a threshold of about 12–13° to detect a change in align-ment for any reason. Despite its problems, our magnified scoring improves on this.

RESULTS

The developmental results on accommodation and convergence behaviour were reported in Hainline *et al.* (1992). To summarize these results briefly, infants of all age, and naive adults, fail to show the expected linear relationship between accommodative demand and response, with non-linear accommoda-tion functions being the rule rather than the exception. Standard non-linear fits to these functions provided parameters for evaluating accommodative response. Accommodation to these targets appears nearly adult-like for most subjects after 2–3 months of age. Before that age, accommodation is much more variable, both between- and within-infants. Below 2 months of age, many infants (about 50%) fail to vary accommodation at all, showing flat accommo-dative functions, usually at a level of 3–4 dioptres of accommodation; this is not so close as the 19 cm (approximately 5 dioptres) of resting accommodation described by Haynes *et al.* (1965) but is reminiscent of those data. At the same time, about 30% accommodated appropriately for near targets but failed to relax their accommodation properly for far targets. A final 20%, including even 1-month-old infants, accommodated appropriately, similar to older infants and adults.

The group convergence data for 653 infants from Hainline *et al.* (1992) have been replotted in Fig. 15.2. In this figure, convergence is shown by more posit-ive values, divergence by more negative ones. The curves for the two youngest ages are plotted. The cross-hatched area shows the range of convergence values found in infants from 61 days to 1 year. The adult slope is higher than that seen in infants because the adults' larger interpupillary distances require a greater convergence angle for close targets. The convergence angle axis has negative values because of angle lambda, which, when negative, means that the fovea is temporal to the optic axis; the intercept of the group convergence curve represents twice the average angle lambda.

Fig. 15.3 presents the data on the systematic change in angle lambda more clearly; here, lambda was calculated from measurements of pupil centre and first Purkinje image, for individual infants who both converged and accom-modated linearly with demand. This shows that angle lambda and thus the appearance of exotropia when young infants are fixating, decreases consist-ently with age (Riddell *et al.* 1994). An extrapolation from the linear portion of our curve to the newborn period yields an estimate of angle lambda at birth of about 8° in each eye, which agrees well with the 8.2° reported by Slater and Findlay (1972). Further examination of the difference in angle lambda between the two eyes of infants finds that on average, angle lambda is approximately

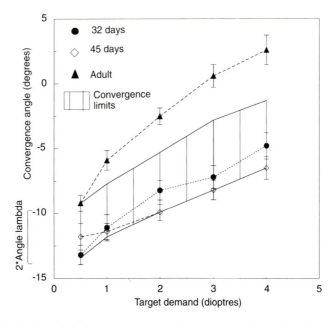

Fig. 15.2 Graph showing the average range of convergence for infants from 60 days to 1 year (hatched area) when converging on targets placed at 0.5 to 4 dioptres from the infant. The average responses for infants of 27–36 days (filled circles), infants of 37–60 days (open diamonds) and adults (filled triangles) are also plotted. The youngest infants do not show appreciably different convergence than the older infants. The adults show a steeper convergence as a result of their wider inter-pupillary distance (IPD). On this plot, convergence is shown as positive and divergence as negative. The offset from zero gives an estimate of twice the average angle lambda.

symmetrical; the mean difference across age is zero, although there is greater variability at young ages. Whether this is a real effect or caused by the greater problems in collecting clean data from the youngest infants remains to be explored further. Certainly, these data do not support the contention of either extreme asymmetrical or unilateral exotropias in young infants.

By analysing the convergence data from this sample of infants, it was also possible to verify empirically across a reasonable range of ages during infancy an observation about eye growth that had previously been believed to be true only from theoretical analyses. Wick and London (1980) argued from data on the relative growth of various structures of the infant eye that the Hirschberg ratio is on average constant from infancy to adulthood, thus justifying the use of the same scale factor to estimate infant eye turns. Based on our data (Riddell *et al.* 1994), it was possible to verify empirically that an average Hirschberg ratio of about 12–13°/mm (or 20–22 prism dioptres/mm) is an appropriate factor to use to estimate eye rotation in both infants and adults.

The data also support the conclusion that convergence for these static targets is a more regular and controlled process than described in earlier accounts of

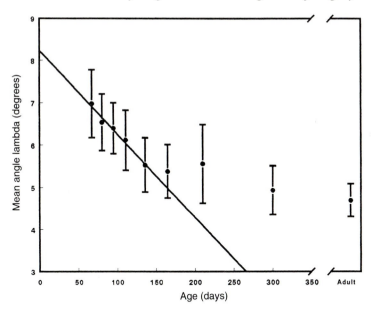

Fig. 15.3 Plot of average angle lambda for eight age groups of infants and for adults. A linear regression has been calculated over the linear portion of the curve. This extrapolates back to an angle lambda of 8.24 for newborn infants, a value that is similar to previous estimates.

infant eye alignment and convergence. They also suggest that, in early infancy, the linkages between accommodation and vergence, normally seen in older children and adults, may not be operating, or if they are operating, they have very different gains, below 2 months of age. Recently, the authors have been re-examining the finer details of the vergence data, to evaluate how well individual infants maintain consistent vergence in this situation. Compared with the great variability observed for accommodation, the regularity and appropriateness of convergence at 1 and 2 months are striking. In most of the cases, the individual convergence functions are as linear as the group functions. The data are in marked contrast with reports of major ocular alignment problems or poor convergence that some have reported.

In the remainder of this paper, vergence data from infants in the first 2 months of life will be discussed; after this age, in this situation, convergence does not change much with age. Examples are presented to support the contention that, in most cases, vergence for such static targets even early in life is appropriate and visually guided, not the coarse open-loop system proposed by Archer and colleagues. At this stage, our data presentation will be more qualitative than quantitative. Appropriate quantitative analysis needs to be performed to support our observations and this is underway; however, a descriptive analysis of infant behaviour is consistent with the existing published work in this area.

When preparing for these analyses, the films from 154 infants of 60 days and under were observed carefully. Unfortunately, both because of the difficulty of getting good data from infants under 1 month, and also because parents are often reluctant or too busy to bring very young infants out to an infant vision laboratory, there are fewer data for infants 30 days and younger than in the intervals between 31–45 and 46–60 days. Data from an additional 55 infants, evenly distributed across the age groups, were not included, in most cases because there were data on too few targets, but occasionally because the child had been obviously sleepy or crying or because the pictures were unscoreable as a result of poor film or picture quality.

Fig. 15.4 illustrates how the data were treated. In Fig. 15.4a is shown data from a 38-day-old demonstrating excellent convergence. The dotted line through the filled symbols is the linear fit to the binocular convergence data. The open diamonds and triangles represent the angular position of the right and left eyes on each trial. The solid line represents the ideal convergence for this infant's specific IPD. Appropriateness of convergence is gauged by comparing the slope of the ideal response with that from the linear regression to the binocular data. The ideal response line has been plotted using an age-appropriate average for the intercept value (twice the average angle lambda for that age group); discrepancies in the intercepts between the ideal and actual binocular response lines reflect individual differences in angle lambda. Note that for this infant, the binocular convergence regression line is parallel to the ideal response line, and the intercept value is close to the age average. The points for the right and left eyes plot almost on top of one another, signifying similar angle lambdas for the two eyes, and the slope for each is about half that for the total convergence.

As with these data, the binocular convergence data were in most cases well fit by a linear function, suggesting that departures from linearity may be especially significant if substantiated (see later discussion). Response for the individual eyes does not always look so regular; however, some of the variability in data from the individual eyes stems from mispositioning of the head with respect to the target. To illustrate the importance of the head position, Fig. 15.4b shows convergence data from a different 38-day-old infant. For this child, the head was off-centre to the left for the 2 dioptre and 3 dioptre targets, resulting in apparent overconvergence of the left eye and underconvergence for the right. Owing to this compensation, the binocular response has a slope very close to that expected for ideal convergence. This result means that convergence when the infant is off-axis for the target must be visually driven, not open-loop. Mispositioning the infant even slightly off the target axis could lead to incorrectly diagnosing a tropia, unless the total convergence of both eyes relative to the target plane is considered. The appropriate binocular convergence, including adjustment for head position, also shows that infants must be using a consistent area of retina to point the two eyes to the different targets.

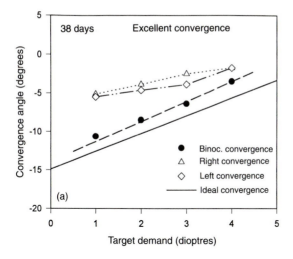

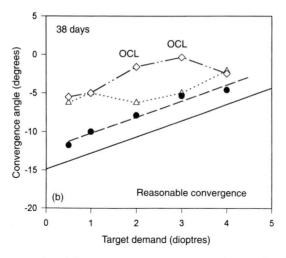

Fig. 15.4 (a) An example of the convergence response of an individual 38-day-old infant showing excellent convergence. The convention for the axes is described in the caption for Fig. 15.2. This infant has a linear binocular convergence response (filled circles), which is closely fit by the ideal response calculated for the IPD of this infant (solid line). Note that the binocular convergence is well fit by the ideal response and that the responses for the individual eyes (open symbols) are linear with a slope that is close to half of that for the binocular response. (b) Convergence data from another 38-day-old infant, showing reasonable convergence, particularly binocularly. The individual responses for the left and right eye are less linear but reflect an ocular response to off-axis head position. At 2 and 3 dioptres, there is a large difference in the eye position between the left and right eyes. Here, the infant was positioned off-centre to the left of the target, resulting in relative over-convergence of the left eye and under-convergence of the right. OCL, off-centre left.

As a preliminary attempt to understand these data, each individual infant's performance was qualitatively classified into one of five categories:

1. **No convergence** was scored for an essentially flat convergence curve across targets. Although the accommodation data are not displayed here, most of these subjects also showed no evidence of accommodation either. It is possible that these 'flat' infants were simply not attending to the targets, although their eyes were open.

2. **Consistent misalignment** was scored if there was evidence that for all targets, one eye or both eyes were consistently misaligned, despite the resulting binocular convergence, and this could not be attributed to poor head position.

3. **Intermittent misalignment** was scored if the infant showed one or two targets with an obvious misalignment, or if there was evidence of an alternating eso- or exotropia. For both the 'misalignment' categories, it is sometimes possible to say with certainty which is the fixating and which the non-fixating eye, so that we can be sure whether the misalignment was exo- or esotropia. However, in some cases, particularly if the fixating eye alternates across pictures, it is more difficult to tell. It is our impression that exotropias were more common than esotropias in our data, but a more quantitative analysis is needed to verify this observation.

4. **Reasonable convergence** was scored if the binocular convergence was appropriate and well-fit by a linear function; however, the data from the individual eyes showed some irregularity. If no extenuating factors were operating (i.e. equal angle lambdas, properly centred head position, and good convergence), the response of the individual eyes should have a slope half that of the binocular curve, and the data from each eye should plot on top of each other, within measurement error. Often, the curves from the individual eyes 'bounced around', although the binocular convergence was quite good. As discussed already, in many of these cases, inspection of the position of the infant's head with respect to the target and the camera showed that the behaviour of the individual eyes was a sensible response to head mispositioning. The effect of head position is not equal across targets; indeed, head mispositioning matters less for the distant targets than it does for the near targets, which require a larger convergence response.

Reasonable alignment was scored in an infant if head position explained most of the variability or if the difference between the two eyes' convergence was less than 4–5° and the binocular response was correct. Departures larger than this tended to be classified as 'intermittent misalignment'; however, the magnitude of these discrepancies has not yet been quantified. Sometimes, it was not possible to detect poor positioning, or the discrepancies between the individual eyes were opposite to that which would have compensated for the head position. This may have been caused by larger than usual measurement error on a given trial; for instance, at times, the pupil margins were hard to see, possibly affecting measurement. On some of these trials, the infants may have

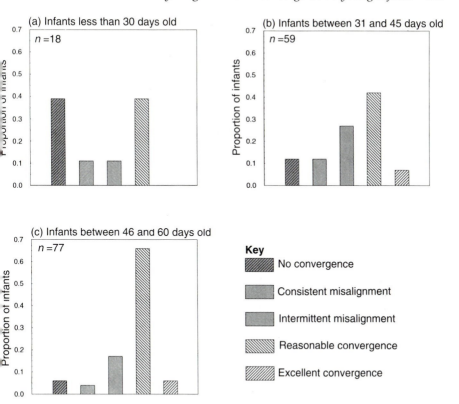

Fig. 15.5 The proportion of infants at different ages by category of convergence response (the categories are fully described in the text): (a) infants less than 30 days; (b) infants between 31 and 45 days; and (c) infants between 46 and 60 days.

been looking at different parts of the dolls. Other cases may be real intermittent microtropias.

5. **Excellent convergence**, the final category, was characterized by clean, linear binocular convergence, and linear response curves for each eye with approximately equal angle lambda in the two eyes.

Fig. 15.5 shows the distribution of these categories of behaviour for three age groups in our sample of infants 60 days and younger. Only in the youngest group was there a high proportion of flat curves, which most probably reflects the influence of state; in most of these cases, the accommodation data also showed no change with target distance, giving no evidence that the stimuli were having any effect on visual behaviour. There are few infants showing these flat functions after 30 days. Another interesting point is that flat functions are much more common than constant or occasional eye turns, which, even in the youngest group, account for less than 20% of the sample. Even at the youngest ages, some reasonable proportion (around 40%) of the infants are showing reasonable convergence. The absence of any of the youngest infants in the 'excellent' classification is more probably because of our difficulty in holding these floppier infants correctly in the apparatus than because of any intrinsic limitation of the infants themselves. Many of our pictures from this age group show badly positioned heads, a problem to which greater attention should be given in the future.

In the second age group (31–45 days), the proportion of infants showing reasonable convergence was about the same (around 40%); however, fewer infants were completely non-responsive (i.e. 'flat'). About 30% showed some difficulty in convergence and alignment, either consistently for all targets or for a few targets. In the next few weeks (46–60 days), performance improved considerably, so that some 70% of the infants showed reasonable or excellent performance. Constant errors were rare, although around 20% showed some evidence of misalignment on at least some targets. Our impression is that after this age, things only get better.

Fig. 15.6(a) shows a typical 'diamond' pattern for the behaviour of the individual eyes; one eye seems more converged on some targets, the other eye on others. For this 27-day-old infant, head position appeared to explain the diamond pattern at 3 dioptres, but not at 1 or 4 dioptres. Possibly, the infant was looking at different parts of the target (which would have a greater effect at near than at far targets). Despite the irregularities in the responses of the individual eyes (for whatever reason), the binocular vergence response is very well fit by a linear function with the expected slope. Fig. 15.6(b) illustrates a case of intermittent misalignment, for a 36-day-old. A linear convergence response for all targets farther than 4 dioptres is found, but the slope of the convergence response function was steeper than expected. At the nearest target the infant suddenly shows a marked left exotropia. In this case, one had the impression that the infant could not converge further, so suddenly the convergence breaks. The importance of relating the performance of each eye to the binocular performance is illustrated by the data in Fig. 15.6(c), which also show a deviation in each eye's performance at 3 dioptres; in this case, the data can be attributed to a head rotation with the result that the binocular response is appropriate for the target distance.

A common pattern, found most often in the youngest babies, is a flat convergence response, as in Fig. 15.7(a) for a 19-day-old. This infant was not changing convergence appropriately with either eye, resulting in a flat response. A likely explanation, especially for this age, is lack of attention to the targets. Lest we leave the impression that babies of this age do not show appropriate convergence, Fig. 15.7(b) is a plot of data from a 17-day-old infant who showed reasonable convergence (although with data from only three targets), and even compensation for a tilt at 0.5 dioptres.

Not all babies show such reasonable convergence responses. Sometimes, the misalignment is consistent across all targets. In Fig. 15.8(a), a 44-day-old baby shows a grossly non-linear convergence response characterized by a systematic separation between the curves for the left and right eyes. This child appears to

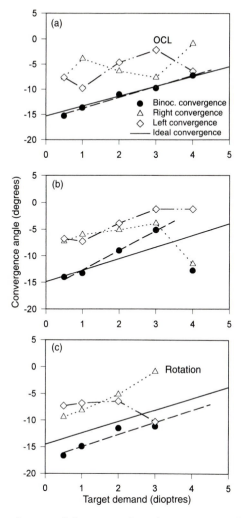

Fig. 15.6 Examples of some of the categories of convergence described in Fig. 15.5. (a) Reasonable convergence is shown from a 27-day-old, showing a pattern that we describe as a 'diamond', with one eye being more converged for one or two targets and the other eye being more converged for others. The data in this case can only partially be explained in terms of mispositioning of the head, at 3 dioptres. For the 1 and 4 dioptre targets, head position seemed appropriate; it is possible that the infant was converged at the appropriate plane but looking to the left of the target. (b) An example of the convergence response described as 'intermittent misalignment' in a 36-day-old infant. The slope of the regression line indicates some over-convergence for the targets from 0.5 to 3 dioptres. At 4 dioptres, the left eye diverges, resulting in an inappropriate binocular response. (c) An example of reasonable convergence in a 48-day-old infant. Note that this infant also shows an apparent divergence of the left eye at 3 dioptres. However, in this case, this is matched by an over-convergence in the right eye, an appropriate adjustment for the rotation of the head with respect to the target observed in the pictures. The binocular response is linear for all targets.

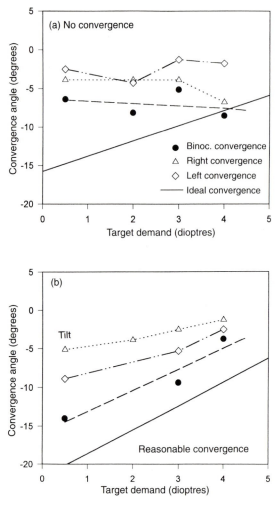

Fig. 15.7 Examples of the convergence responses from some of the youngest infants tested. (a) An example of what is described as a 'flat' response in a 19-day-old infant. The convergence is inappropriate at all target distances. (b) An example of reasonable convergence response in a 17-day-old infant. The difference between the position of the right and left eye at 0.5 dioptres is accounted for by a head tilt. Otherwise, the responses show a reasonable fit to a linear function.

have a constant left esotropia. Occasionally, a pattern of convergence insuf-ficiency is seen, with increasing divergence for near targets. Fig. 15.8(b) shows an extreme case of this for a 30-day-old infant. The exotropia seen in the left eye gets substantially worse as target distance decreases, with a resulting flat binocular convergence function.

Whether these are consistent patterns across age is unclear. In a few cases, the infants were tested more than once. Sometimes, on a second testing, no

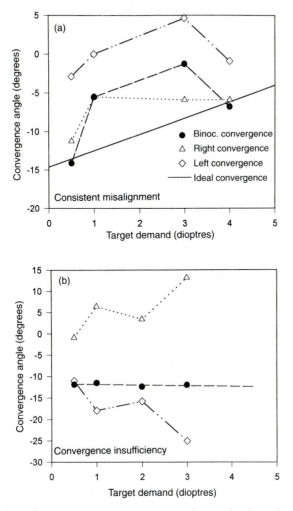

Fig. 15.8 Examples of inappropriate convergence, observed relatively infrequently in this sample of infants. (a) 'Consistent misalignment' in a 44-day-old infant. In this example, the binocular response is very non-linear, and inappropriate at all target distances. Across all targets, there is a consistent difference in the position of the left and right eyes with the left eye consistently over-converged. It appears that this infant has a constant right esotropia. (b) Convergence insufficiency in a 30-day-old infant, in whom the eyes appear to become increasingly diverged with decreasing target distance. Note that the binocular response in this infant is flat.

problems were revealed. In a few cases, infants continued to have problems of convergence. Clearly, this is an area where more systematic longitudinal testing would be of benefit; currently we are trying to re-test more of our subjects.

CONCLUSION

In these data, evidence is presented that many normal infants possess a mechanism to produce appropriate binocular convergence to static targets as early as the first month of life. Although newborns were not tested, other workers have tested them and reported that newborns too can align their eyes on static targets in depth, if they are paying attention. Unlike some earlier studies, our conclusions are based on carefully scored photographs, measuring the position of the corneal reflection relative to the pupil in both eyes simultaneously. While this method is the basis of the familiar observational Hirschberg test, there is the added benefit of a permanent, magnified record that can be carefully analysed for each eye separately and for the eyes together. Usually the Hirschberg test is performed for one eye at a time. If fixation shifts from moment to moment, the observer can have difficulty correcting estimates of alignment for these shifts. The influence of head position needs to be measured in our set-up more precisely; however, the data suggest that even the youngest infants are able to shift their binocular alignment to adjust for changes in the position of the head with respect to the target. Along with the close resemblance between the slope of the convergence response curve to the convergence demand curve, this is evidence that these behaviours are under visual control. The visuomotor system is not 'open loop' even at 1 month of age, far before the emergence of stereopsis.

The data agree with some of the observations of eye alignment reported earlier. Like Horwood (1993), in our study most normal infants can show good alignment, at least when they are interested in the targets. Episodes of both esotropia and exotropia have been found, but of much smaller angle and less frequently than reported by Sondhi *et al.* (1988) and Archer *et al.* (1989). Further analysis to estimate exact proportions of misalignment at each age is required. Even without those measures, however, it is clear the data are in striking disagreement with the Nixon *et al.* (1985) and Archer *et al.* (1989) findings about the very high proportion of large exotropias for normal infants before 6 months of age. Despite trying several different scenarios to understand what they might have been seeing, there is no satisfactory explanation of why those data differ so much from ours. We suspect some combination of problems with the subjective measurement used, the infants' fleeting attention and their exact distance and position with respect to the experimenter. It seems unlikely that, as Horwood suggests, merely lack of interest in the experimenter's face would explain what they report as the rule.

How might infants be controlling their convergence under these circumstances? Should we be surprised at this result in respect to infants' poor visual acuity, the lack of binocular functions such as stereopsis, and the presumed lack of distinctive cortical ocular dominance columns? We may be focusing too much on the precise, acute spatial vision that we are familiar with as adults, giving too much emphasis to the fovea and binocularity as represented by stereopsis. One possibility that we and others (Schor 1990) have entertained is that early vergence is controlled separately in the two eyes. If each eye uses a consistent retinal locus with which it points at a target, then nearer targets will require each eye to turn inwards, giving the appearance of convergence but not controlled by a binocular process, in the usual sense of that term.

Alternatively, there could be some early form of cortical binocular processing that predates stereopsis that is sensitive to objects at different distances. Cues to the distance of interesting targets may come from accommodative or proximal vergence. In our infant data, there are no signs of any significant connection between accommodation and convergence until at least 2–3 months of age, which probably disconfirms that it is accommodative vergence. Closer analysis of accommodation/convergence linkages is currently underway. Proximal vergence is driven by the perceived distance of the object. Estimates of relative object distance can be derived from monocular parallax. However, the infant's head is stabilized during testing so that it is unlikely that significant motion parallax is available, although it cannot be ruled out completely. A final possibility is that the response seen is driven by crude disparity detectors, too gross to be detected by the tests of stereopsis used with infants to date but sufficient to position the eyes appropriately.

One candidate as a primitive cortical mechanism for this early vergence control was described in passing by Held (1988): a mechanism that signals registration of images by maximizing firing rate. With such a mechanism in place, the eyes could be aligned reasonably precisely much of the time, allowing the conditions for the emergence of cells coded for eye-of-origin, which can add the sign of the disparity to information about the size of the difference in images between the two eyes. The more primitive alignment process may be induced by the disparity of retinal images falling on non-corresponding peripheral retinal locations. This process would be more dependent on peripheral retina and consequently on sensitivities to lower spatial frequencies, both of which are more mature than corresponding foveal functions in the infant.

Panum's area (the area of sensory fusion in front and behind the convergence plane, effectively a dead-zone during which we have single vision despite retinal disparities) is broader both in the periphery and for lower spatial frequencies (Ogle *et al.* 1949). Within the limits of our measurement, and probably also of infant vision, a mechanism such as this could align the eyes reasonably well, if there was some time for trial and error correction. This might not be a problem for an attractive stationary target; however, the calculations could be more than an infant can manage for dynamic stimuli. Also if the sign of the discrepancy had to be arrived at by trial and error, rather than by a mechanism that codes for the direction of the disparity, infants would, as reported, have trouble with moving targets. The search process would never be able to correctly 'tune in' a convergence movement for a target moving in depth, at least until it came to rest at one distance. The most common clinical test for vergence with infants is to ask the infant to follow an approaching or receding target, which may be why many clinicians do not report vergence appearing until a later age.

Whether this is the correct explanation for these data remains to be established by further experimentation. We continue to be surprised by how well very young infants manage their visual/motor performance. This surprise probably stems from the common tendency to view the infant visual system as 'deficient', even in the normal case. Visual development is rapid and complex. While clearly not adult-like, the sensory and motor functions present early in life may be more than sufficient to 'bootstrap' the coarse forms of binocular fusion, both motor and sensory, commonly observed in young infants. This might be based on use of peripheral parts of the retina.

Data such as these do not answer any questions about what goes wrong for children who develop strabismus early in life, although they do imply that eye alignment problems probably represent the loss of some normal orthotropic controls, rather than a failure for a normal orthotropia to develop gradually. Given the complexity of the sensory and motor connections that are being established early in infancy, the causes of developmental eye alignment problems are almost certainly multiple. Some non-mutually exclusive candidates include problems in forming the linkages between sensory and motor retinal maps; relationships between accommodation and convergence (AC/A and CA/C ratios); and problems with the development of motion sensitivity mechanisms including the pursuit system. Such sensory-motor relationships are complex, and it will take time and some real creativity to design experiments that will answer these questions with infants.

ACKNOWLEDGEMENTS

We would like to thank the staff of the Infant Study Center, both past and present, who were responsible for testing the babies and organizing the data. Without them, our research would not be possible. This research was completed with the support of NIH Grant EY-03957, and PSC-CUNY Faculty Research Award Program grants 669455, 662226, and 663218 to the first author.

REFERENCES

Abramov, I., Gordon, J., Hendrickson, A., Hainline, L., Dobson, V., and LaBossiere, E. (1982). The retina of the newborn human infant. *Science*, **217**, 265–7.

Abramov, I., Hainline, L., and Duckman, R. (1990). Screening infant vision with paraxial photorefraction. *Optometry and Visual Science*, **67**, 538–45.

Archer, S. M. (1993). Detection and treatment of congenital esotropia. In *Early visual development: normal and abnormal,* (ed. K. Simons), pp. 349–63. Oxford University Press, New York.

Archer, S. M., Sondhi, N., and Helveston, E. M. (1989). Strabismus in infancy. *Ophthalmology*, **96**, 133–7.

Aslin, R. M. (1977). Development of binocular fixation in human infants. *Journal of Experimental Child Psychology*, **23**, 133–50.

Baitch, L. and Srebro, R. (1990). Binocular interactions in sleeping and awake human infants. *Investigative Ophthalmology and Visual Science*, **31** (suppl.), 251.

Banks, M. S. and Bennett, P. J. (1988). Optical and photoreceptor immaturities limit the spatial and chromatic vision of human infants. *Journal of the Optical Society of America*, **5**, 2059–79.

Birch, E. E. (1993). Stereopsis in infants and its developmental relationship to visual acuity. In *Early visual development: normal and abnormal*, (ed. K. Simons), pp. 224–36. Oxford University Press, New York.

Birch, E. E., Gwiazda, J., and Held, R. (1982). Stereoacuity for crossed and uncrossed disparities in human infants. *Vision Research*, **22**, 507–13.

Birch, E. E., Gwiazda, J., and Held, R. (1983). The development of vergence does not account for the onset of stereopsis. *Perception*, **12**, 331–6.

Braddick, O., Wattam-Bell, J., Day, J., and Atkinson, J. (1983). The onset of binocular function in human infants. *Human Neurobiology*, **2**, 65–9.

Chavasse, B. F. (1939). *Worth's squint or the binocular reflexes and the treatment of strabismus.* Blakiston, Philadelphia.

Crawford, M. L. J. and von Noorden, G. K. (1979). The effect of short-term experimental strabismus on the visual system of *Macaca mulatta*. *Investigative Ophthalmology and Visual Science*, **18**, 496–505.

Crawford, M. L. J. and von Noorden, G. K. (1980). Optically induced concomitant strabismus in monkeys. *Investigative Ophthalmology and Visual Science*, **19**, 1105–9.

Dobson, V. and Teller, D. Y. (1978). Visual acuity in human infants: a review and comparison of behavioural and electrophysiological studies. *Vision Research*, **18**, 1469–83.

Eizenman, M., Skarf, B., and McCulloch, D. (1989). Development of binocular vision in infants. *Investigative Ophthalmology and Visual Science*, **30** (suppl.), 313.

Graves, A., Trotter, Y., and Fregnac, Y. (1987). Role of extraocular muscle proprioception in the development of depth perception in cats. *Journal of Neurophysiology*, **85**, 816–31.

Hainline, L. (1978). Developmental changes in scanning of face and nonface patterns by infants. *Journal of Experimental Child Psychology*, **25**, 90–115.

Hainline, L. (1993). Conjugate eye movements in infants. In *Early visual development: normal and abnormal*, (ed. K. Simons), pp. 47–79. Oxford University Press, New York.

Hainline, L. and Abramov, I. (1992). Assessing visual development: is infant vision good enough? In *Advances in infancy research*, Vol. 7, (ed. C. Rovee-Collier and L. P. Lipsitt), pp. 39–102. Ablex, Norwood, New Jersey.

Hainline, L., Riddell, P. M., Grose-Fifer, J., and Abramov, I. (1992). Development of accommodation and convergence in infancy. *Behavioural Brain Research*, **49**, 33–50.

Haith, M. M., Berman, R., and Moore, M. (1977). Eye contact and face scanning in early infancy. *Science*, **198**, 853–5.

Haynes, H., White, B. L., and Held, R. (1965). Visual accommodation in human infants. *Science*, **141**, 528–30.

Hein, A. and Diamond, R. (1983). Contribution of eye movement to the representation of space. In *Spatially oriented behavior*, (ed. A. Hein and M. Jeannerod), pp. 119–32. Springer, New York.

Held, R. (1985). Binocular vision: behavioural and neural development. In *Neonate cognition: beyond the blooming, buzzing confusion*, (ed. J. Mehler and R. Fox), pp. 37–44. Erlbaum, Hillsdale, New Jersey.

Held, R. (1988). Normal visual development and its deviations. In *Strabismus and amblyopia*, (ed. G. Lennerstrand, G. K. von Noorden, and E. C. Campos), pp. 247–57. Macmillan, London.

Held, R. (1993). Two stages in binocular development. In *Early visual development: normal and abnormal*, (ed. K. Simons), pp. 250–7. Oxford University Press, New York.

Hickey, J. L. and Peduzzi, J. D. (1987). Structure and development in the visual system. In *Handbook of infant perception*, Vol. 1, (ed. P. Salapatek and L. B. Cohen), pp. 1–42. Academic Press, New York.

Horwood, A. (1993). Maternal observations of ocular alignment in infants. *Journal of Pediatric Ophthalmology and Strabismus*, **30**, 100–5.

Katz, L., Eizenman, M., and Skarf, B. (1991). VEP measurements of cortical binocularity in adults and infants using dichoptic checkerboards. *Investigative Ophthalmology and Visual Science*, **32** (suppl.), 964.

Kiorpes, L. and Kiper, D. C. (1991). Peripheral contrast sensitivity during development in macaque monkeys. *Investigative Ophthalmology and Visual Science*, **32** (suppl.), 1044.

Krinsky, S., Hainline, L., and Scanlon, M. (1990). In pursuit of smooth pursuit: a repeated excursion approach. *Infant Behavior and Development*, **13**, 462a.

LeVay, S., Wiesel, T. N., and Hubel, D. H. (1980). The development of ocular dominance columns in normal and visually deprived monkeys. *Journal of Comparative Neurology*, **161**, 1–51.

Ling, B. C. (1942). A genetic study of sustained visual fixation and associated behaviour in the human infant from birth to six months. *Journal of Genetic Psychology*, **61**, 227–77.

Maurer, D. (1975). The development of binocular convergence in infants. Doctoral dissertation, University of Minnesota, 1974. *Dissertation Abstracts*, **35**, 6136-B.

Nixon, R. B., Helveston, E. M., Miller, K., Archer, S. M., and Ellis, F. D. (1985). Incidence of strabismus in neonates. *American Journal of Ophthalmology*, **100**, 798–801.

Ogle, K. N., Mussey, F., and Prangen, A. (1949). Fixation disparity and the fusional processes of binocular single vision. *American Journal of Ophthalmology*, **32**, 1069–87.

Packer, O., Hendrickson, A. E., and Curcio, C. (1990). Developmental redistribution of photoreceptors across the *Macaca nemestrina* (pigtail macaque) retina. *Journal of Comparative Neurology*, **298**, 472–93.

Piaget, J. (1952). *The Origins of Intelligence in Children*. Norton, New York.

Reinecke, R., Sterling, R., and Wizov, S. (1991). Accuracy of judgements of the presence or absence of eccentric (non-primary) gaze and the presence or absence of strabismus. *Binocular Vision Quarterly*, **6**, 189–96.

Riddell, P. M., Hainline, L., and Abramov, I. (1994). Measurement of the Hirschberg test in human infants. *Investigative Ophthalmology and Visual Science*, **35**, 538–43.

Schor, C. M. (1990). Visuomotor development. In *Principles and practice of pediatric optometry*, (ed. A. A. Rosenbloom and M. W. Morgan), pp. 66–90. Lippincott, Philadelphia.

Shimojo, S., Bauer, J. A., O'Connell, K. M., and Held, R. (1986). Pre-stereoptic binocular vision in infants. *Vision Research*, **26**, 501–10.

Skarf, B., Katz, L. M., Bachynski, B., and Eizenman, M. (1992). Two-stage development of fusion and stereopsis in human infants: a VEP study. *Investigative Ophthalmology and Visual Science*, **33** (suppl.), 1353.

Slater, A. M. and Findlay, J. M. (1972). The measurement of fixation position in the newborn baby. *Journal of Experimental Child Psychology*, **14**, 349–64.

Slater, A. M. and Findlay, J. M. (1975). Binocular fixation in the newborn baby. *Journal of Experimental Child Psychology*, **20**, 248–73.

Sondhi, N., Archer, S. M., and Helveston, E. M. (1988). Development of normal ocular alignment. *Journal of Pediatric Ophthalmology and Strabismus*, **25**, 210–11.

Stager, D. R. and Birch, E.E. (1986). Preferential looking acuity and stereopsis in infantile esotropia. *Journal of Pediatric Ophthalmology and Strabismus*, **23**, 160–5.

Teller, D.Y. and Movshon, J. A. (1986). Visual development. *Vision Research*, **26**, 1481–90.

Thelan, E. (1989). Self organization in developmental processes: can systems approaches work? In *Systems and development: The Minnesota symposium on child psychology*, Vol.22, (ed. M. R. Gunnar and E. Thelan), pp. 77–117. Erlbaum, Hillsdale, New Jersey.

Thorn, F., Gwiazda, J., Cruz, A., Bauer, J., and Held, R. (1994). Eye alignment, sensory binocularity, and convergence in young infants. *Investigative Ophthalmology and Visual Science*, **25**, 544–53.

Trotter, Y., Fregnac, Y., and Buisseret, P. (1987). The period of susceptibility of visual cortical binocularity to unilateral proprioceptive deafferentiation of extroacular muscles. *Journal of Neurophysiology*, **58**, 795–815.

Tyler, C. W. (1990). A stereoscopic view of visual processing streams. *Vision Research*, **30**, 1877–95.

von Noorden, G. K. (1984). Infantile esotropia: a continuing riddle. *American Orthoptic Journal*, **34**, 52–62.

von Noorden, G. K. (1988*a*). Current concepts of infantile esotropia. *Eye*, **2**, 343–57.

von Noorden, G. K. (1988*b*). A reassessment of infantile esotropia. *American Journal of Ophthalmology*, **105**, 1–10.

Wick, B. and London, R. (1980). The Hirschberg Test: analysis from birth to age 5. *Journal of the American Optometric Association*, **51**, 1009–10.

Wickelgren, B. (1967). Convergence in the human newborn. *Journal of Experimental Child Psychology*, **5**, 74–85.

Wilson, H. R. (1988). Development of spatiotemporal mechanisms in infant vision. *Vision Research*, **28**, 611–28.

Worth, C (1903). *Squint: its causes, pathology, and treatment*. Bale, Sons and Danielson, London.

Yuodelis, C. and Hendrickson, A. (1986). A qualitative and quantitative analysis of the human fovea during development. *Vision Research*, **26**, 847–55.

16

Eye–head relations in neonates and young infants

I. Carchon and H. Bloch

SUMMARY

A basic issue is to determine whether the probability of obtaining eye–head coupling depends upon the stimulus location in the visual field. The present experiment investigated the effect of target direction on both oculomotor activity and head coupling in a pursuit task. Two age groups were compared: neonates (3 days old) and young infants (45 days old). Horizontal eye movements were measured from EOG recordings and were also recorded by a video camera. A second camera filmed head movements. The data show that pursuit is more extended when the target moves from the periphery to the centre (P→C) at both ages. In most cases, smooth pursuit is performed in the central region of the visual field (0–24°), regardless of whether the starting point of the target is central or peripheral. To analyse eye–head coupling, the portion of smooth pursuit performed with ipsilateral head movements was examined. There was more smooth pursuit in the 45-day-old infants than in the neonates, and more in the centre-to-periphery (C→P) condition than in the periphery-to-centre condition.

INTRODUCTION

The existence and the nature of oculocephalic relations in very young infants is a topic of long-standing debate: Roucoux *et al.* (1983) argued that, because of foveal immaturity, the head must intervene very early in visual pursuit. Hence young infants would perform large saccades similar to those observed in afoveate animals. In this account, the role of infant head movements would differ greatly from its later role in child and adult visual perception.

Regal *et al.* (1983) observed sequential patterns of eye–head coupling as early as the first month of life; generally a head movement following an eye saccade and, less frequently, an eye saccade following a head rotation. They interpreted these data as showing that the young infant's ocular activity in a pursuit task is mainly saccadic. However, other researchers have reported that visual pursuit can include some portions of smooth eye movements. Smooth eye movements in young infants were described at least 30 years ago by Dayton and Jones (1964) and confirmed by Kremenitzer *et al.* (1979).

More recently, we showed that head movements in 45-day-old infants are more frequently coupled with smooth eye movements than with saccadic displacement (Bloch and Carchon 1992; Carchon and Bloch 1993). These findings run counter to the explanation given by Roucoux *et al.* (1983). In the same study, our data indicated that neonates did not use their heads, although their pursuit appeared to be composite, that is, made up of small portions of smooth pursuit but primarily of saccades. Smooth pursuit must be increased and stabilized in order for the head to be used in visual activity.

The basic issue is to determine which situational features, such as position of a target in the visual field, favour smooth eye movements. Since peripheral vision is more mature at birth than central vision (Mann 1964; Abramov *et al.* 1982), the neonate cannot be expected to follow a target exclusively with smooth eye movements.

The visual field is still small at birth (Tronick 1972; Harris and Mac Farlane 1974; Mohn and van Hof-van Duin 1986; Sireteanu, Chapter 2, this volume). Thus there should be smooth pursuit of targets in the central region of the visual field more easily than in eccentric regions. Smooth eye movements make maintenance of central fixation possible by holding spatial coordinates constant. This requires head participation, because, as Bishop (1970) has shown, the eye has no detector of its own position. Thus smooth eye movement is likely to be observed when the starting point of a mobile target is easily fixated and corresponds to the median plane of the subject's head (i.e. corresponds to what is called the orthostatic position). Note that if the target trajectory starts from an eccentric position, it would be captured by peripheral vision and would result in saccadic pursuit up to the vicinity of the centre.

The aim of the present experiment was to investigate the effect of target direction. For this purpose, a target trajectory from centre (0°) to the periphery (48°) was compared with a trajectory from periphery (48°) to the centre (0°) for both oculomotor activity and head coupling. The hypotheses were the following:

(1) Pursuit of a target should be more extended when the target moves from the periphery (P) to the centre (C) than when the target moves from centre to the periphery, because it requires more peripheral vision.

(2) Smooth pursuit should occur more frequently when the target moves from centre to the periphery than from the periphery to the centre.

(3) Head movements should accompany smooth pursuit more often when the target moves from the centre to the periphery than in the opposite way. Smooth pursuit was predicted to increase in the first month of life. Accordingly, centre to periphery head movements should tend to be more pronounced in 45-day-olds than in neonates.

METHOD

Subjects

Eight newborns (4 boys and 4 girls) with an average age of 3 days (±1 day) and 11 infants (6 boys and 5 girls) aged 45 days (±5 days) were tested in the Maternity Unit of the International Hospital of the University of Paris. All met standard criteria for normal delivery, Apgar scores (10) and a state of quiet alertness.

Stimulus

The target was a light cross of 5° in angular subtense. It was formed by nine red and six green diodes. The target was attached to the lens of a camera, placed at the subject's eye line. The distance of the target from the subject's eye was 40 cm. The camera was operated by an electric motor, producing an horizontal translation of exactly 48°, with an angular velocity of 10°/s. Small variations could affect velocity from one trial to another. However, the velocity was constant over each trial. Two conditions were tested:

(1) C→P condition: the target moved 48° from the centre to the right periphery (no condition to the left periphery was employed because no differences between left to right or right to left were observed in a preliminary experiment);

(2) P→C condition: the target started at 48° in the right periphery and moved to the centre.

Experimental set-up

The experimental set-up is depicted in Fig. 16.1. The baby was seated comfortably in a slightly inclined seat adapted to his/her size, in a neutral grey enclosure. The target was viewed through a horizontal slot facing the subject.

Data recording

Ocular activity was recorded by two independent devices, as described by Finocchio *et al.* (1990):

(1) A video camera 1 (Sony CCD 445, 8 mm) supported the stimulus and filmed the eye movements.

(2) To obtain a finer measure of ocular motility, horizontal eye movements were measured from EOG recordings. Miniature electrodes (BBCOM 3-01-2020-60) measuring 4 mm in diameter (contact with silver chloride) were placed at the outside corners of each eye, horizontal to the pupil. A third ground electrode was positioned on the subject's forehead. No visible discomfort was observed from these electrodes.

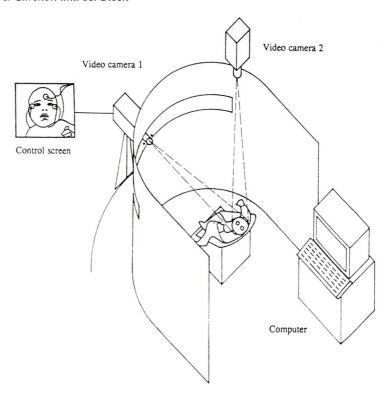

Fig. 16.1 Diagram of the experimental set-up. Eye and head movements filmed by two independent video cameras.

(3) A second camera 2 (of the same type) was placed above the subject's head and filmed head movements. Two reflective self-adhesive dots were placed on the infant's head (one on the vertex and the other behind in line with the first one) and served as markers for measuring the angle of head rotation with reference to the sagittal axis.

Procedure

The experimenter put the baby in the infant seat and attached the electrodes. A trial began when the subject was in a quiet alert behavioural state, and the baby's gaze was fixed on the target. At least two trials in each direction were obtained for each subject.

Data reduction

Analysis of EOG signals

A method similar to the one used by Finocchio *et al.* (1990) was employed. This consisted in overlaying the data from the video recording of eye movements with the EOG signal data. The study by Finocchio *et al.* on 2- and 3-month-old infants shows that the EOG signal is linear up to ±20° of eccentricity.

Video analysis of eye movements

Eye movement data from video images were analysed in 500 ms frames to locate the time periods when the infant's eyes were on the target. This analysis is descriptive.

Video analysis of head movements

Video images (from camera 2) were converted with a digital video system interfaced with a computer,[1] and thus served to code the X and Y coordinates of the two dots frame by frame, and to measure head angle from the vertical geographic position.

The system accuracy permits appreciation of a deviation of 1° in the horizontal plane. However, a head rotation was defined if the movement was above a threshold criterion of 5° of amplitude.

Timing correspondences between the filtered EOG and video data were used to plot a graph for each trial and each subject. Each graph showed the target course, EOG outline, head angle, and what we call the 'theoretical curve' of the eyes, on the same amplitude scale. The 'theoretical curve' was obtained by measuring the algebraic difference between the angular position of the target and the angular position of the head. It thus represents perfect pursuit, that is, the position of the eyes for and only for, a constant and continuous pursuit of the target. Two categories in eye movements were distinguished:

(1) the saccade is a jump, a deviation of the eye with a threshold criterion amplitude of 5° or more, and a velocity of more than 10°/s;
(2) when the eyes remained on the target before or after a saccade that was considered as 'smooth pursuit'.

Comparison of these four curves provided a picture of the association between head and eye movements during each trial. Computations of amplitude, frequency and duration parameters are based on these data.

RESULTS

The mean extent of pursuit

First, the sum of pursuit time for a trial and for each individual was extracted from video recorder analysis, by two independent observers. The following equation yielded the extent of pursuit (E):

$$E = V \times t$$

where V is the velocity of the target per second and t is the total pursuit

---

[1] The digital video computer system was developed by C. Kervella, CNRS engineer in the laboratory.

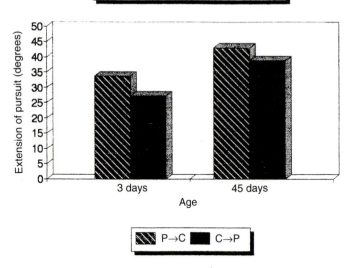

Fig. 16.2 Graph of the extent of pursuit of an object according to the direction of target for 3-day-old and 45-day-old neonates. Target directions: from periphery to centre (P→C) and from centre to periphery (C→P).

duration. **The average extent of pursuit** in degrees is given for each group, in each condition in Fig. 16.2. Fig. 16.2 shows that the extent of pursuit was slightly larger in the P→C condition than in the C→P condition and for both ages. In the P→C condition, neonates detected the target in 10 out of 18 trials at around 18° from the starting point (48°). Then, their eyes remained on the target up to the centre. In the C→P condition, the target was lost before the target reached 32° (at about 27°).

As shown by Tronick (1972), target movement seems to be easily detectable by the newborn in the peripheral field.

Features of ocular activity

The form of ocular activity was initially examined using the following two criteria:

(1) the proportion of smooth pursuit (Fig. 16.3);
(2) the number and direction of ocular saccades (Figs 16.4 and 16.5).

Fig. 16.3 shows the proportion of smooth pursuit according to the duration of the target course.

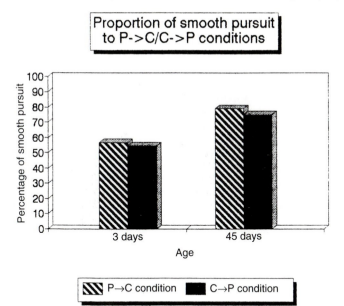

Fig. 16.3 Graph showing the percentage of smooth pursuit according to the target course (P→C and C→P) in 3-day-old and 45-day-old neonates.

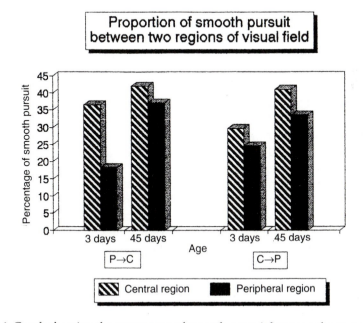

Fig. 16.4 Graph showing the percentage of smooth pursuit between the two regions of the visual field: a central one from 0 to 24°, and a peripheral one from 24 to 48°.

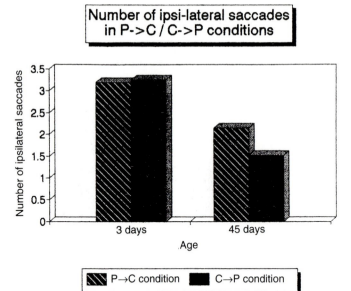

Fig. 16.5 Number of ipsilateral saccades for P→C and C→P in 3-day-old and 45-day-old neonates.

Strikingly, as shown in Fig. 16.3, a high proportion of smooth eye movements was observed, even in 3-day-olds. The proportion increased in 45-day-olds. For both ages, the proportion of smooth pursuit was a little more prominent in the P→C condition but the difference was negligible.

The environmental visual field (i.e. the field of the target course) was bisected in order to compare pursuit in a central region and in a peripheral one. The central region is defined by the space from 0–24° and a peripheral region beyond 24° up to 48° (Fig. 16.4).

In newborns, as shown in Fig. 16.4, smooth pursuit accompanied the target course more often in the central region than in the peripheral one. The difference between these two regions was significant for the P→C condition (Student t test = 3.27 d.f. = 7 $p < 0.02$) but not for the C→P condition. No significant difference was found in the two conditions for the 45-day-old babies who presented smoother pursuit than the neonates.

Hypothesis 2 on the more frequent relation between the presence of smooth pursuit in the C→P condition than in P→C condition was thus partially confirmed. In all cases, whatever the starting point of the target, smoother pursuit occurred when the target was in the central region of the visual field. These results suggest that smooth pursuit related to the spatial

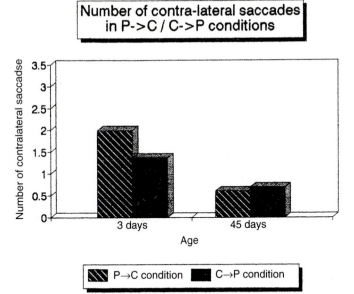

Fig. 16.6 Number of contralateral saccades for P→C and C→P in 3-day-old and 45-day-old neonates.

coordinates, which themselves are related to the orthostatic position of the head.

To assess the features of oculomotor activity, the number of ocular saccades during pursuit was measured per trial and per subject. Since pursuit time varied across subjects and trials, the number of saccades was calculated with respect to the same pursuit time value. For example, subject X tracked the target for 60% of the total trial duration and made two saccades. This number of saccades was then scaled for the total trial duration, in this case $(2 \times 100)/60 = 3$ saccades.

The comparison between Figs 16.5 and 16.6 shows that saccades were performed in the direction of the target movement more frequently than in the opposite direction. The number of saccades decreased from 3 to 45 days. Neonates produce more saccades than the 45-day-olds in accordance with the literature (Aslin and Salapatek 1975; Aslin 1987), which indicates that the saccadic component of pursuit decreases with age.

The number of ipsilateral saccades differed with the direction of the target and was slightly larger in P→C than C→P condition, only for neonates, because in the C→P condition pursuit was less eccentric, as indicated in the first paragraph.

Table 16.1 The maximal amplitude of the head rotation according to the direction of the target (P→C and C→P) for both ages.

Age	P→C	C→P
3 days old	9.4	19.5
45 days old	18.1	17

Characteristics of head movements

Since the head did not always return to its initial position, the maximal angular deviation (in degrees) was calculated to obtain a measure of the range of head movements (Table 16.1).

As shown in Table 16.1, 45-day-olds used their heads more systematically than newborns. This is consistent with an increase of pursuit and with increasing control of the head. Neonates moved their heads less when the target position was not centred.

As already noted, head rotations were included if they were above a threshold criterion of 5° of amplitude, performed in the horizontal plane. The number of ipsi- and contralateral rotations was calculated on the same basis as the number of saccades, that is, scaled to the total trial duration (Figs 16.7 and 16.8).

In 45-day-olds, head movements in the direction of the target (ipsilateral rotations) were clearly more numerous than head movements in the opposite direction (contralateral rotations). (For P→C condition Student t test = 5.02, d.f. = 21, and $p < 0.001$; for C→P condition $t = 4.18$, d.f. = 20, and $p < 0.001$). In 3-day-olds, when the target moved from the centre to the periphery, there were as many ipsilateral head rotations as contralateral. When the target moved from the periphery to the centre, ipsilateral head rotations were less numerous but the difference was not significant. However, the head participates more in the C→P than in the P→C condition.

The coupling of eye and head

According to Mitkin (1987), eye-head pursuit is seen as a more mature form of pursuit than ocular pursuit. It has been assumed that eye-head pursuit emerges in relation to the onset of smooth ocular movements. To test this hypothetical relationship, smooth pursuit, regardless of when it occurred, was compared with smooth pursuit coupled with ipsilateral head rotations, in both conditions (Fig. 16.9 for P→C condition and for C→P condition).

As shown in Fig. 16.9, smooth pursuit can be performed with or without head movements. In 3-day-olds, only a small portion of smooth pursuit was associated with ipsilateral head rotations. Head rotations were significantly more coupled with smooth pursuit in 45-day-olds.

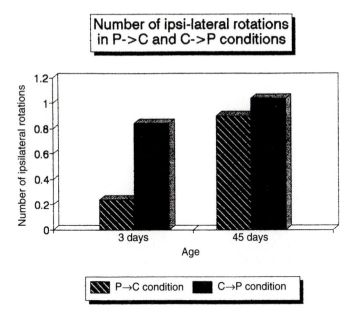

Fig. 16.7 Number of ipsilateral rotations for P→C and C→P in 3-day-old and 45-day-old neonates.

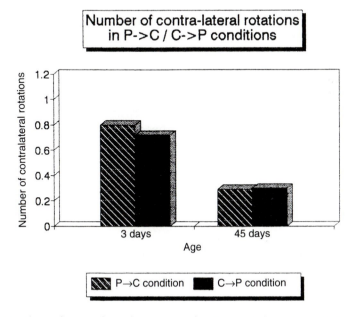

Fig. 16.8 Number of contralateral rotations for P→C and C→P in 3-day-old and 45-day-old neonates.

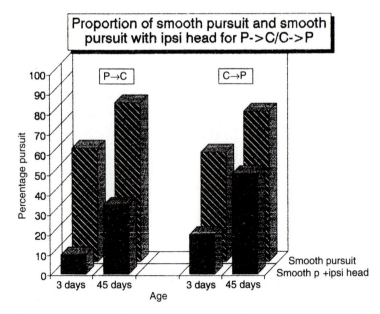

Fig. 16.9 Percentage of smooth pursuit compared with smooth pursuit with ipsilateral head rotations for P→C and C→P in 3-day-old and 45-day-old neonates.

The head accompanied pursuit more often in the C→P condition than in the P→C condition at both ages. This difference in conditions was more clearcut in the 45-day-olds.

Thus, the strong and determinant relation between the onset of smooth pursuit and eye-head coupling as suggested by Mitkin, is not confirmed in this experiment. However, it does not mean that smooth pursuit would not be a condition for the onset of such a coordination.

Fig. 16.10 shows the proportion of smooth pursuit coupled with ipsilateral head rotations in the two regions of the environmental visual field (central and peripheral regions). 45-day-olds coupled head with smooth pursuit even in the peripheral region when the target started from the periphery. This suggests that they tended to read a stable position that enabled them to maintain the spatial coordinates invariant.

CONCLUSION

The findings of our study show that the extent of visual pursuit is greater when the target moves from the periphery to the central visual field but, in this direction of motion, more saccades are observed than in the opposite direction. The first hypothesis is thus confirmed.

This result can be attributed to the optimization of the situation: the size of the target was large enough to be salient, the target distance was small, and its

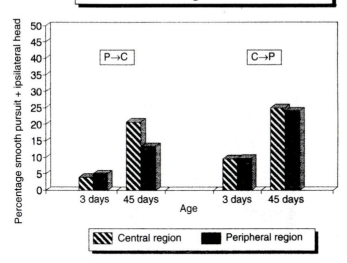

Fig. 16.10 Percentage of smooth pursuit with ipsilateral head rotations between the two regions of the visual field: a central region (from 0 to 24°), and a peripheral region (from 24 to 48°).

velocity was slow. This velocity (around 10°/s) had been shown by Roucoux *et al.* (1982) to promote very early pursuit activity. Furthermore, as pointed out by Tronick (1972) detection of an eccentric movement may have also enhanced pursuit.

Contrary to expectation (hypothesis 2), the amount of smooth pursuit does not differ in the two conditions. Furthermore, this smooth pursuit was coupled more with ipsilateral head rotations in the C→P condition than in the P→C at both ages. These data suggest that the C→P condition favours oculocephalic smooth pursuit, while the P→C condition favours ocular pursuit alone. This difference was still present in 45-day-olds, who used their heads more systematically than did the 3-day-olds. This confirms our hypothesis concerning the more probable coupling of the head with smooth ocular movements in the C→P condition.

The findings are discrepant with the position adopted by Roucoux *et al.* (1983) concerning a foveal saccadic pursuit and the role of the head in early visual behaviour. Rather the data suggest that central vision is functional in neonates (Mac Farlane *et al.* 1976; Lewis *et al.* 1978; Lewis and Maurer 1980; Atkinson 1984; Yuodelis and Hendrickson 1986).

From birth to the second month, considerable changes take place in visual activity. One of these consists in increased participation of the head. This implies greater control of head motility before the infant is able to hold its head upright.

ACKNOWLEDGEMENTS

We would like to thank the laboratory engineer, Claude Kervella, who built the video system for analysis of head rotations and for all the EOG treatment. We would also like to thank the director of the Maternity Unit, Dr H. Cohen, who authorized testing in this unit, the nurses for their help and kindness, and all the babies and their parents for having participated in this study. Mr K. Knoblauch is thanked for his help in polishing our English.

REFERENCES

Abramov, I., Gordon, J., Hendrickson, A., Hainline, L., Dobson, V., and Laboissiere, E. (1982). The retina of the newborn human infant. *Science*, **271**, 265–7.

Aslin, R. N. (1987). *Motor aspects of visual development in infancy*. In *Handbook of infant perception, from sensation to perception*, Vol. 1., (ed. P. Salapatek and L. Cohen), Academic Press, New York.

Aslin, R. N. and Salapatek, P. (1975). Saccadic localization of visual pattern targets by the very young human infant. *Perception and Psychophysics*, **17**(3), 293–319.

Atkinson, J. (1984). *How does infant vision change in the first months of life*, Continuity of neural functions from prenatal to postnatal life, (ed. H. F. R. Prechtl), Spastics International Medical Publications and Blackwell Scientific, Oxford.

Bishop, P. O. (1970). Beginning of form vision end binocular depth discrimination in cortex. In *The neurosciences second study program*, pp. 471–85. Rockefeller University Press, New York.

Bloch, H. and Carchon, I. (1992). On the onset of eye-head coordination in infants. *Behavioural Brain Research*, **49**, 85–90.

Carchon, I. and Bloch, H. (1993). Fonctionnement oculaire et coordination oculo-céphalique: méthode de traitement du signal électro-oculographique chez le nouveau-né et le nourrisson de 6 semaines. *Psychologie Française*, **38**, 1.

Dayton, G. O. and Jones, M. H. (1964). Analysis of characteristics of fixation reflex in infants by use of direct current electrooculography. *Neurology*, **14**, 1152–6.

Finocchio, D. V., Preston, K. L., and Fuchs, A. F. (1990). Obtaining a quantitative measure of eye movements in human infants: a method of calibrating the electro-oculogram. *Vision Research*, **30**, 1119–28.

Harris, P. and Mac Farlane, A. (1974). The growth of the effective visual field from birth to seven weeks. *Journal of Experimental Child Psychology*, **18**, 340–8.

Kremenitzer, J. P., Vaughan, H. G., Kurtzberg, D., and Dowling K. (1979). Smooth pursuit eye movements in the newborn infant. *Child Development*, **50**, 442–8.

Lewis, T. L. and Maurer, D. (1980). Central vision in the newborn. *Journal of Experimental Child Psychology*, **26**, 475–80.

Lewis, T. L., Maurer, D., and Kay, D. (1978). Newborn's central vision: whole or hole? *Journal of Experimental Child Psychology*, **26**, 193–203.

MacFarlane, A., Harris, P., and Barnes, I. (1976). Central and peripheral vision in early infancy. *Journal of Experimental Child Psychology*, **21**, 532–8.

Mann, I. (1964). *The development of human eye*. British Medical Association, London.

Mitkin, A. (1987). *Eye movements and visual functions in infancy*. Proceedings of the IXth Biennial Meeting of International Society for the Study of Behavioural Development, pp. 80–90. Tokyo.

Mohn, G. and van Hof-van Duin, J. (1986). Development of binocular and monocular visual fields of human infants during the first year of life. *Clinical Vision Science*, **1**, 51–64.

Regal, D. M., Ashmead, D. H., and Salapatek, P. (1983). The coordination of eye and head movements during infancy: a selective review. *Behavioural Brain Research*, **10**, 125–32.

Roucoux, A., Culée, C., and Roucoux, M. (1982). Gaze fixation and pursuit in head free human infants. In *Physiological and pathological aspects of eye movements*, (ed. Roucoux and Crommelinck), pp. 23–31, W. Junk Publishers, The Hague.

Roucoux, A., Culée, C., and Roucoux, M. (1983). Development of fixation and pursuit eye movements in human infants. *Behavioural Brain Research*, **10**, 133–9.

Tronick, E. (1972). Stimulus control and the growth of the infant's effective visual field. *Perception and Psychophysics*, **11**, 373–6.

Yuodelis, C. and Hendrickson, A. (1986). A qualitative and quantitative analysis of the human fovea during development. *Vision Research*, **26**, 847–56.

17

Development of binocularity and its sexual differentiation

Richard Held, Frank Thorn, Jane Gwiazda, and Joseph Bauer

SENSORY BINOCULARITY

By now it appears that the chronology of development of binocular vision has been established. The essential findings are reviewed in recent articles by Birch (1993), Held (1991), and Held (1993). Several different testing procedures all fail to find any evidence for stereopsis prior to approximately 6 weeks of age, although infants are quite capable of making other sorts of visual discrimination at, and prior to, this age. The average age of onset of a selective response to binocular disparity is between 12 and 14 weeks. Almost all infants have acquired it by 6 months of age. Following an abrupt onset—from absent when tested during 1 week to present during the next—of selective response to coarse disparity, stereoacuity rises rapidly (Birch *et al.* 1982; Held *et al.* 1980). Several theories of the neuronal substrate of this process have been proposed and some have led to further insights into binocular development, as discussed in the abovementioned reviews.

Studies of interocularly rivalling stimuli have revealed aspects of binocular development. Using a two-alternative forced-choice procedure, Birch *et al.* (1985) have shown that interocularly fusible stimuli, such as in-phase checkerboards, become preferred over rivalling stimuli, such as out-of-phase checkerboards, at approximately the same age at which stereoptic stimuli become discriminated. In these experiments, it appears that maturation of binocularity makes the rival grating aversive.

The strong evidence for post-natal delay in onset of stereopsis and response to binocular rivalry raises the question of how binocular stimuli are perceived prior to the onset of stereopsis. The following experiments suggest that a primitive form of binocularity exists before stereopsis.

Dynamic interocularly counterphased stimuli are reported to produce significant evoked responses before such responses are evoked by stereoptic stimuli (Eizenman *et al.* 1989). This finding is in accord with the results of Shimojo *et al.* (1986) who report that interocularly orthogonal gratings are preferred to interocularly parallel gratings before the age of onset of stereopsis, although the preference is dramatically reversed at the age of onset of stereopsis. The prestereoptic preference for interocularly orthogonal gratings is believed to result

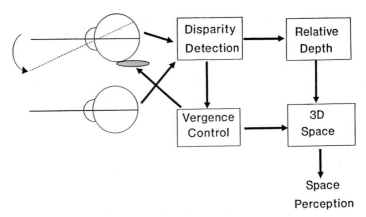

Fig. 17.1 Flow-chart for disparity detection and consequences. When disparity signals become available, they will affect vergence control at the same time as allowing stereopsis. (From Held 1993.)

from a primitive, additive process in which the orthogonal gratings are fused in order to produce the appearance of a grid. It is made plausible by the finding that an ordinary grid display is preferred to a grating display of similar dimensions (Shimojo *et al.* 1986). This preference remains until aversion to rivalry has its onset at which time the preference completely reverses. Several other examples of binocular combination confirm the existence of this primitive binocular process followed by an abrupt transition to mature binocularity (Held 1993; Shimojo 1993).

The very sharply delineated transition in time from primitive to mature binocularity has proven to be a useful marker. It also suggests an equally abrupt change in the underlying neuronal mechanism for binocular vision. To account for it, we proposed a neuronal model of the transition from primitive to mature binocularity in terms of segregation of the ocular dominance columns in layer four of the visual cortex (Held 1985, 1991, 1993; Shimojo *et al.* 1986). Alternative explanations have also been proposed as discussed in Held (1993).

MOTOR CONTROL

In addition to the abovementioned development of sensory binocularity, changes in the control of movements that depend upon binocular disparity and three-dimensional discrimination may be expected to develop simultaneously (Fig. 17.1). Control of vergence, in particular, might be expected to improve once information about binocular disparity is available. Disparity information is one of the drivers of vergence movements as shown in Fig. 17.1. In this diagram the two eyes are depicted with their optic nerve outputs feeding into a disparity detection module. The latter, in turn, sends signals to a vergence control module, which activates the extraocular musculature (shaded oblong) that produces vergence change. The disparity detection module also outputs to a relative depth module, which, in turn, outputs to a three-dimensional space module whose metric is co-determined by the state of vergence of the eyes.

Aslin showed that infants of 1 and 2 months of age fail to follow a stimulus moving slowly in depth but begin to do so at 3 months (Aslin 1977). Only during their fourth month are they capable of following a step change in depth. More recently, Mitkin and Orestova (1988) reported an abrupt increase in the number of adequate vergence responses between 12 and 15 weeks of age. Granrud (1986) reported that, after the onset of stereopsis, 4-month-old infants showed a significantly increased number of reaching responses to the nearer of two objects. While these results are consistent with our contention that changes in motor control should occur simultaneously with sensory binocularity, better confirmation requires simultaneous observations of both sensory and motor aspects of binocularity in the same subjects. To this end the following experiment was performed.

METHOD

A large group of infants was serially tested on both a sensory task (preference for fusible binocular patterns) and a contingent motor task (dynamic convergence) in order to determine ages of onset of the two tasks and their temporal relationship (Thorn *et al.* 1994). Convergence was tested by presenting a small internally illuminated toy, in an otherwise darkened room, at a distance of 50 cm from the infant's face. Once the toy was fixated, it was moved slowly towards the bridge of the nose to within 12 cm. Full convergence was established when the toy was pursued by convergence throughout the approach. The age of onset of sensory binocularity was established by the shift of preference to the binocularly fused stimulus in the fusion-rivalry procedure comparing fusible with interocularly orthogonal gratings as already discussed.

RESULTS

The results (Fig. 17.2) show that the courses of development of the two forms of binocularity run in parallel within a week of each other. When the individual data are plotted on both variables, the scatterplot (Fig. 17.3) yields a highly significant Pearson correlation of 0.59. The authors conclude that the development of mature binocularity, disparity sensitivity in particular, indeed enhances the control of vergence movements.

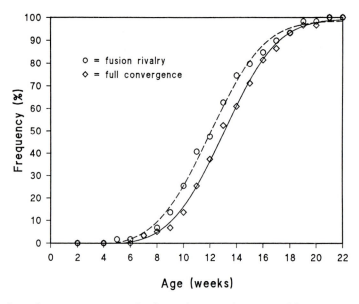

Fig. 17.2 Cumulative proportion of infants showing the onset of full convergence and binocular fusion preference as a function of age. (Adapted from Thorn *et al.* 1994.)

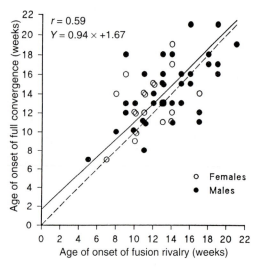

Fig. 17.3 Scatterplot for age of onset of full convergence and binocular fusion preference as a function of age and sex. (From Thorn *et al.* 1994.)

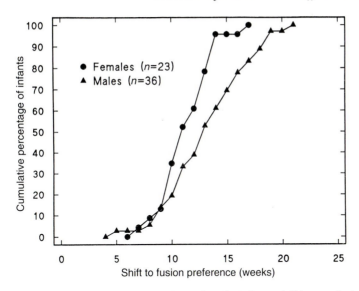

Fig. 17.4 Cumulative percentage of female and male infants shifting to fusion preference as a function of age.

Sex differences

The distribution of points in Fig. 17.3 suggests that the mean age of onset on both dimensions differs between the sexes with females having a slightly earlier age of onset. Further analyses of the outcomes of this experiment are portrayed in Fig. 17.4, showing the distribution of ages of shift to fusion preference, and in Fig. 17.5 showing the distribution of ages of onset of full convergence.

An analysis of variance of these data shows significant sex differences (females earlier), fusion preference slightly but significantly earlier than onset of convergence, and no significant interaction between the two. This finding further confirms our conclusion that the onset of disparity sensitivity enhances control of vergence since the same relation holds when the data are broken down into the two subclasses. It adds a new case to the array of sex differences that have been found to occur in infantile development. A brief review of these findings follows.

DISCUSSION

Our first observation of a sex difference was found upon analysis of data dealing with measures of vernier acuity from the experiments of Shimojo *et al.* (1984) and Shimojo and Held (1987) as reported by Held *et al.* (1984) (Fig. 17.6). Significant superiority of females over males in terms of acuity appeared at 2,

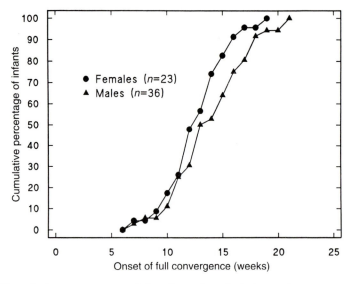

Fig. 17.5 Cumulative percentage of female and male infants showing onset of full convergence as a function of age.

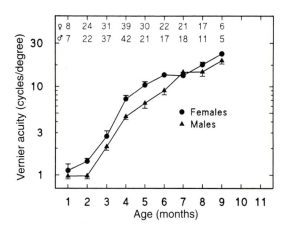

Fig. 17.6 Mean and standard error of vernier acuity and number of subjects measured at each point for females and males as a function of age.

4, 5, and 6 months of age but not later. Our large sample of infants tested for grating acuity during the first year was then checked and no significant differences were found between the sexes at any age as shown in Fig. 17.7 (Held *et al.* 1984). The lack of a difference in grating acuity serves as a control against different rates of behavioural development since the same behaviours are involved in both tests. Moreover, this initial finding of a difference in vernier but not grating acuity suggests that the former threshold might reflect a degree of

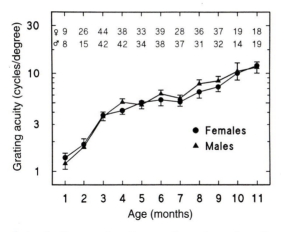

Fig. 17.7 Mean and standard error of grating acuity and number of subjects measured at each point for females and males as a function of age.

cortical processing not required for the latter threshold. In turn, this suggested that sex differences in binocular processes in which the interocular interaction is presumed to occur only in cortex should be tested.

Analysis of the data of Birch *et al.* (1985) and Shimojo *et al.* (1986) revealed significant sex differences in the onset of fusion preference (Bauer *et al.* 1986). These differences were replicated in the experiment already discussed (see Fig. 17.4). The data reported in Held *et al.* (1980) and Birch *et al.* (1982) on the onset of stereopsis also revealed sex differences. Although stereoacuity and vernier acuity (defining the vernier offset as one-half a grating cycle) are initially less than grating acuity, they increase at a more rapid rate than grating acuity during development. Consequently, it is possible to define a criterion of hyperacuity as a certain degree of superiority of the former over the latter and to determine the age of reaching this criterion. By analysing data on stereoacuity measured at the same age as grating acuity in individual subjects we managed to calculate the age at which infants achieve a one-half octave superiority of stereoptic acuity over grating acuity, with the resulting function shown in Fig. 17.8. This figure also shows a similar analysis of data on vernier acuity. In a later experiment (Gwiazda *et al.* 1989), a new group of infants was tested for both the onset age of fusion preference and of coarse stereopsis. The two test measurements were highly correlated ($r = 0.79$) and both showed the familiar age advantage for females.

These substantial differences between the sexes are found in the two processes that exhibit hyperacuity—stereoptic and vernier acuity. Such processes presumably involve more cortical computation than grating acuity, which is partially constrained by the grain of the retinal receptors. Consequently, another presumed cortical process was tested—orientational selectivity. A procedure that allowed comparison of the threshold changes produced by

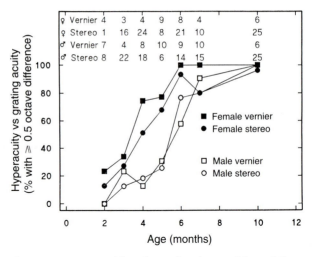

Fig. 17.8 Cumulative percentage of females and males reaching a 0.5 octave superiority of stereoacuity and vernier acuity over grating acuity as a function of age with number of subjects measured at each point.

masking gratings displaced by varied angles from a test grating was developed. By 1 or 2 months of age, a difference appeared between the masking efficacy of gratings at different angles (Held *et al.* 1989; Yoshida *et al.* 1990). However, to date, no significant sex differences have been found between sensitivities during the age of acquisition. If this result should be substantiated it would be an important exception to the hypothesis that the sex differences result from a dimorphism related to cortical development. Perhaps only certain cortical processes exhibit this dimorphism.

In addition to the above two other results should be mentioned. The first is a report of a significant sex difference in the development of the precedence effect in auditory direction finding, occurring at about the same age as that of stereopsis (Muir *et al.* 1989). The second is a report of a small but significant difference in contrast sensitivity favouring female infants at 6 months of age (Peterzell 1992). It is doubtful that a difference in contrast sensitivity could explain our sex differences.

Finally, the testosterone hypothesis should be mentioned. When searching for a possible sexual dimorphism in young infants, we found evidence in the literature that, in their earliest months, males show significant levels of serum testosterone that are absent in females. If this hormone should modulate some aspect of neuronal function of the developing visual system it might be a source of the differences observed by us. At one time, tests of the age of onset of mature binocularity in male infants were made in an attempt to correlate it with assays of testosterone levels. We reasoned that the higher the level of testosterone, the more delayed should be the onset of binocularity. Initially, a correlation was thought to exist (Held *et al.* 1988); however, later it was discovered that our assays were unreliable. The intriguing question remains: how to explain the sex differences by some dimorphic neuronal process occurring only during the first semester of life.

ACKNOWLEDGEMENTS

The authors thank Eileen Birch and Shinsuke Shimojo for their contributions to this paper including data collection, data analyses, and permission to include their results.

The research of the authors has been supported by National Institutes of Health grants 2R01-EY01191 and 5P30-EY02621.

REFERENCES

Aslin, A. N. (1977). Development of binocular fixation in human infants. *Journal of Experimental Child Psychology*, **23**, 133–50.

Bauer, J., Shimojo, S., Gwiazda, J., and Held, R. (1977). Sex differences in the development of binocularity in human infants. *Investigative Ophthalmology and Visual Science*, **27** (suppl.), 265.

Birch, E. (1993). Stereopsis in infants and its developmental relationship to visual acuity. In *Early visual development: normal and abnormal,* (ed. K. Simons), pp. 224–36. Oxford University Press, New York.

Birch, E. E., Gwiazda, J., and Held, R. (1982). Stereoacuity development for crossed and uncrossed disparities in human infants. *Vision Research*, **22**, 507–13.

Birch, E. E., Shimojo, S., and Held, R. (1985). Preferential looking assessment of fusion and stereopsis in infants aged 1 to 6 months. *Investigative Ophthalmology and Visual Science*, **26**, 366–70.

Eizenman, M., Skarf, B., and McCulloch, D. (1989). Development. of binocular vision in infants. *Investigative Ophthalmology and Visual Science*, **30** (suppl.), 313.

Granrud, C. E. (1986). Binocular vision and spatial perception in 4- and 5-month-old infants. *Journal of Experimental Psychology: Human Perception and Performance*, **12**, 36–49.

Gwiazda, J., Bauer, J., and Held, R. (1989). Binocular function in human infants: correlation of stereoptic and fusion-rivalry discriminations. *Journal of Pediatric Ophthalmology and Strabismus*, **26**, 128–32.

Held, R. (1985). Binocular vision—behavioural and neural development. In *Neonate cognition: beyond the blooming buzzing confusion,* (ed. J. Mehler and R. Fox), pp. 37–44. Lawrence Erlbaum Associates, Hillsdale, New Jersey.

Held, R. (1991). Development of binocular vision and stereopsis. In *Vision and visual dysfunction,* (ed. D. Regan and J. R. Cronly-Dillon), Vol. 9, pp. 170–8. Macmillan, London.

Held, R. (1993). Two stages in the development of binocular vision and eye alignment. In *Early visual development: normal and abnormal,* (ed. K. Simons), pp. 250–7. Oxford University Press, New York.

Held, R., Birch, E. E., and Gwiazda, J. (1980). Stereoacuity of human infants. *Proceedings of the National Academy of Sciences*, **77**, 5572–4.

Held, R., Shimojo, S., and Gwiazda, J. (1984). Gender differences in the early development of human visual resolution. *Investigative Ophthalmology and Visual Science*, **25** (suppl.), 220.

Held, R., Bauer, J., and Gwiazda, J. (1988). Age of onset of binocularity correlates with level of plasma testosterone in male infants. *Investigative Ophthalmology and Visual Science*, **29** (suppl.), 60.

Held, R., Yoshida, H., Gwiazda, J., and Bauer, J. (1989). Development of orientation selectivity measured by a masking procedure. *Investigative Ophthalmology and Visual Science*, **30** (suppl.), 312.

Mitkin, A. and Orestova, E. (1988). Development of binocular vision in early ontogenesis. *Psychologische Beitrage*, **30**, 65–74.

Muir, D. W., Clifton, R. K., and Clarkson, M. G. (1989). The development of a human auditory localization response: a U-shaped function. *Canadian Journal of Psychology*, **43**, 199–216.

Peterzell, D. (1992). A longitudinal study of individual differences in the contrast sensitivity functions of 4-, 6- and 8-month-old human infants. Doctoral dissertation, University of Colorado. *Dissertation Abstracts International*, **53**, 1084B. University Microfilms No. 9220443.

Shimojo, S. (1993). Development of interocular vision in infants. In *Early visual development: normal and abnormal*, (ed. K. Simons), pp. 201–23. Oxford University Press, New York.

Shimojo, S. and Held, R. (1987). Vernier acuity is less than grating acuity in 2 and 3-month-olds. *Vision Research*, **27**, 77–86.

Shimojo, S., Birch, E. E., Gwiazda, J., and Held, R. (1984). Development of vernier acuity in infants. *Vision Research*, **24**, 721–8.

Shimojo, S., Bauer, J. A., O'Connell, K. M., and Held, R. (1986). Pre-stereoptic binocular vision in infants. *Vision Research*, **26**, 501–10.

Thorn, F., Gwiazda, J., Cruz, A., Bauer, J., and Held, R. (1994). The development of eye alignment, convergence, and sensory binocularity in young infants. *Investigative Ophthalmology and Visual Science*, **35**, 544–53.

Yoshida, H., Gwiazda, J., Bauer, J., and Held, R. (1990). Orientation selectivity is present in the first month and subsequently sharpens. *Investigative Ophthalmology and Visual Science*, **31** (suppl.), 8.

18

Dioptric blur, grating visual acuity, and stereoacuity in infants

Paulette P. Schmidt, Ivan C. J. Wood, Sarah Lewin, and Helen Davis

INTRODUCTION

In the assessment of visual function, visual and stereo acuity measurement play important roles in diagnosing vision problems and in monitoring the effects of clinical treatments. Grating-acuity measurement determined by preferential-looking methods is the most widely available tool for assessment of visual function in infants and toddlers. Yet questions have been raised about the sensitivity of grating acuity in the detection and quantification of vision problems in these populations (Orel-Bixler and Norcia 1988; Thorn and Schwartz 1990; Schmidt 1991). Visual acuity may be measured binocularly and monocularly but requires monocular measurements to determine the presence of unilateral blur (Schmidt 1993). Stereoacuity is the perception of depth as a consequence of cortical recognition of horizontal retinal disparity between the two eyes. It is a form of hyperacuity and is measured binocularly. Stereopsis is the result of activating cortical binocular cells with identical but disparate images (Hubel and Wiesel 1970). Disrupted or discordant binocular vision during human infancy results in amblyopia and/or suppression thereby interrupting stereopsis (von Noorden 1985). The development of stereopsis has important implications for both understanding human visual development and the clinical treatment of visual anomalies.

Several investigators have compared stereotest sensitivity with blur; however, those results were all obtained with real-depth tests or two-dimensional line stereo stimuli. Earlier investigations in which the sensitivity of visual and stereo acuity were compared with blur used real-depth tests (one in which the test object is physically moved out the plane of one or more objects) and line stereograms to measure stereoacuity (a test in which the figures seen monocularly appear in depth when viewed through polarizing or anaglyphic lenses). Using a Howard-Dolman type apparatus (a real-depth test), Fry and Kent (1944) showed that stereoacuity decreased more than visual acuity as 'plus lens' blur was induced binocularly. Wood (1983), using the same apparatus, demonstrated that monocular blur produced a greater increase on stereo threshold than binocular blur. Ogle (1962), Lit (1968), Stigmar (1971), and Donzis *et al.* (1983) each demonstrated that line stereogram tests were more

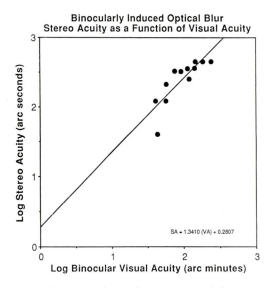

Fig. 18.1 Stereoacuity as a function of visual acuity. A model was tested for the relative sensitivity of stereo and visual acuity to blur (SA = slope × VA + intercept). A slope greater than one (m = 1.341) shows that the subjects' sensitivity to the effects of binocular optical blur is revealed by RDE stereoacuity more readily than by visual acuity. For direct comparison of values, log stereo and visual acuity were used.

sensitive to unilateral than bilateral symmetrical changes in Snellen visual acuity in the 20/20 to 20/40 range of acuity while Levy and Glick (1974) showed that for monocularly induced blur, monocular Snellen acuity and binocular stereoacuity for line stereograms were linearly related. Westheimer and McKee (1980) found that monocular blur of line stereograms reduced stereoacuity at least as much as visual acuity at low amounts of blur, and even more so when the magnitude of blur is higher.

Schmidt (1989; 1992; 1993) demonstrated that random-dot stereoacuity is sensitive to monocular and binocular blur over a 12 dioptre range of optically induced blur. In four adult subjects, stereoacuity was found to be more sensitive to binocular blur than Bailey-Lovie visual acuity, and it was especially sensitive to monocular blur whereas Bailey-Lovie acuity was not. Each subject had stereo and visual acuity threshold estimates measured from 0 to ±6.0 dioptres of optically induced blur in 0.50-dioptre increments (Fig. 18.1). A model was tested for the relative sensitivity of stereoacuity (SA) and visual acuity (VA) to binocularly induced optical blur (SA = slope × VA + intercept). The summary data in Fig. 18.1 show how the subjects' sensitivity to the effects of binocular optical blur is revealed by Random Dot E stereoacuity (RDE) more readily than by visual acuity. Stereo and visual acuity are not entirely independent variables, therefore principle axis analysis [$y - \bar{y} = m(x - \bar{x})$, then $y = mx - m\bar{x} + \bar{y}$, which $= mx + b$ where $b = \bar{y} - m\bar{x}$] was used. The results show that the slope is greater than one ($m = 1.341$) with an intercept of $b = 0.281$. Therefore, stereoacuity declines consistently in response to increasing amounts of binocular optical blur and at a faster rate than visual acuity.

The sensitivity to binocular blur shows the potential value of Random Dot Stereo-test (RDS) in detecting refractive blur in addition to suppression, abnormal fusion and amblyopic blur. For two subjects, blur was also induced monocularly and visual and stereo acuity were measured under binocular viewing conditions. With blur in only one eye (a condition approximating refractive anisometropic amblyopia), RDE stereoacuity deteriorated even more rapidly, the slope was 3.774 (Schmidt 1993). Initial results by Schmidt (1992) and Schmidt and White (1993) of similar experiments conducted with anisometropic amblyopes, further show the sensitivity to blur of selected random-dot stimulus parameters. Schmidt's work supports the greater sensitivity of RDS to both binocular and monocular blur and further demonstrates that for certain RDS stimuli monocularly induced optical blur causes stereothresholds to decrease more rapidly than binocularly measured visual acuity.

The random dot stereoacuity (RDSA) measurement particularly provides a single binocular test requiring equal visual acuity in each eye and functional binocular disparity detection (Schmidt 1992; Schmidt and White 1993). Therefore clinical measures of random-dot stereoacuity in infancy could be particularly useful in the diagnosis, management and treatment of vision problems such as amblyopia, refractive error and strabismus, which interrupt binocular vision.

Since the appreciation of random-dot stereopsis depends upon the combination of visual information processed independently by each eye through the visual pathways to a single binocular percept in the visual cortex, random-dot stereoacuity is reduced or absent in conditions that interrupt binocular function such as anisometropia, strabismus, organic or functional amblyopia and other more subtle interruptions of neural development (Petrig *et al.* 1981; Hubel and Livingstone 1987; Livingstone *et al.* 1987).

HISTORICAL REVIEW OF STEREOACUITY DEVELOPMENT AND METHODS OF TESTING IN INFANCY

Studies of the onset and development of stereoacuity indicate that stereoacuity is first measurable between 3–5 months of age (Fox *et al.* 1980; Held *et al.* 1980; Shea *et al.* 1980; Petrig *et al.* 1981; Birch *et al.* 1982; Teller 1983; Archer *et al.* 1986; Gwiazda *et al.* 1989).

Onset of stereopsis

Fox *et al.* (1980) reported that the onset of stereopsis (Table 18.1) occurs in children between 3.5 and 6 months of age. Using random-element stereograms,

Table 18.1 Literature reviewed.

Authors	Year	Stereo test used	Ages tested and norms (arc minutes)	n	Experimental design/ population tested
Fox, Aslin, Shea and Dumais	1980	Unique to laboratory random-element, dynamic	3.5–4.5 months 45' and 134' No norms	17	2AFC/Normals
Held, Birch and Gwiazda	1980	Unique to laboratory line stereogram	16 weeks = 58' 20 weeks = 1'	16	2AFC/Normals
Fox, Aslin, Shea and Dumais	1980	Unique to laboratory random-element, dynamic	4 months, 6 months and 12 months No norms	10	2AFC/Normals
Gwiazda, Bauer and Held	1989	Unique to laboratory line stereogram	2 weeks–22 weeks No norms	17	2AFC/Normals
Romano, Romano and Puklin	1975	Titmus	1.5–13 years Some norms (see Table 18.2)	321	4AFC/Normals
Petrig, Julesz, Kropf et al.	1981	Unique to laboratory random-element, dynamic	7–48 weeks No norms	17	VEPs/Normals
Birch and Hale	1989	Unique to laboratory random-element, static	19–60 months Some norms (see Table 18.2)	76	OPL and 2AFC/Normals
Ciner, Schanel-Klitsch et al.	1991	Unique to laboratory random-element, static	18–65 months Some norms (see Table 18.3)	180	OPL and 2AFC/Normals

they measured stereoacuity of 45′ (arc minutes) at 15 weeks. Held *et al.* (1980), measured stereoacuities of 58′ at 16 weeks and of 1′ at 20 weeks, using line stereograms. Petrig *et al.* (1981) demonstrated that random-dot stereopsis can be measured at 10–19 weeks of age using visual-evoked potentials, after cortical binocularity develops. Gwiazda *et al.* (1989) tracked the development of line stereopsis in 17 infants and showed correlation between the onset of stereopsis and the shift in fixation preference from rivalrous patterns to fusible patterns. Females showed an earlier onset for both fusion preference (females, 9.9 weeks; males, 13.8 weeks) and stereopsis (females, 9.1 weeks; males, 12.1 weeks).

Development of stereopsis

Birch *et al.* (1982) used line stereograms to show that detection of crossed disparities precedes uncrossed disparities but that both develop at the same rate, suggesting the existence of separate binocular mechanisms subserving each. Birch and Hale (1989) demonstrated grating and stereo acuity development with operant preferential looking procedures using projected, polarized static random-dot figures. In all age groups, the median stereoacuity was superior to the mean grating acuity by a factor of 1.54–2.58 (Table 18.2; see also Table 18.1).

Romano *et al.* (1975) conducted the pioneering work of stereoacuity development in children aged 2–9 years using a widely available clinically used line stereogram. Steady improvement was seen in the scores on the Titmus stereotest from 2–9 years of age (see Table 18.2). However, the Titmus stereotest is a line stereogram making these stereoacuity norms difficult to compare with values from a random-dot stereogram, since children with known vision problems show measurable stereoacuity on line stereotests owing to monocular depth cues (Julesz 1986). Notably, only children with evidence of normal binocular vision were included in the study. Therefore, evidence is lacking that the Titmus test successfully discriminates between those with normal binocular vision and those with binocular vision anomalies. Interestingly, stereoacuity values for the Titmus test are poorer than those reported by Ciner *et al.* (1991) using RDS targets for children of similar ages.

Ciner *et al.* (1991) used projected static random-dot targets and revealed a steady improvement in stereoacuity with increased age from 250 arc seconds (″) to 60″. Cut-off values of acceptable stereoacuity for the different age groups are shown in Table 18.2.

Table 18.2 summarizes the results of the three studies that reported age-related stereoacuity measurements in young children. Romano *et al.* (1975) and Ciner *et al.* (1991) reported minimum stereoacuities obtained from subjects tested in each age category. Yet, minimum stereoacuities differ greatly between line (3000″) and random-dot (100–60″) stereopsis for children 36–60 months of age. The other study reported median values related to age. Median random-dot stereoacuity was 77″ (19–24 months) while minimum random-dot stereocuity was 250″ (18–23 months). Both Birch and Hale (1989) and Ciner *et al.* (1991) used RDS stimuli unique to research settings. Studies where age-related

Table 18.2 Stereoacuity as a function of age. Few studies provide stereoacuity norms for young children. Romano *et al.*'s early study results show behavioural measures of stereoacuity threshold for line stereo stimuli. Most recently, Birch *et al.* and Ciner have used random-dot stimuli for children of similar ages, i.e. between 36 and 60 months.

Age (months)	Titmus (seconds of arc)[a] Romano *et al.* (1975)	RDS (seconds of arc)[a] Birch *et al.* (1989)	RDS (seconds of arc)[a] Ciner (1991)
18–23		77 (19–24)[b]	250
24–29		68 (25–30)[b]	225
30–35		40 (31–36)[b]	125
36–41		40 (37–48)[b]	100
42–47			100
48–53		40 (49–60)[b]	100
54–59			60
36–60	3000		
60–65			60
60-66	140		
66–72	100		
72–84	80		
84–96	60		
over 96	40		

[a] Stereoacuity results are reported as minimum (Romano, Ciner) or median (Birch) values for age; RDS values are from stimuli unique to the lab (Birch used RDS stimuli from Simons 1981 studies), i.e. not available for widespread use.
[b] Birch *et al.* used slightly different age categories, shown in parentheses.

stereoacuity norms are reported show some corresponding ages but the results vary for similarly aged children and are not comparable because stereoacuities are not reported in the same way. Finally, only children with evidence of normal binocular vision were included in the three studies.

Whereas behavioural tests using forced-choice preferential-looking methods of assessment confirm that depth perception, as determined by line stereo targets, begins to develop between 4 and 6 months of age and is generally mature between the ages of 3 and 5 years, local (line) stereopsis provides monocular cues to depth that enable strabismics and others to display false levels of stereoacuity when none exist (Cotter and Scharre 1987; Baitch *et al.* 1991) Normed values for infants do not exist and are very limited for 2–5-year-olds.

It was the purpose of this study to determine whether: (i) preferential-looking measures of RDSA could be made in a clinically useful way in infancy (ii) preliminary age-related stereoacuity norms could be determined in infants with normal visual development; and (iii) the effect of dioptric blur produced by the infant optical system for stereo and grating stimuli, used in testing the visual capability of infants, could be determined.

EXPERIMENT 1

Full-term infants ($n = 120$) from birth to 18 months of age were selected randomly from the birth records of the Hazel Grove Community Health Clinic, Stockport, UK, and invited to participate in this project. Experiments 1 and 2 address stereoacuity measurements in 6–12-month-old infants.

Subjects

Seventy-six infants 6–12 months of age were categorized as visually normal on the basis of preferential-looking acuity, refractive state, ocular health and orthoptic assessment of eye alignment.

Methods

Estimates of grating visual acuity (TAC) and modified Lang random-dot stereoacuity (M-LRDSA) thresholds were collected on the 76 infants whose vision was developing normally. Visual acuity, refractive error, ocular alignment (by cover test, Hirschberg reflexes as well as 20 dioptre base-in and base-out prism fusion) and stereoacuity were each determined by individual examiners. Each examiner was masked from the outcome on the other evaluations. Infants were pseudorandomly directed to an examining station on the basis of the order of their arrival at the clinic.

Photographic random-dot stimuli were modified from commercially available Lang stereotests (M-LRDSA) creating one stimulus with an embedded figure (a cat) and a matched random-dot pattern with no three-dimensional figure. The stimuli were attached behind apertures in silver crescent board number 620. The dimensions, spacing, and centre peephole were similar to the commercially available Teller acuity cards.

The stereo stimuli were adapted for use in a preferential-looking paradigm that required no glasses for disparity appreciation. RDS stimuli were selected to assure that resultant stereoacuity measurements were the consequence of binocular disparity detection and not based on monocular cues as can occur with line stereograms (Donzis *et al.* 1983; Julesz 1986).

The plane of the M-LRDSA testing card was held parallel to the face plane of the viewing infant. In a 2AFC preferential-looking paradigm, M-LRDSA was determined in visually normal 6–12-month-olds using a modified descending staircase procedure (Schmidt 1994) in a way similar to Gwiazda *et al.* (1980). Operant preferential-looking techniques were used with auditory reinforcement for correct responses. Stimulus disparities ($n = 6$) ranged from 1200 to 201 arc seconds (") disparity in equal 0.15 log interval steps and were created by

Table 18.3 Mean M-LRDSA stereo and TAC visual acuity in infants.

Age (months)	$\overline{X}_{\text{M-LRDSA}}$ σ (arc seconds)	Number	Testability	$\overline{X}_{\text{TAC}}$ σ (cycles/degree)
6 ± 1	960 ± 264	18	69.2% (18/26)	4.29 ± 1.51
9 ± 1	683 ± 247	24	75.0% (24/32)	5.36 ± 1.13
12 ± 1	443 ± 149	16	88.0% (16/18)	6.68 ± 1.05

varying the testing distance from 0.5 to 2.5 m. Stereoacuity was judged to be the finest disparity at which the position of the stereo stimulus was identified correctly on more than 75% of the presentations. Stereo stimulus (cat) position (right or left) was pseudorandomized for presentation and order remained consistent for all subjects.

Results

Seventy-six per cent ($n = 58$) of the infant subjects were testable on the M-LRDSA. While 100% completed binocular grating acuity estimates, the percentage of infants able to complete both monocular TAC measurements was approximately 72% despite the shorter testing time. All threshold values were related to a 50 cm viewing distance for ease of comparison. The mean estimates of stereo threshold by age (Table 18.3) for a 50 cm viewing distance were:

(1) 6 months = 960″ (σ = ±264″);
(2) 9 months = 683″ (σ = ±247″);
(3) 12 months = 443″ (σ = ±149″).

Grating acuity threshold estimates were within expected age norms (Table 18.3) and for a 50 cm viewing distance were:

(1) 6 months = 4.29 cycles/degree (c/d) (σ = ±1.51 c/d);
(2) 9 months = 5.36 c/d (σ = ±1.13 c/d);
(3) 12 months = 6.68 c/d (σ = ±1.05 c/d).

Retest on M-LRDSA was completed on 41 of the testable subjects. A paired t-test showed no significant difference ($t = 0.91, p = 0.36, n = 41$) between repeated measures of stereothreshold. Stimulus (cat) position (right or left) was re-randomized for the series of retest trials. Consistently better stereoacuities and less variability occurred as age increased. A review of the clinical and vision science literature indicates the changes in stereoacuity documented in this study are the first reported efforts at establishing random-dot stereoacuity norms in infants younger than 18 months of age. Therefore limited comparisons can be made. Two subjects aged 15 and 19 months were documented (350–400″) by Ciner *et al.* (1991) while Birch and Hale (1989) reported (median = 77″) for 13/23 (56.5%) 19–24-month-olds who were testable.

As part of the orthoptic test of eye alignment, a 20 prism dioptre base-in and base-out test was completed. Interestingly, infants unable to overcome a 20 prism dioptre base-out showed markedly lower stereoacuities than those able to do the test.

Novel age-related M-LRDSA thresholds have been demonstrated in infants using a 2AFC preferential-looking procedure with a RDS test requiring no glasses for disparity detection and for which the results are repeatable. Corresponding binocular TAC acuity thresholds were also documented. Stereoacuity improves faster than grating acuity over this age range.

EXPERIMENT 2

The dioptric blur produced by the infant optical system for various stimuli used in testing the visual capability of infants has not been documented previously. A series of infant model eyes were developed by us using a computer program to determine the size of the refractive blur circle for the stereo and grating acuity thresholds obtained from the random sample of 6–12-month-old infants in Experiment 1 (O'Keefe and Coile 1988).

Methods

Pupil sizes were measured videographically while subjects fixated a target at 50 cm. Dynamic retinoscopy was used to determine the lag of accommodation (accuracy of accommodation focus with respect to the fixation for the plane of regard of the target). High-contrast fixation targets similar to visual and stereo acuity targets were used for measurement of pupil size and accommodation. Blur ratios were then determined for visual and stereo acuity stimuli to provide information about the comparative visibility of the grating and random-dot stimuli. A series of model eyes for the neonate, 3-, 6-, 9- and 12-month-old infants were generated from sparse model eye, ultrasonic, corneal, lens and refractive measurement using the 'Schemeye' computer program (Yorke and Mandell 1962; Larsen 1971; Hill and Fry 1974; Lotmar 1976; Blomdahl 1979; Hirano *et al.* 1979; Enoch and Hammer 1983; Moore 1987; Wood and Hodi 1992). The sizes of the blur circle diameters and basic heights of the retinal images were determined for both M-LRDSA and TAC grating threshold stimuli for each 6-, 9- and 12-month-old infant model eyes. Estimates of grating and stereo thresholds were taken from Experiment 1. Blur ratio was defined as the relative size of the blur circle to the height of the blurred retinal image (Hill and Fry 1974; Bennett and Rabbetts 1989). Therefore, visibility increases as the blur ratio decreases.

Retinal image height was calculated for each pattern based upon the size of the age-related visual or stereo acuity threshold and respective dimensions of grating period, cat, cluster or individual pixel. Cluster for the random-dot stereo stimuli was defined as the smallest area at the edge of the embedded figure required to enable disparity detection by an adult with normal binocularity. Use of the cluster dimension resulted from personal conversation with Professor Bela Julesz who developed random-dot stereograms and discussions with Professor Glenn A. Fry regarding analysis of the effects of blur on the retinal image.

Results

Model eye parameters essential to blur ratio calculations are shown in Fig. 18.2. The blur ratios for each of the TAC and M-LRDSA patterns (e.g. grating, cluster, pixel, cat) are shown in Table 18.4 for the mean pupil size at each given age and for a testing distance of 50 cm. Blur ratios decrease as infant age increases. Lag of accommodation values indicates that the residual retinal blur cannot be attributed to inaccurate focus. For all ages, mean lag of accommodation was positive and within normal adult ranges (+0.25 to +0.75). The accommodative lag values measured indicate infants focus in the plane of the target. Values of +0.25 to +0.75 dioptres represent the lens power used to compensate for a physical constant, the physical placement of the fixation target at a distance closer to the eye by the thickness of the retinoscope. Values different from these indicate accommodative errors in response to the plane in which the target is located. The blur ratios shown in Table 18.4 slowly decrease with age, increased eye size and threshold stimulus size.

DISCUSSION

Seventy-six infants with normally developing vision had grating visual acuity and random-dot stereoacuity measured. The results show that the behavioural measures of grating acuity fell within established age norms and that behavioural measures of stereoacuity were collectable in 6–12-month-old infants, mean stereoacuity values and deviations decreased with increased infant age and the results were repeatable. Stereoacuity improved more rapidly (53.8% change) than resolution acuity (35.8%) over this age range. The change in M-LRDSA was measurable using modified Lang stereo stimuli without glasses in 58 (76%) of the full-term infants. Monocular TAC acuities required to detect amblyopia were possible in 72% of the infants. Random-dot stereo stimuli were selected to assure that resultant stereoacuity measurements were the consequence of binocular disparity detection and not based on monocular cues, as can occur with line stereograms.

Blur ratios were calculated for grating stimuli in infants whose TAC thresholds were consistent with established norms and whose vision was found to be developing normally. Correspondingly, blur ratios for three aspects of the M-LRDSA stimuli were also calculated. The resultant blur ratios predicted by the developing infant (6–12-month-olds in this study) optical systems and retinal cone mosaic are not markedly different than those

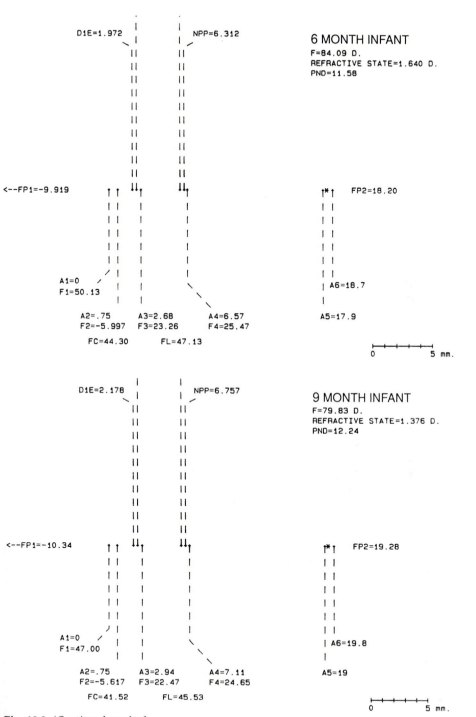

Fig. 18.2 (*Continued overleaf*)

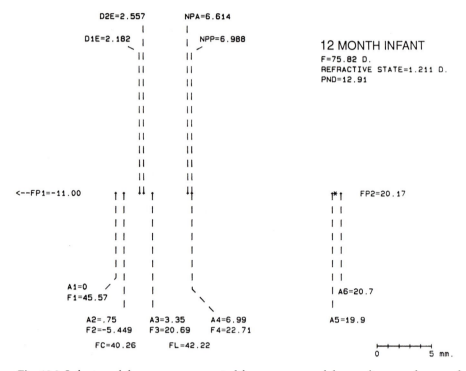

Fig. 18.2 Infant model eyes were generated from sparse model eye, ultrasound, corneal, lens and refractive measurements obtained from the literature for neonates and infants. Model eyes for 6-, 9- and 12-month-old infants are shown here.

F = power; D = dioptres;

F1 = Power (D) of anterior cornea;

F2 = Power (D) of posterior cornea;

F3 = Power (D) of anterior lens;

F4 = Power (D) of posterior lens;

FC = Power (D) of total cornea;

FL = Power (D) of total lens;

A = Position (mm) of structure (from front of eye);

A1 = Position (mm) of anterior corneal surface;

A2 = Position (mm) of posterior corneal surface;

A3 = Position (mm) of anterior lens surface;

A4 = Position (mm) of posterior lens surface;

A5 = Position (mm) of retina;

A6 = Position (mm) of sclera;

FP1 = Position (mm) of anterior focal point;

FP2 = Position (mm) of posterior focal point;

PND = Posterior nodal distance;

NPP = Nodal principle point;

D1E = Distance (mm) of entrance pupil from cornea.

Table 18.4 Blur ratios for threshold grating and random-dot stimuli.

Age (months)	TAC	M-LRDSA			Pupil size (mm)	Accommodative Lag (dioptre equivalent sphere)
		Cluster	Pixel	Cat		
6 ± 1	0.425	0.268	0.740	0.021	4.1 ± 0.99	0.37 ± 0.73
9 ± 1	0.377	0.255	0.665	0.019	3.7 ± 0.73	0.37 ± 0.56
12 ± 1	0.266	0.170	0.498	0.016	4.1 ± 0.50	0.16 ± 0.71

established for adults with 4 mm pupil diameters (adult blur ratios: 0.4–0.5) (Bennett and Rabbetts 1989). These results suggests that optical limits are approached more closely as age increases. While most discussions of acuity development conclude that the limiting factors are rarely optical, Wood and Davis (1994) have shown recently that optical limitations have an effect after 9 months of age. For children with ≥+3.75 dioptres of hyperopia or ≥+1.00 dioptres of astigmatism, TAC grating acuity was reduced compared with infants of the same age with smaller refractive errors. Our results and those of Wood and Davis (1994) suggest optical factors may limit visual development in the older infant. Blur ratios for the cluster pattern in the stereogram correspond most closely to those for gratings and may provide a theoretical basis for stimulus detection. One can speculate from the results that infants may make disparity judgements on the basis of the cluster pattern in the random-dot stereogram.

A review of the clinical and vision science literature indicates the changes in stereoacuity documented in this study are novel results. Therefore limited comparisons can be made. Traditionally, decreased acuteness of central vision, visual acuity loss, has been the most frequently occurring sign of vision problems in children. Birch and Hale (1989) have demonstrated in young children that disparity detection, a hyperacuity task, is superior to grating and recognition acuity tasks by a factor of at least 1.5. Additionally, questions about the effectiveness of grating acuity (discrimination acuity) in detecting blurred vision, amblyopia, caused by the effects of spurious resolution are unresolved (Campbell and Green 1965; Jenkins *et al.* 1983; Thorn and Schwartz 1990). Therefore, by establishing age-referenced norms for RDS tests without monocular cues to depth and higher sensitivity to blur, fusion loss or suppression than visual acuity, the tests would be potentially effective in determining normal cortical development of binocularity, binocular depth perception skills and whether optical, neural and motor components of both eyes are indeed functioning normally.

CONCLUSIONS

(1) Novel age-related modified Lang random dot stereoacuity (M-LRDSA) thresholds have been demonstrated in infants using a 2AFC preferential-looking procedure with a random-dot stereotest requiring no glasses for disparity detection.
(2) Estimates of stereothreshold among these infants were repeatable.
(3) Dioptric blur ratios show reasonable agreement between the cluster size characteristic of the random-dot stimulus pattern and grating size for threshold M-LRDSA and grating acuity (TAC) values.
(4) Comparisons of the blur ratio results for cluster and grating aspects of stereo and grating acuity targets suggest that infants may make disparity judge-ments on the basis of the cluster pattern in the random-dot stereogram.

ACKNOWLEDGEMENTS

The authors wish to express their thanks for partial support of this invest-igation to NIH EY0882501 to Dr Schmidt, University of Manchester Institute of Science and Technology, Department of Optometry and Vision Sciences, and the Hazel Grove Health Clinic staff. Dr Schmidt wishes to thank The Ohio State University, College of Optometry for support of this project.

This study was funded in part by grant EY0882501 from the National Eye Institute and The University of Manchester Institute of Science and Technology to Paulette P. Schmidt while an invited summer Visiting Research Professor at UMIST.

REFERENCES

Archer, S., Helveston, E., Miller, K., and Ellis, F. (1986). Stereopsis in normal infants and infants with congenital esotropia. *American Journal of Ophthalmology*, **101**, 591–6.

Baitch, L. W., Ridder III, W. H., Harwerth, R. S., and Smith III, E. L. (1991). Binocular beat vep's: losses of cortical binocularity in monkeys reared with abnormal visual experience. *Investigative Ophthalmology and Visual Science*, **32**, 3096–103.

Bennett, A. G. and Rabbetts, R. (1989). The schematic eye. In *Clinical visual optics*, 2nd edn. pp. 249–74. Butterworths, London.

Birch, E. and Hale, L. (1989). Operant assessment of stereoacuity. *Clinical Vision Science* **4**, 295–300.

Birch, E. E., Gwiazda, J., and Held, R. (1982). Stereoacuity development for crossed and uncrossed disparities in human infants. *Vision Research*, **22**, 507–13.

Blomdahl, S. (1979). Ultrasonic measurements of the eye in the newborn infant. *Acta Ophthalmologica*, **57**, 1048–56.

Campbell, F. W. and Green, D. G. (1965). Optical and retinal factors affecting visual resolution. *Journal of Physiology (London)*, **181**, 576–93.

Ciner, E. B., Schanel-Klitsch, E., and Scheiman, M. (1991). Stereoacuity development in young children. *Optometry and Vision Science*, **68**, 533–6.

Cotter, S. and Scharre, J. (1987). The Lang stereotest: performance by strabismic, amblyopic and visually normal patients. *American Journal of Optometry and Physiological Optics*, **64**, 68P.

Donzis, P. B., Pappazzo, A., Burde, R. M., and Gordon, M. (1983). Effect of binocular variations of Snellen's visual acuity on Titmus stereoacuity. *Archives of Ophthalmology*, **101**, 930–2.

Enoch, J. M. and Hamer, R. D. (1983). Image size correction of the unilateral aphakic infant. *Ophthalmic Paediatrics and Genetics*, **2**, 153–65.

Fox, R., Aslin, R. N., Shea, S. L., and Dumais, S. T. (1980). Stereopsis in human infants. *Science*, **207**, 323–4.

Fry, G. and Kent, P. R. (1944). The effects of base-in and base-out prisms on stereoacuity. *American Journal of Optometry and The Archives of the American Academy of Optometry*, **21**, 492–507.

Gwiazda, J., Wolfe, J. M., Briss, S., Mohindra, I., and Held, R. (1980). Quick assessment of preferential looking acuity in infants. *American Journal of Optometry and Physiological Optics*, **57**, 420–7.

Gwiazda, J., Bauer, J., and Held, R. (1989). Binocular function in human infants: correlation of stereo-optic and fusion-rivalry discriminations. *Journal of Pediatric Ophthalmology and Strabismus*, **26**, 128–32.

Held, R., Birch, E., and Gwiazda, J. (1980). Stereoacuity in human infants. *Proceedings of the National Academy of Sciences of the United States of America*, **77**, 5572–4.

Hill, R. M. and Fry, G. A. (1974). Retinal blur circle calculations based on the Hughes Schematic Eye for the rabbit. *Vision Research*, **14**, 1037–8.

Hirano, S., Yakamoto, Y., and Takayama, H. (1979). Ultrasonic observation of eyes in premature babies. *Acta Ophthalmologica*, **83**, 1679–93.

Hubel, D. H. and Livingstone, M. S. (1987). Segregation of form, color, and stereopsis in primate area 18. *Journal of Neuroscience*, **7**, 3378–415.

Hubel, D. H. and Wiesel, T. N. (1970). Stereoscopic vision in macaque monkey. Cells sensitive to binocular depth in area 18 of the macaque monkey cortex *Nature*, **225**, 41–2.

Jenkins, P. F., Prager, T. C., Mazow, M. L., Allen, S. B., and Russek, M. G. (1983). Preliterate vision screening: a comparative study. *American Orthoptic Journal*, **33**, 91–8.

Julesz, B. (1986). Stereoscopic vision. *Vision Research*, **26**, 1601–12.

Larsen, J. S. (1971). The sagittal growth of the eye Parts I, II, III. *Acta Ophthalmologica*, **49**, 239–62, 427–40, 441–53.

Levy, N. S. and Glick, E. B. (1974). Stereoscopic perception and Snellen visual acuity. *American Journal of Ophthalmology*, **78**, 722–4.

Lit, A. (1968). Presentation of experimental data. *Journal of the American Optometric Association*, **39**, 1098–9.

Livingstone, M. S. and Hubel, D. H. (1987). Psychophysical evidence for separate channels for the perception of form, color, movement, and depth. *Journal of Neuroscience*, **7**, 3416–68.

Lotmar, W. (1976). A theoretical model for the eye of the newborn infants. *Graefe's Archive for Clinical and Experimental Ophthalmology*, **198**, 179–85.

Moore, B. D. (1987). Mensuration data in infant eyes with unilateral congenital cataracts. *American Journal of Optometry*, **64**, 204–10.

Ogle, K. N. (1962). Spatial localization through binocular vision. In *The eye IV. Visual optics and optical space sense*, (ed. H. Davson), pp. 289–90. Academic Press, New York.

O'Keefe, L. P. and Coile, D. C. (1988). A basic computer program for schematic and reduced eye construction. *Ophthalmic and Physiological Optics*, **8**, 97–100.

Orel-Bixler, D. and Norcia, A. (1988). Predicting optotype acuity from grating acuity in strabismus or anisometropia. *Investigative Ophthalmology and Visual Science*, **29**, 10.

Petrig, B., Julesz, B., Kropfl, W., Baumgartner, G., and Ankiker, M. (1981). Development of steropsis and cortical binocularity in human infants: electrophysiological evidence. *Science*, **213**, 1402–5.

Romano, P. E., Romano, J. A., and Puklin, J. E. (1975). Stereoacuity development in children with normal binocular single vision. *American Journal of Ophthalmology*, **79**, 966–71.

Schmidt, P. P. (1989). Sensitivity of RDE stereoacuity and Snellen acuity to optical blur. *Investigative Ophthalmology and Visual Science*, **30** (suppl.), 303.

Schmidt, P. (1991). Effectiveness of vision-screening in pre-school populations with preferential-looking cards used for assessment of visual acuity. *Optometry and Vision Science*, **68**, 210–19.

Schmidt, P. (1992). Stereoacuity testing in amblyopia. *Investigative Ophthalmology and Visual Science*, **33**, 1339.

Schmidt, P. (1993). Sensitivity of stereoacuity and visual acuity to optically induced blur. *Optometry and Vision Science*, **71**, 466–71.

Schmidt, P. P. (1994). Visual acuity measurement in exceptional children. *Journal of the American Optometric Association*, **66**, 627–33.

Schmidt, P. and White, R. F. (1993). Stereoacuity in children with refractive anisometropic amblyopia. *Investigative Ophthalmology and Visual Science*, **33**, 864.

Shea, S., Fox, R., Aslin, R., and Dumais, S. (1980). Assessment of stereopsis in human infants. *Investigative Ophthalmology and Visual Science*, **19**, 1400–4.

Stigmar, G. (1971). Blurred visual stimuli: II. The effect of blurred visual stimuli on vernier and stereo acuity. *Acta Ophthalmologica*, **49**, 364–79.

Teller, D. Y. (1983). Scotopic vision, color vision, and stereopsis in infants. *Current Eye Research*, **2**, 199–210.

Thorn, F. and Schwartz, F. (1990). Effects of dioptric blur on Snellen and grating acuity. *Optometry and Vision Science*, **67**, 3–7.

von Noorden, G. K. (1985). Amblyopia: a multidisciplinary approach. *Investigative Ophthalmology and Visual Science*, **26**, 1704.

Westheimer, G. and McKee, S. P. (1980). Stereoscopic acuity with defocused and spatially filtered images. *Journal of the Optometric Society of America*, **70**, 772–8.

Wood, I. C. J. (1983). Stereopsis with spatially-degraded images. *Ophthalmic and Physiological Optics*, **3**, 337–40.

Wood, I. C. J. and Davis, H. (1994). Infant acuity screening and cycloplegic refraction. *Optometry and Vision Science, Amsterdam Academy Europe Scientific Program Book*, **May**, **1**, 221–2.

Wood, I. C. J. and Hodi, S. (1992). Longitudinal refractive change in infancy. *Investigative Ophthalmology and Visual Science*, **33**, 971.

Yorke, M. A. and Mandall, R. B. (1962). A new calibration system for photokeratoscopy: Part II. Corneal contour measurements. *American Journal of Optometry and Physiological Optics*, **46**, 818–22.

19

Evaluation of sensory visual development based on measures of oculomotor responses

Cathy Buquet and Jacques R. Charlier

INTRODUCTION

During the past 30 years, studies of oculomotor responses greatly contributed to the evaluation of sensory visual functions in non-verbal children. These developments result from a better understanding of the oculomotor behaviours of infants and from the introduction of objective techniques for measuring their eye movements. For this reason, the foundations of methods based on eye movement responses to study the detection and discrimination of visual stimuli will firstly be reviewed. Second, the various techniques that are available today for measuring eye movements in children will be presented. Third, how these developments have been applied to the evaluation of sensory visual functions will be summarized.

There is no ambition to make a thorough analysis of all these subjects. They involve so many scientific disciplines as far apart as neurophysiology, psychology, system engineering, and medicine, that this could only be devised as a collaborative work of specialists from these various disciplines. Therefore our purpose will be to provide a framework with references to the different reviews made in each of these specialties.

MEASURING SENSORY VISUAL FUNCTIONS WITH OCULOMOTOR RESPONSES

The rationale behind the use of oculomotor responses for testing sensory visual functions is based on the fact that the oculomotor system is driven, at least partially, by visual input information.

Oculomotor responses found in young infants

Visual stimuli can elicit a wide variety of eye movement responses at the earliest ages (Maurer and Lewis 1979). Newborn infants can fixate a stationary

292   *Cathy Buquet and Jacques R. Charlier*

stimulus (Bryan 1930). They can make saccades in the direction of stimulus localized in the periphery (Tronick 1972). They can track a stimulus in motion (Beasley 1933). They also present optokinetic nystagmus (OKN) to a moving repetitive pattern (McGinnis 1930).

How do these responses reflect the information processing that takes place at the sensory level? At the present time, there are no clear-cut answers to this fundamental question. Many issues are still a matter of debate and the actual knowledge on the different processes involved and their maturation is fragmentary.

Mechanisms involved in the oculomotor responses

The oculomotor responses obtained from young infants are different, in many aspects, from those obtained from attentive adult subjects. In young infants, fixations present dispersions that are considerably larger than adults. When viewing simple geometric forms, they make slower, hypometric saccades (Aslin 1985; Hainline *et al.* 1984). They track a smoothly moving target with mainly saccadic movements and only some short episodes of smooth pursuit (Kremenitzer *et al.* 1979). Their OKN shows a tonic deviation in the direction of the field movement (Kremenitzer *et al.* 1979) and a temporo-nasal asymmetry under monocular viewing conditions (Atkinson and Braddick 1981). The mechanisms responsible for these immature oculomotor behaviours have not yet been identified clearly. It is likely that the developments of sensory, motor and attention mechanisms contribute together to the maturation of these oculomotor responses (Aslin 1981). The reduced performances of infants with respect to the spatial, temporal and velocity attributes of the visual stimulus may affect their oculomotor responses. Other factors such as the sensorimotor controls and the mechanical properties of the oculomotor 'plant', including viscosity, frictions and inertia may also be involved. Selective attention is also likely to play a major role: numerous attention-preference studies have demonstrated that infants are capable of some, low-level degree of attention by using their sensorimotor apparatus to select among the available input information (Haith 1978). Even if the effect of attention on infants' oculomotor responses has not been demonstrated, it is worth noting that infants' eye movements resemble strikingly those of non-attentive adults (i.e. adults who stare at the stimulus rather than look at it or who perform passive rather than active viewing). In inattentive adults, the quick phase of OKN becomes the primary component, resulting in a mean ocular deviation in the direction from which the movement is coming (Carpenter 1988). The velocity of saccades is reduced (Becker 1991). Also the gain of visual pursuit decreases and its phase augments (Pola and Wyatt 1991).

It is very important, for practical reasons, to control attention phenomena since they make examination techniques less sensitive and less reliable by introducing large variations in their results. If such precautions are not taken, the absence of oculomotor response is difficult to interpret, as it may result from several causes (Aslin 1985) such as a lack of detection of the visual stimulus by sensory processes, a failure in programming an oculomotor response, or an absence of attention.

For this reason, different approaches that have been attempted to reduce or control the influence of attention phenomena will now be reviewed. In the following section, the possibility of using oculomotor responses that are independent from attention mechanisms shall be studied. Following this, the question of controlling the state of wakefulness in order to perform visual tests under optimal conditions will be reviewed. The influence of attention on estimations of sensory visual processing will then be analysed and, in a final paragraph, the possibility of maintaining an optimal level of attention by reinforcement techniques providing rewards to the subjects according to their performance will be discussed.

Oculomotor responses that are independent from attention mechanisms

Numerous physiological and anatomical studies suggest that the oculomotor system is fundamentally split into two mechanisms named by Carpenter (1991), namely, gaze-shifting and gaze-holding. These mechanisms process specific visual information, velocity and position, respectively, and imply specific neurological centres.

The gaze-shifting mechanism is the consequence of the non-uniformity of the spatiotemporal properties of the visual system across the retina. It acts to form the image of a visual stimulus over the fovea, where the spatial resolution is much higher than anywhere else on the retina. This is accomplished either by fast, saccadic movements when a visual stimulus is detected in the periphery or by slow, tracking movements when the displacement of the stimulus relative to the fovea is small. It is important to note here that, although the macular region is not mature in young infants, it presents a higher spatial resolution than the peripheral retina (Sireteanu *et al.* 1984).

The gaze-holding mechanism acts to maintain the retinal image of a visual stimulus still and so avoids the degradation of spatial information resulting from motion. Such optokinetic responses are evoked by movements of the visual scenery. There is much evidence that the gaze-holding and gaze-shifting mechanisms are differently affected by attention: 'the response to target motion is continuously variable as a function of attention, whereas the response to target position is switched on when a deliberate effort is made to look at the target' (Pola and Wyatt 1991).

Oculomotor responses that imply movement of the stimulus are less dependent on attention than others that are static. In fact, optokinetic responses cannot be completely suppressed in the absence of a stationary target. Furthermore, they cannot be initiated voluntarily in the absence of a moving target. According to Kowler (1990), these results 'make it quite sensible to regard smooth eye movements as a sensorimotor reflex, operating under the control of the stimulus rather than free will'. It should be noted, however, that optokinetic responses cannot be obtained when a subject is sleeping, even when his or her pupil is directed toward the stimulus (Gardner and Weitzman 1967), which demonstrates the need for a minimum level of wakefulness. Nevertheless, most studies performed on babies have demonstrated the presence of optokinetic responses in almost all of them (McGinnis 1930; Gormann *et al.* 1957).

The use of these responses as a mean of testing sensory visual functions has been criticized (Fantz *et al.* 1962) on the basis that optokinetic responses may not involve retinogeniculo-cortical pathways and structures. If this judgment is true, the sensory visual performances of subjects estimated from these responses would be much lower than what would be obtained if the cortical processes were involved (Pasik and Pasik 1980). In fact, recent studies indicate that optokinetic responses involve both cortical and subcortical components (Kowler 1990).

It is probable that when the subjects' arousal level is low their performances correspond to subcortical processes and that optimal performances can only be achieved if cortical processes, which are under the control of attention are involved (Bushnelle *et al.* 1981). On this basis, it may be concluded that optimal estimations of sensory visual functions cannot be obtained from oculomotor responses independently of attention mechanisms.

Control of the state of wakefulness

It is worthwhile to mention that several environmental conditions are required in order to maintain a suitable state of wakefulness in infants. Such conditions involve, for example, the amount of ambient light and posture (Grenier 1981). Furthermore, infants are known to exhibit cyclic patterns of sleep and wakefulness. Scales have been developed in order to grade these different states of behaviour by Brazelton (Horowitz and Brazelton 1973) and by Prechtl (Prechtl *et al.* 1973).

Several studies have shown that responses to sensory stimuli are more reliable and reproducible when the test is performed in a specific behavioural state, for example, in Prechtl's state III (calm awakeness with opened eyes, absence of large body movements and regular respiration).

Influence of attention mechanisms on estimations of sensory visual processing

It has been shown previously that attention mechanisms play a key role in the elaboration of the oculomotor responses to visual stimulation. If the influence of these mechanisms is not identified, there is no guarantee that the subject's sensory threshold can be estimated reliably from oculomotor responses. Some examples of the influence of attention will first be given. These demonstrate the need to take its effect into account in the design of the evaluation procedures, as well as in the interpretation of the results. The possibility of estimating the level of attention as an attempt to provide reliability criteria for these interpretations will then be considered.

Our first example will be concerned with the analysis of fixation duration. The idea that infants spend more time fixating a portion of space where they locate a stimulus that captures their attention was introduced by Chase (1939) and developed by Fantz (1956; Fantz *et al.* 1962). It was later popularized under the name of preferential looking. Subsequent studies demonstrated that this measure is affected greatly by the novelty and the familiarity of the stimulus (Saayman *et al.* 1964). Many infants seem to prefer novel stimuli but some may actually favour stimuli that are familiar. Therefore duration of fixation is influenced by the attractivity of the stimulus in an uncontrolled manner and cannot be used as a reliable indicator of sensory visual processing.

Our second example will deal with the analysis of gaze-orientation responses. The preferential-looking technique evolved with the replacement of duration of fixation as a measure of preference by the estimation of gaze orientation toward the stimulus (i.e. a peripheral localization task). This approach was named forced-choice preferential looking (Teller *et al.* 1974) indicating the use of a forced-choice paradigm to eliminate observer biases in the evaluation of gaze-orientation responses: the observer determines on which side of a screen the stimulus is presented by looking at the infant's eye movements. This technique has since had a wide diffusion for research and clinical applications, such as the assessment of visual acuity, with consistent results across many laboratories and with other techniques (Vital-Durand and Hullo 1989). However, these responses have been shown to be affected by ill-defined characteristics of the stimulus described as complexity, salience or conspicuousness (Berlyne 1958). Furthermore, Held *et al.* (1979) have shown that infants do not exhibit preference to stimuli presented near threshold.

These two examples illustrate the fact that attention mechanisms may cause large variations of the oculomotor responses to a given visual stimulus. The same problem affects other oculomotor responses such as OKN and visual pursuit. Nevertheless, there is an important difference: these latter responses cannot be produced in the absence of a moving target, whereas fixations and saccades can be made with an empty visual field (Kowler 1990). In any case, the problem of interpreting the absence of oculomotor response in the presence of a stimulus remains unsolved with all oculomotor responses. There is no guarantee that the subject demonstrates his or her maximum sensitivity level and there is no evidence that the infant sensory threshold is reached (Teller 1985). It is therefore important to estimate the level of attention of subjects for the interpretation of oculomotor responses. A well-trained experimenter may be able to do so but such an evaluation is highly dependent on individual skill and experience.

Another possibility is to use features of the oculomotor response that characterize the attention level. For example Charlier and Buquet (1995), in an experiment involving the pursuit of a pattern stimulus by young infants, have shown that infants with reduced spatial discrimination do not present smooth pursuit or have reduced visual pursuit gains. They suggest that this quality of visual pursuit might be influenced by the attention level; however, further research is needed to substantiate this hypothesis. Other possible indicators of attention level may be thought of for other oculomotor responses, such as, for example, the dispersion of fixations or the latency of saccadic responses (Hainline *et al.* 1984; Hainline and Harris 1990).

Operant procedures to maintain attention

Another approach is to maintain attention by reinforcing the infants' behaviour according to the appropriateness of their responses. Operant-conditioning techniques are often needed for the examination of infants after the age of 5 months since they get bored very fast by repetitive stimulations. Rewards such as the appearance of an animated toy or the gift of food cereals have been used successfully (Mayer and Dobson 1980).

A major difficulty in applying these techniques is that there are large variations of behaviour between subjects, which result from factors such as age and sex, as well as cognitive and cultural development. Their application may be again highly dependent on the individual skill and experience of the experimenter. Feedback techniques based on an automated analysis of the 'quality' of the oculomotor responses may improve this approach considerably and are possibly a promising orientation for future research.

TECHNIQUES FOR MEASURING EYE MOVEMENTS

Several arguments demonstrate the need for an objective recording of oculomotor responses in children. Direct viewing of a subject's eyes does not allow a precise determination of the gaze orientation. It is dependent upon the observer's skill and does not provide an objective documentation. Furthermore, it is unsuitable for the analysis of dynamic responses.

Our purpose is not to make an exhaustive description of the numerous techniques that have been proposed for measuring eye movements. Such descriptions can be found elsewhere (Young and Sheena 1975; Maurer 1975; Aslin 1985). Rather, the major requirements that have to be met in order to make recordings from infants will be presented together with an estimate of how these requirements are fulfilled by the techniques presently available.

A suitable sensor for infants' eye movements would be non-invasive, easy to implement, easy to calibrate, highly reliable and available at an accessible cost. Other technical specifications will depend upon the type of eye movements studied. The analysis of fixations and slow movements, such as pursuit requires absolute measurements and can be made with rather low sampling rates (e.g. 5 measures/s), whereas the analysis of fast movements, such as saccades, requires higher sampling rates.

Another important consideration is the ability of the technique to separate eye movements from head movements. For the evaluation of sensory visual

Table 19.1 Summary of standard techniques for measuring eye movements and their effectiveness/drawbacks in infants.

	Electro-oculography	Magnetic coils	Limbus reflectance	Hirschberg principle
Invasiveness	Skin electrodes—risk of skin abrasion	Contact lenses blurring effect and risk of corneal abrasion	Goggles—visual field limitation	No
Horizontal measurements	Yes	Yes	Yes	Yes
Vertical measurements	Unreliable (eyelid movements contamination)	Yes	Unreliable (masking of iris margin by eyelids)	Yes
Measurement reference	Head	Fixed	Head	Fixed
Analysis of fixations and slow movements	Unreliable (electrode drift, head movements)	Yes	Limited (head movements)	Yes
Analysis of fast movements	Limited (30 Hz effective bandwidth due to noise)	Yes	Yes	Limited (60 Hz sampling frequency)

functions, it is necessary to evaluate the correlation between the oculomotor response and the position and movement of the visual stimulus. Techniques that make measurements relative to the head are unsuitable for the evaluation of fixations and slow eye movements relative to a visual target, except if the head is kept steady, which cannot be achieved in infants within a suitable range.

Specific adaptations have to be made to the techniques designed for adults in order to obtain recordings from infants, since most infants will grasp any object at a reachable distance in their visual field and, after the age of 5 months, many will not tolerate anything touching their eyes or head.

Table 19.1 gives a summary of these characteristics, the specifications of which will now be discussed.

The electro-oculography technique

Electro-oculography (Marg 1951) was probably the first technique used for recording eye movements in infants (Dayton *et al.* 1964). It consists of measuring differences in electric potential between electrodes placed on the skin around the eye.

These potentials result from the electric field between the retina and the cornea of the eye and are modulated by rotations of the eye relative to the head. They are affected by several artefacts, such as drifts of the electrode potential and heterogeneities of the bioelectric field (Zao *et al.* 1952), which impede absolute measurements and reduce considerably its reliability along the vertical and oblique axis.

The magnetic coils technique

The magnetic coils technique (Robinson 1963) is frequently used, because of its accuracy and sensitivity, in eye movement research on animals or adult humans. It is based upon electric currents induced in a small coil by a magnetic field. These currents are modulated by rotations of the eye relative to the magnetic field. The small coil is usually embedded within a scleral lens with small wires making the connection to the recording apparatus. This arrangement is extremely difficult to apply and potentially harmful for infant subjects.

The limbus reflectance technique

The limbus reflectance technique (Torok *et al.* 1951) comprises the measurement of the amount of light reflected by the border of the iris. The variation of reflectance between the iris and sclera produces a modulation of this signal by movements of the eye. This technique does not allow eye movements to be separated from head movements. As a result of the masking of the iris margin by the eyelids, it is limited to horizontal eye movements.

Techniques based on Hirschberg's principle

Methods based on Hirschberg's principle (Hirschberg 1885) measure the position of the image of a light source over the cornea (corneal reflex) relative to the pupil.

These measurements do not require contact with the subject and are not sensitive to translation movements of the head. They are directly related to the gaze direction by the geometry of the eye anterior chamber. As a consequence, they allow an isotropic and absolute evaluation of the angular eye rotation. Without any calibration, locus of fixation can be estimated with an absolute precision better than 5° (Buquet and Charlier 1994).

Owing to these interesting characteristics, this method was used in early studies of infant fixations (Fantz 1956) with the instrumentation available at that time, namely photographic recordings. However, the measurement rate was not quite fast enough to allow the analysis of successive fixations.

The advent of cinematography allowed higher sampling rates and a suitable temporal resolution. Nevertheless, the analysis of these recordings was

xtremely time consuming (1 minute of recording at a sampling rate of 30 Hz
epresents 1800 images to score!).

Recent technological developments of near-infrared video sensors, electron-
cs and microprocessors have permitted the increase of sampling rate and the
utomated analysis of these eye images, first 'off-line' (Haith 1969) and there-
fter in 'real time' (Merchant *et al.* 1974; Charlier 1980; Aslin 1981; Hainline
981).

At present, the performance of video sensors and image processors is still
imited and an optimal precision can only be achieved with a camera viewing
ield of about 25 mm. It is therefore necessary to track the recorded eye in order
ɔ maintain its image on the sensor and compensate the body movements of the
ubject (Hainline 1981; Buquet *et al.* 1992).

APPLICATION TO THE EVALUATION OF SENSORY VISUAL FUNCTIONS

he different possibilities offered by the oculomotor responses obtained in
nfants for the evaluation of each of the main sensory functions will now be
iscussed. Any visual function can be studied with almost any oculomotor
esponse, given the choice of an appropriate stimulus. For example, an eye
racking response can be elicited by a moving grating, allowing the evaluation
ɔf spatial discrimination or by a moving stereogram for the determination
ɔf stereopsis. However, there are many constraints to be met, advantages
nd drawbacks for each solution that will be discussed in the following
ɔaragraphs.

Visual acuity

efore reviewing the various methods that have been proposed for the
stimation of visual acuity, the authors would like to stress two important
ɔoints. The first is that the best spatial discrimination can only be obtained with
ɔecific spatio-temporal properties of the stimulus. In human adults, spatial
iscrimination decreases sharply when the stimulus is projected away from the
entral part of the retina and when its retinal image is in motion (Carpenter
988).

The second point worth mentioning is the difficulty of obtaining a 'pure'
isual stimulus, in other words one that is really testing what it is supposed to
est. The problems that are most frequently encountered are the contamination
ɔf high spatial frequency gratings with lower frequency components, mis-
natches of luminance between a local stimulus and its background and ap-
ɔarent edges where the grating is delineated from the background (Schor and
Narayan 1981; Robinson *et al.* 1988). Such problems have explained erroneous

results in several past studies and are often difficult to solve, even with today's technologies.

Attempts to estimate visual acuity have been made with all the oculomotor responses that have been described in infants. These responses include OKN, visual exploration and visual tracking of a moving target.

Optokinetic nystagmus

Optokinetic nystagmus (OKN) is a rhythmic oculomotor response that occurs when a subject is watching a repetitive pattern in motion at a constant speed. It is made up of a characteristic succession of slow and fast movements in opposite directions.

OKN responses have occasioned many studies in the 1950s and 1960s and have been the object of several reviews (Reinecke and Cogan 1958; Delthyl *et al.* 1968; Goddé-Jolly and Larmande 1973). They have since been almost abandoned as their results were often found unreliable in infants.

Two major approaches have been described: induced nystagmus and nystagmus arrest.

In induced nystagmus, visual acuity is estimated as the smallest separation between the bars of a grating in motion that can elicit a nystagmic response. This approach permits evaluations of visual acuity that are consistent with those obtained with other techniques for infants with ages up to 2 months (Gunther 1948; Gormann *et al.* 1957). So far as we know, reliable results have not been obtained in older subjects. There are several reasons that may account for this. The first is that it is technically extremely difficult to realize a 'pure' stimulus with high spatial frequencies covering a large visual field. A second reason is that, as the spatial frequency of the grating is increased, its velocity has to be reduced so that the temporal repetition of bars does not exceed the critical frequency of fusion (Collewijn 1991). As an example, the velocity of a grating of 5 cycles/degree, suitable for estimating the visual acuity of a 5-month-old child, has to be reduced to less than 4°/s in order to keep the repetition rate under 40 Hz. Such a velocity is probably too low to maintain attention and elicit an optokinetic response involving the cortical processes.

The second approach, nystagmus arrest, is based upon the finding by Dodge and Fox (1928) that the optokinetic movement generated by a large moving grating can be easily inhibited by fixation of a target superimposed on the stripes. This observation was later applied by Ohm (1932; 1956) to realize objective estimations of visual acuity in adults by measuring the threshold of nystagmus arrest obtained by adjusting the visibility of a target. The major problem with this technique is that the selection between tracking the moving grating and fixating the target is governed by selective attention (Kowler *et al.* 1984) and so the subject has to be instructed to fixate the target. Therefore, it is not surprising that studies in infants have obtained unreliable results (Delthyl *et al.* 1968).

Visual exploration

The exploration of a static visual scene is made through a succession of eye fixations and saccades. In infants, these changes of fixation do not operate randomly but respond to visual information from the peripheral retina (Aslin 1985). In adults, they are controlled by complex perceptual and cognitive functions that probably already have some effect at the earliest ages.

One implementation of visual exploration for the assessment of visual acuity is the preferential-looking technique. In the usual set-up, the infant is placed in front of a screen, which comprises two zones, one with a grating of a given spatial frequency and the other being uniform. The two zones are luminance matched and separated by a visual angle of about 20° from border to border. The test is based upon the fact that subjects direct their gaze toward the stimulus that they find most interesting. This implies that they are able to detect the stimulus before they can exert a preference. This is possible only if the stimulus is brought in the macular area where the spatial discrimination is higher than in the periphery (and becomes more and more so with age). The projection of the stimulus on the macular area can be obtained by chance, if enough time is given to the subject to scan through the visual scene. If the infant is old enough, he or she can be conditioned with operant techniques to scan through the two areas of interest.

A third solution proposed by Brown and Yamamoto (1986) consists of attracting fixation on the stimulus presented at the centre of the scene before displacing it toward the periphery. This solution is quite similar to the tracking approach that will be presented in the next paragraph.

Visual tracking of a moving target

Visual tracking is made by a set of ocular movements that aim to keep the image of a moving target on the macular area. These movements include slow movements called smooth pursuit and fast saccadic movements that occur when the gain of smooth pursuit is insufficient or when smooth pursuit is absent.

The first attempts to use visual tracking as a measure of visual acuity in infants have been made by using moving objects of decreasing sizes. Such objects included steel wires fitted on the swinging arm of a metronome (Schwarting 1954) or polystyrene balls (Sheridan 1963). However, in these situations, it is not clear whether the response is affected by a local change in stimulus luminance or by a change in stimulus resolution. A solution to this problem has been proposed for measurements of acuity in adults by Goldmann (1943) and later by Millodot and Harper (1969). It consists of a moving grating of limited size, with a luminance matching that of the background.

This latter approach was first tested on young infants by Delthyl *et al.* (1968) who used the Goldmann apparatus and later by Atkinson and Braddick (1983). These preliminary studies were based on direct observations of the oculomotor responses. The application of the electro-oculographic technique (Charlier *et al.*

1987) and of a technique based upon the Hirschberg principle (Buquet *et al.* 1992) allowed a more precise analysis of the oculomotor responses obtained with small moving gratings. This latter study reported high success rate in eliciting visual tracking: 82% of babies at birth, 98% at 2 months and 100% at 4 months.

The use of tracking oculomotor responses for the assessment of visual acuity raises several questions. A first question is the appropriateness of moving targets for a spatial discrimination task. It may be worthwhile to remember that under normal viewing conditions, there is not such thing as a static stimulus. The oculomotor system continuously exerts visual tracking to achieve a precise compensation of body and head movements.

A second question concerns the velocity limit imposed by the critical frequency of fusion, a problem that was mentioned previously with OKN responses. Actually the velocity of the retinal image of the stimulus is low when the eye is tracking the stimulus continuously. The problem arises when the stimulus is put in motion and it can be solved by increasing velocity progressively.

Evaluation of other sensory visual functions

Oculomotor responses have also been used for the assessment of many other sensory visual functions. Visual field has been studied by detecting gaze shifting responses to peripheral targets (Tronick 1972; Harris and MacFarlane 1974). Colour discrimination has been evaluated with OKN (Anstis *et al.* 1987), light adaptation with preferential looking (Dannemiller and Banks 1983) and stereopsis with the visual pursuit of a random-dot stereogram (Fox *et al.* 1980; Simons and Moss 1981) and with forced-choice preferential looking (Birch *et al.* 1985). These techniques have been used only for research purpose and are still not available to the clinic.

CONCLUSION

In this review, the major problems involved with the evaluation of infants sensory visual functions with oculomotor responses have been outlined. At present, very promising results have been obtained in research laboratories, however, there is still no widespread application of these techniques in the clinical world. One major barrier is the extremely high level of expertise that is needed to conduct the examinations and to interpret their results. There is some hope for future improvements of the present status by a better understanding of the neurophysiology of sensory and attentional processes. Other possible evolutions may come from the technological development of eye-movement sensors adapted to infants. Such techniques allow more objective and precise analysis of oculomotor responses and might be used to ensure a better control of attention effects.

REFERENCES

Anstis, S., Cavanagh, P., Maurer, D., and Lewis, T. (1987). Optokinetic technique for measuring infants' response to color. *Applied Optics*, **26**, 1510–16.

Aslin, R. N. (1981). Development of smooth pursuit in human infants. In *Eye movements: cognition and visual perception*, (ed. D. F. Fischer, R. A. Monty, and J. W. Senders), pp. 31–53. Lawrence Erlbaum, Hillsdale, New Jersey.

Aslin, R. N. (1985). Oculomotor measures of visual development. In *Measurement of audition and vision in the first year of postnatal life: a methodological overview*, (ed. N. A. Krasnegor), pp. 391–417. Abex Publishing Corporation, Norwood, New Jersey.

Atkinson, J. and Braddick, O. (1981). Development of optokinetic nystagmus in infants: an indicator of cortical binocularity? In *Eye movements: cognition and visual perception*, (ed. D. F. Fischer, R. A. Monty, and J. W. Senders), pp. 53–64. Lawrence Erlbaum, Hillsdale, New Jersey

Atkinson, J. and Braddick, O. (1983). Assessment of visual acuity in infancy and early childhood. In *Early visual development normal and abnormal*, (ed. L. Hyvarinen and E. Lindstedt), pp. 18–26. *Acta Ophthalmologica* Supplementum 157, Scriptor, Copenhagen.

Beasley, W. C. (1933). Visual pursuit in 109 white and 142 negro newborn infants. *Child Development*, **4**, 106–20.

Becker, W. (1991). Saccades. In *Vision and visual dysfunction. Eye movements*, (ed. R. H. S. Carpenter), pp. 95–137. Macmillan, London.

Berlyne, D. E. (1958). The influence of the albedo and complexity of stimulus on visual fixation in the human infant. *British Journal of Psychology*, **49**, 315–18.

Birch, E. E., Shimojo, S., and Held, R. (1985). Preferential looking assessment of fusion and stereopsis in infants aged 1–6 months. *Investigative Ophthalmology and Visual Science*, **26**, 366–70.

Brown, A. M. and Yamamoto, M. (1986). Visual acuity in newborn and preterm infants measured with grating acuity card. *American Journal of Ophthalmology*, **102**, 245–53.

Bryan, E. S. (1930). Variations in the responses of infants during the first ten days of life. *Child Development*, **1**, 56–77.

Buquet, C. and Charlier, J. (1994). Quantitative assessment of the static properties of the oculo-motor system with the photo-oculographic technique. *Medical Biological Engineering and Computing*, **32**, 197–204.

Buquet, C., Desmidt, C., Charlier, J., and Querleu, D. (1992). Evaluation des capacités de discrimination spatiale des enfants nouveau-nés par la poursuite visuelle de tests structurés. *Comptes Rendus de l'Académie des Sciences, Paris*, **314**, Série III, 133–40.

Bushnelle, M. C., Goldberg, M. E., and Robinson, D. L. (1981). Enhancement of visual responses in monkey cerebral cortex I: modulation in posterior parietal cortex related to selective visual attention. *Journal of Neurophysiology*, **46**, 755–72.

Carpenter, R. H. S. (1988). The use of eye movements. In *Movements of the eye. 2nd edn*, (ed. R. H. S. Carpenter), pp. 1–11. Pion, London.

Carpenter, R. H. S. (1991). The visual origin of ocular motility. In *Vision and visual dysfunctions. Eye movements*, (ed. R. H. S. Carpenter). pp. 1–9. Macmillan, London.

Charlier, J. R. (1980). A new instrument for automatic subjective and objective perimetry. *Medical Progress Through Technology*, **7**, 125–9.

Charlier, J. R. and Buquet, C. (1995). Effect of the pursuit gain on the spatial discrimination performance of a moving target in infants.

Charlier, J. R., Nguyen, D. D., Hugeux, J. P., Querleu, D., Dewavrin, D., Hache, J. C., and Defoort, S. (1987). A new technique for the clinical evaluation of visual functions in human neonates. In *Advances in Diagnostic Visual Optics*, (ed. A. Fiorentini, D. L. Guyton, and I. M. Siegel), pp. 176–80. Springer, Berlin.

Chase, W. (1939). Color vision in infants. *Journal of Experimental Psychology*, **20**, 203–22.

Collewijn, H. (1991). The optokinetic contribution. In *Vision and visual dysfunctions. Eye movements*, (ed. R. H. S. Carpenter), pp. 45–70. Macmillan, London.

Dannemiller, J. L. and Banks, M. S. (1983). The development of light adaptation. *Vision Research*, **23**, 599–609.

Dayton, G. O., Jones, M. H., Aiu, P., Rawson, R. A., Steele, B., and Rose, M. (1964). Developmental study of coordinated eye movements in the human infants. *Archives of Ophthalmology*, **71**, 865–70.

Delthyl, S., Sourdille, J., and Perdriel, G. (1968). Appréciation des fonctions visuelles chez l'enfant de 2 à 6 ans. Rapport annuel de la société d'ophtalmologie de Paris. *Bulletin des Sociétés d'Ophtalmologie de France*.

Dodge, R. and Fox, J. C. (1928). Optic nystagmus. *Archives of Neurology and Psychiatry*, **20**, 812–23.

Fantz, R. L. (1956). A method to study early visual development. *Perception and Motor Skills*, **6**, 13–15.

Fantz, R. L., Ordy, J. M., and Urdelf, M. S. (1962). Maturation of pattern vision in infants during the first six months. *Journal of Comparative and Physiological Psychology*, **55**, 907–17.

Fox, R., Aslin, R. N., Shea, S. L., and Dumais, S. T. (1980). Stereopsis in human infants. *Science*, **207**, 323–4.

Gardner, M. and Weitzman, E. (1967). Examination for optokinetic nystagmus in sleep and waking. *Archives of Neurology*, **16**, 415–20.

Goddé-Jolly, D. and Larmande, A. (1973). Le nystagmus optocinétique en ophtalmologie. In *Les nystagmus*, (ed. D. Goddé-Jolly and A. Larmande), pp. 1278–1352. Rapport de la société française d'ophtalmologie. Masson and Cie, Paris.

Goldmann, H. (1943). Objektive Sehcharfenstimmung. *Ophthalmologica*, **105**, 240–52.

Gormann, J. J., Cogan, D. G., and Gellis, S. S. (1957). An apparatus for grading the visual acuity on the basis of optokinetic nystagmus. *Pediatrics*, **19**, 1088–92.

Grenier, A. (1981). La motricité libérée par fixation manuelle de la nuque au cours des premières semaines de la vie. *Archives Françaises de Pédiatrie*, **38**, 557–61.

Gunther, G. (1948). Ein Gerat zur objektiven Prufung der zentralen Sehrshafe. *Graefe's Archiv für Ophthalmologie*, **148**, 430–42.

Hainline, L. (1981). An automated eye movement recording system for use with human infants. *Behavior Research Methods and Instrumentation*, **13**, 20–24.

Hainline, L., Turkel, J., Abramov, I., Lemerise, E., and Harris, C. M. (1984). Characteristics of saccades in human infants. *Vision Research*, **24**, 177–80.

Hainline, L. and Harris, C. M. (1990). Does foveal immaturity influence the infant's consistency of point of regard? In *From eye to mind: information acquisition in perception search and reading*, (ed. R. Groner, G. d'Ydewalle, and R. Parham), pp. 81–90. Elsevier, Amsterdam.

Haith, M. M. (1969). Infrared television recording and measurement of ocular behaviour in the human infant. *American Psychologist*, **24**, 279–83.

Haith, M. M. (1978). Visual competence in early infancy. In *Handbook of sensory physiology VIII*, (ed. R. Held, H. Leibowitz, and H. L. Teuber), Springer, Berlin.

Harris, P. and MacFarlane, A. (1974). The growth of the effective visual field from birth to seven weeks. *Journal of Experimental Child Psychology*, **18**, 340–8.

Held, R., Gwiazda, J. E., Brills, S., Mohindra, I., and Wolfe, J. (1979). Infant visual acuity is underestimated because near threshold gratings are not preferentially fixated. *Vision Research*, **19**, 1377–9.

Hirschberg, J. (1885). Uber die Messung des Schieldgrades und die Dosierung der Schieloperation. *Zentrabl Prakt. Augenheild*, **8**, 325.

Horowitz, F. D. and Brazelton, T. B. (1973). Research with the Brazelton neonatal scale. *Clinics in Developmental Medicine*, **xx**, 48–61.

Kowler, E. (1990). The role of visual and cognitive processes in the control of eye movements. In *Eye movements and their role in visual and cognitive processes*, (ed. E. Kowler), pp. 1–70. Elsevier, Amsterdam.

Kowler, E., Van Der Steen, J., Tamminga, E. P., and Collewijn, H. (1984). Voluntary selection of the target for smooth eye movement in the presence of superimposed, full field stationary and moving stimuli. *Vision Research*, **24**, 1789–98.

Kremenitzer, J. P., Vaughan, H. G., Kurtzberg, D., and Dowling, K. (1979). Smooth pursuit eye movements in the newborn infants. *Child Development*, **50**, 442–8.

McGinnis, J. M. (1930). Eye movements and optic nystagmus in early infancy. *Genetic Psychology Monographs*, **8**, 321–430.

Marg, E. (1951). Development of electro-oculography—standing potential of the eye in registration of eye movement. *Archives of Ophthalmology*, **45**, 169.

Maurer, D. (1975). Infant visual perception: methods of study. In *Infant perception: from sensation to cognition, Vol I: Basic visual processes*, (ed. L. B. Cohen and P. Salapatek), pp. 1–76. Academic Press, New York.

Maurer, D. and Lewis, T. L. (1979). A physiological explanation of infants' early visual development. *Canadian Journal of Psychology*, **33**(4), 232–51.

Mayer, D. L. and Dobson, V. (1980). Assessment of vision in young children: a new operant approach yields estimates of acuity. *Investigative Ophthalmology and Visual Science*, **19**, 566–70.

Merchant, J., Morissette, R., and Portefield, J. L. (1974). Remote measurement of eye direction allowing subject motion over one cubic foot of space. *IEEE Transactions on Biomedical Engineering*, **21**, 309–17.

Millodot, M. and Harper, P. (1969). Measure of visual acuity by means of eye movements. *American Journal of Optometry*, **46**, 938–45.

Ohm, J. (1932). Ueber ein Einfluss gespiegelter Marken au den optokinetischen Nystagmus. *Graefe's Archiv für Ophthalmologie*, **128**, 67–79.

Ohm, J. (1956). Optokinetic and optostatic reactions in children. *Klinische Monatsblat Augenheilk*, **129**, 235–52.

Pasik, T. and Pasik, P. (1980). Extrageniculostriate vision in primates. In *Neuro-ophthalmology, Vol. 1*, (ed. S. Lessell and J. T. W. Van Dalen), pp. 95–119. Excerpta Medica, Paris.

Pola, J. and Wyatt, H. J. (1991). Smooth pursuit: response characteristics, stimuli and mechanisms. In *Vision and visual dysfunction. Eye movements*, (ed. R. H. S. Carpenter), pp. 138–56. Macmillan, London.

Prechtl, H. F. R., Theorell, K., and Blair, A. W. (1973). Behavioural state cycles in abnormal infants. *Developmental Medicine and Child Neurology*, **15**, 606–14.

Reinecke, R. D. and Cogan, D. G. (1958). Standardization of objective visual acuity measurement. Optokinetic nystagmus *vs* Snellen acuity. *Archives of Ophthalmology*, **60**(3), 418–21.

Robinson, D. A. (1963). A method of measuring eye movements using a search coil technique in a magnetic field. *IEEE Transactions in Biomedical Electronics*, **10**, 137–45.

Robinson, J., Moseley, M. J., and Fielder, A. R. (1988). Grating acuity cards: spurious resolution and the 'edge artefact'. *Clinical Vision Sciences*, **3**, 285–8.

Saayman, G., Ames, E. W., and Moffet, A. (1964). Response to novelty as an indicator of visual discrimination in the human infant. *Journal of Experimental Child Psychology*, **1**, 189–98.

Schor, C. M. and Narayan, V. (1981). The influence of field size upon the spatial frequency response of optokinetic nystagmus. *Vision Research*, **21**, 985–94.

Schwarting, B. H. (1954). Testing infants vision: an apparatus for estimating the visual acuity of infants and young children. *American Journal of Ophthalmology*, **38**, 714–15.

Sheridan, M. (1963). Vision screening in very young and handicapped children. *British Medicine*, **2**, 453–60.

Simons, K. and Moss, A. (1981). A dynamic random-dot stereogram-based system for strabismus and amblyopia screening of infants. *Computers in Biology and Medicine*, **11**, 33–46.

Sireteanu, R., Kellerer, R., and Boergen, K. P. (1984). The development of peripheral visual acuity in human infants: a preliminary study. *Human Neurobiology*, **3**, 81–5.

Teller, D. Y. (1985). Psychophysics of infant vision: definitions and limitations. In *Measurement of audition and vision in the first year of postnatal life: a methodological overview*, (ed. N. A. Krasnegor), pp. 127–43. Abex, Norwood, New Jersey.

Teller, D. Y., Morse, R., Borton, R., and Regal, D. (1974). Visual acuity for vertical and diagonal gratings in human infants. *Vision Research*, **14**, 1433–9.

Torok, N., Guillemin, V., and Barthony, J. M. (1951). Photo-electro-nystagmography. *Annals of Oto-Rhino-Laryngology*, **60**, 917.

Tronick, E. (1972). Stimulus control and the growth of the infant's effective visual field. *Perception and Psychophysics*, **11**, 373–6.

Vital-Durand, F. and Hullo, A. (1989). La mesure de l'acuité visuelle du nourrisson en six minutes: les cartes d'acuité de Teller. *Journal Français d'Ophtalmologie*, **12**, 221–5.

Young, L. R. and Sheena, D. (1975). Survey of eye movement recording methods. *Behaviour Research Methods and Instrumentation*, **7**, 397–429.

Zao, Z. Z., Gelbin, J., and Rémond, A. (1952). Le champ électrique de l'oeil. *Semaine des Hôpitaux de Paris*, **28**, 1506–13.

Part IV
Perception, the brain, and clinical applications

The knowledge of how vision develops in infancy, both normally and in pathology, leads on to wider issues and applications. On the one hand, the visual system exists to provide a channel for learning about objects and events. Knowing something of the information delivered by the early stages of visual processing, one faces the question of how the infant makes use of it in perception. On the other, our research on visual development needs to be justified in terms of what it can provide the visually impaired child in terms of diagnosis, therapy, and rehabilitation.

The first two chapters in this section show some of the possibilities in the study of infant visual perception. Slater, in Chapter 20, shows that even the limited spatial information available to the newborn can be organized to make a range of form discriminations possible but that the visual cognition of the world of objects requires an extended developmental process. This process rests on the specialization of brain areas from an early age, strikingly shown in the dissociations of functions between different hemispheres that are presented by de Schonen and her colleagues in Chapter 21.

The next chapters move on to techniques that can be applied in the diagnosis and prognosis of pathology. Visual evoked potentials, the subject of Chapter 22 by Apkarian, have converged with behavioural measures to provide much of our knowledge of visual development. Here, VEP techniques are exploited for their ability to distinguish specific pathological conditions that affect different parts of the visual pathway. Complementing the VEP as a non-invasive functional probe for brain pathways, magnetic resonance imaging provides a non-invasive means of examining brain structure. To understand these images, one needs to know the functional consequences of the lesions they reveal; Cioni and colleagues (Chapter 23) relate the structural damage resulting from hypoxic and ischaemic conditions around birth, to behavioural measures of visual performance. This approach promises an earlier and more accurate prognosis of the effects of perinatal cerebral insults, which may extend beyond the purely visual effects.

A group of chapters follow that are concerned with therapy. Deprivation amblyopia is the most powerful example of visual neural plasticity, seen at its strongest in the loss of vision in unilateral cataract (Sjöström et al., Chapter 26). Occlusion therapy endeavours to use the same plasticity to reverse the effect, but can be a difficult procedure to manage. Moseley and Fielder (Chapter 24) discuss the evaluation of occlusion, which requires appropriate measures not only of visual outcome but also of how far the occlusion was effectively implemented by the child patients and their families. The animal model explored by Boothe (Chapter 25) reveals the potential power but difficulty of early occlusion: a small variation of the occlusion regime can change from a satisfactory result for both eyes, to a result in which occlusion has created an amblyopia in the treated eye as severe as that caused in the other eye by the original cataract.

Finally, it has to be appreciated that for many kinds of severe visual impairment, there are no specific therapies. This does not mean that scientific knowledge of visual development has nothing to offer such children. Rather, it must be directed to identifying their residual visual capacities, and tailoring a programme of rehabilitation to their individual needs in their family context. Such a programme, outlined in the final chapter by Portalier and Vital-Durand, aims to stimulate the spared capacity, often motion sensitivity, and use it in new ways. This objective challenges us to use the full range of our scientific understanding in ways that are creative for each new patient.

20

The organization of visual perception in early infancy

Alan Slater

INTRODUCTION

The major characteristic of perception, which applies to all the sensory modalities, is that it is organized. With respect to visual perception, the world that we experience is immensely complex, consisting of many entities whose surfaces are a potentially bewildering array of overlapping textures, colours, contrasts and contours, undergoing constant change as their position relative to the observer changes. However, we do not perceive a world of fleeting, unconnected retinal images; rather, we perceive objects that move and change in an organized and coherent manner.

Many organizational principles contribute to the perceived coherence and stability of the visually perceived environment; however, answers to the many questions about their origins and development awaited the development of procedures and methodologies to test infants' perceptual abilities. Many such procedures are now available and, in the last 30 years, many relevant infant studies have been reported. The obvious starting point is the visual world of the newborn baby; vision is unique among the senses in that there is no possibility of its use prior to birth, hence the visual capabilities of the newborn are the innate product of our evolutionary endowment. Many chapters in this volume point to the limitations of the newborn's visual abilities but there is no doubt that the visual system is functioning at birth. As an illustration of this, visual acuity at birth is between 10–30 times poorer than in the adult: adult acuity is about 30 cycles/degree, which represents 6/6 (or 20/20) vision, while that for the newborn is about 1 cycle/degree (20/600 vision) or a little better. Fig. 20.1 shows how a face might look to a newborn baby at a distance of about 30 cm from the eyes: while the image is considerably blurred, there is sufficient information to allow the infant to detect many of its important features. This figure, of course, is achromatic but, in the real world, there will be some chromatic information available to the infant.

In general, studies of infant vision have given rise to conceptions of the 'competent infant', since the perception of young infants has been found to be extremely well organized. While extreme empiricist views of perceptual development can be rejected, the picture of infant visual perception that is emerging is

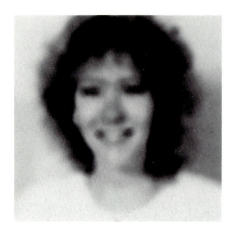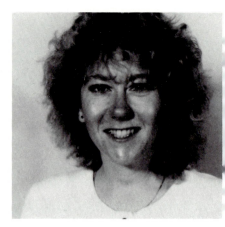

Fig. 20.1 The face as it might appear to (a) a newborn baby and (b) to us.

complex: some aspects of perceptual organization are present at birth, while others show considerable development through infancy. Several types of visual organization that are found in early infancy are discussed here, under the headings, *Shape and size constancy, Form perception, Biomechanical motion, Perception of objects*, and *Perception of faces*.

Shape and size constancy

As objects move, they change in orientation, or slant, relative to an observer. Indeed when they change in distance their retinal image size changes: an adult 10 feet away gives a retinal image that is half the size of that subtended by the same person at 5 feet from the observer. In order for the baby to make sense of these changes some degree of shape and size constancy—perception of objects' real shapes and sizes regardless of changes in orientation and retinal image size—needs to be present in visual perception.

The first evidence for the presence of these constancies in early infancy was presented by Bower (1966). He used a head-turn conditioning procedure and reported that 2-month-olds responded to objects' *real*, rather than *retinal*, shapes and sizes. Even this early an attainment, however, still leaves open the question of whether or not learning is involved: '... even 8 weeks gives a lot of opportunity for visual experience' (Gibson 1970, p. 104). Recent findings argue for the presence of both of these constancies at birth, and these are discussed next.

Slater and Morison (1985) described two experiments on shape constancy and slant perception in the newborn baby. In the first, using a preferential-looking procedure, newborns' preferences for one stimulus (an outline square)

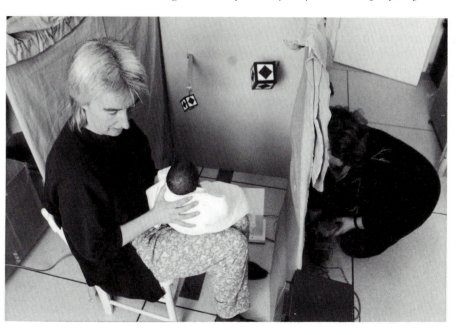

Fig. 20.2 A newborn baby being tested in a size-constancy experiment.

were found to change in a consistent manner with changes in slant, when it was shown paired with an outline trapezium that remained in the fronto-parallel plane relative to the infants: as the orientation of the square shifted progressively away from the frontal plane it became increasingly less preferred. This was a clear demonstration that changes to stimulus slant are detected by newborns, and that such changes can cause highly systematic changes to their looking behaviour. In the second experiment, newborns were desensitized to changes in slant during familiarization trials, and subsequently they strongly preferred a *different* shape when it was shown paired with the familiar shape, the latter being in a different slant than any shown earlier.

Fig. 20.2 shows a newborn baby being tested in experiments on size constancy (Slater *et al.* 1990*b*): the stimuli used in these experiments were cubes, one being half the size of the other. In the first (of two) experiments a preferential-looking procedure was used and the infants were shown several pairings of cubes, which varied in their sizes and distances from them. Highly consistent preferences were found, which could be described in terms of a simple rule: 'Look longest at the stimulus that gives the largest retinal image size, regardless of its distance or real size'. This was convincing evidence that newborns could base their responding on the basis of retinal size alone.

In the second experiment, 12 newborn babies were tested, and each of them was given six familiarization trials with one stimulus (either the small or the large cube), this being a different distance away in each trial. The intention of these trials was progressively to desensitize the infants to changes in the distance (and hence retinal size) of a constant-sized cube, in the hope that this would direct their attention to the cube's real size. After this familiarization period, the small and large cubes were shown at different distances, the smaller being half the distance of the larger one, so that their retinal sizes were the same. In these test trials the familiarized cube was a different distance away (and hence subtended a different retinal image) than any shown before, ensuring that the subjects could not be basing their responses on the test trials on any specific distance or size cues detected during the familiarization trials. Every one of the babies spent more time looking at the novel-sized cube on these trials, indicating that they had detected the stimulus invariant (the real size) from the retinally variable stimulus input presented on the familiarization trials. Several cues may have been available to the infants to allow them to make this discrimination: the patterns of light and shade differed for the cubes at the different distances; accommodation and vergence cues might have specified their different distances; motion parallax would also give distance information.

The findings of these studies demonstrate both a sensitivity to changes in slant and retinal size, and also the ability to perceive objective, real shape and size: that is, shape and size constancy are organizing features of perception that are present at birth. E. J. Gibson (1969, p. 366) seemed to anticipate these findings:

I think, as is the case with perceived shape, that an object tends to be perceived in its true size very early in development, not because the organism has learned to correct for distance, but because he sees the object as such, not its projected size or its distance abstracted from it.

Form perception

The terms 'figure', 'pattern', 'shape', and 'form' are often used interchangeably, and Zusne (1970, p. 1) commented that 'Form, like love, is a many splendored thing … there is no agreement on what is meant by form, in spite of the tacit agreement that there is'. Given this uncertainty, it is worth mentioning that most theories of form perception have been concerned with static, achromatic, two- or three-dimensional figures that can stand as figures in a figure–ground relationship, and it is the infants' detection of, and response to, these types of stimuli that are considered here.

PERCEPTION OF SIMPLE SHAPES

It would be impossible for a functional visual system *not* to respond to at least some variations in stimulus shape, and it is known that newborn babies make a variety of such discriminations. Typical procedures used to demonstrate these abilities include the visual preference method where if infants look more at ('prefer') one stimulus of a pair it indicates discrimination between the pair, and habituation to one pattern and subsequent testing for novelty responses to a new shape or pattern. Some of the findings from the use of these procedures with newborns are as follows:

(1) discrimination between the simple outline shapes of a square, triangle, circle and cross (Slater *et al.* 1983), and between complex abstract shapes (Slater *et al.* 1984);

(2) discrimination between gratings that differ only in orientation (Atkinson *et al.* 1988; Slater *et al.* 1988);

(3) discrimination between acute and obtuse angles, which may be the basic 'building blocks' of form perception (Slater *et al.* 1991*a*).

The findings from these studies are often not easy to interpret. For example, Cohen, in Slater *et al.* (1991*a*) argues that 'the discrimination between acute and obtuse angles shown by newborns might be interpreted in terms of differences in the relative sizes of the "blob" at the apex of the angles, rather than on the angular relationship between the two line segments' (p. 405). It is possible to discriminate, for example, between a square and a triangle on the basis of orientation differences: the square has horizontal and vertical lines, while the triangle has horizontal and diagonal ones. In order for us to be convinced that infants have form perception it would be necessary to demonstrate that they see squares *as* squares, rather than as collections of lines and angles. The virtual impossibility of eliminating alternative, non-form interpretations of stimulus discriminations is the reason why an understanding of the origins of form perception has remained elusive. Other findings are perhaps more convincing in suggesting that form perception is present either at birth or shortly after. These are considered in the next sections.

STIMULUS COMPOUNDS

All visual stimuli contain separate features that occur at the same spatial location, and which the mature perceiver 'binds together' as a whole. With such an ability we see, for example, a red square or a green triangle, while without it we would see redness, squareness, greenness and triangularity as separate, unrelated stimulus properties.

Evidence suggests that newborn babies perceive stimulus compounds rather than processing or detecting only the separate elements or components of the stimuli. An achromatic representation of the chromatic stimuli shown to newborn babies by Slater *et al.* (1991*b*) is shown in Fig. 20.3. The babies were familiarized, on successive trials, to two separate stimuli. For half the infants these were a green diagonal (GD) stripe and a red vertical (RV) stripe—the other babies were familiarized to GV and RD. In the former case, there are two

FAMILIARIZATION

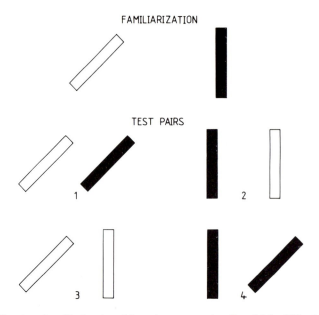

TEST PAIRS

Fig. 20.3 Following familiarization (above) to two stimuli, which differ in colour and orientation, there are four possible test pairings of familiar and novel compounds (below).

novel compounds of these elements—RD and GV. On test trials, the babies were shown one of the familiar compounds paired with one of the novel ones (Fig. 20.3 shows the four possible test pairings), and they showed strong novelty preferences. Note that the novel compounds consisted of stimulus properties that had been seen before, and the novelty preferences are therefore clear evidence that the babies had processed, and remembered, the simple stimulus compounds shown on the familiarization trials.

SUBJECTIVE CONTOURS

Subjective contours are illusory contours that are perceived 'in the absence of any physical gradient of change in the display' (Kanizsa 1979; Ghim 1990). An example of this illusion is pattern (A) in Fig. 20.4, and most adults see the contours of a square, despite the fact that the contours are physically absent. Perception of subjective contours is dependent upon the alignment of the inducing elements, and when this alignment is altered the subjective contour of the square is not seen, as is apparent by looking at patterns (B), (C) and (D), in Fig. 20.4.

Convincing evidence that 3- and 4-month-olds perceive subjective contours was provided in a series of experiments by Ghim (1990), from whose work

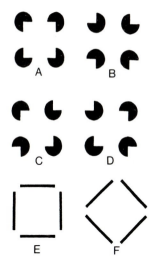

Fig. 20.4 Stimuli used by Ghim (1990). Pattern A (SC) produces subjective contours forming a square. Patterns B, C and D (NSC) do not produce subjective contours. The incomplete lines E and F were used in the test phase of an experiment following habituation to pattern A.

Fig. 20.4 is derived. In one experimental condition, the infants were familiarized either to a pattern containing a subjective contour (SC, pattern A, Fig. 20.4) or to a non-subjective contour (NSC, one of patterns B, C or D). Following this, the infants in the SC group discriminated SC from the NSC pattern, while those in the NSC group did not discriminate between the familiarized pattern and a different NSC pattern. This leads to the conclusion that '... the difference between patterns with and without subjective contours is greater than the differences between patterns without subjective contours' (Ghim 1990, p. 225).

In Ghim's (1990) fourth experiment, infants were familiarized to the SC pattern, and on the test trials they were shown patterns E and F of Fig. 20.4, and they gave a strong novelty preference for the incomplete diamond pattern, indicating that the incomplete squarelike pattern (E, Fig. 20.4) was seen as being similar to the SC pattern. Note that this novelty preference could not have resulted if the infants had only attended to the corners in the SC pattern, since there are no corners in either of patterns E and F (Fig. 20.4). Ghim (1990, pp. 243, 244) suggested that the results:

.. support contentions that the infants filled in the gaps among the aligned elements in the SC pattern, and ... add to our belief that infants have knowledge of the complete form and its components after viewing patterns that produce forms with subjective contours.

CATEGORIES AND PROTOTYPES

In order to reduce, and make sense of, the infinite variety of our perceptions and experiences an important human activity is categorization: categorization occurs whenever two or more perceptually (or conceptually) different stimuli or events are treated as being equivalent, and we allocate them to particular categories in terms of their possession (or absence) of invariant features that define the category. Infants, too, categorize their experiences, and examples of perceptual categorization that are present at birth (discussed earlier) are shape and size constancy. Newborn infants discriminated changes to the slant, and to the distance, of objects but were also able to respond on the basis of the objects' *real* shapes and sizes, independently of their retinal projections. Two aspects of categorization relevant to form perception are discussed here—orientation and form prototypes.

Bomba (1984) familiarized 4-month-olds to several striped patterns, which differed in their orientations but were all obliques (as opposed to being horizontal or vertical). On test trials, the infants generalized what they had seen to a differently oriented oblique (in the sense that they perceived a vertical pattern as novel and a new oblique as familiar). This suggests that the infants were treating the different obliques as members of the same category. For many perceptual categories a *prototype* can be defined as an ideal or average member, and the prototypical member is used both to organize and to define other members of the population and to select new members from incoming stimuli. An 'ideal' prototype might be, for example, a perfect square, with equal length sides and right-angles, and Bomba and Siqueland (1983) showed that 3- and 4-month-olds demonstrate prototypicality effects. In their experiments, the stimuli used were prototypes of a square, a diamond, and a triangle, and various distortions of these figures (for example, the distortions of the square might have unequal length, or slightly bent lines but look more 'square-like' than 'diamond-like' or 'triangle-like'). They found that the infants discriminated between each prototype and its distorted versions but treated the prototype as the 'best' exemplar of the category. Thus, when the babies were familiarized to several 'distorted' exemplars of one of the categories, and later shown one of the distorted versions paired with the previously unseen prototype, they treated the prototype as the familiar stimulus. What they seemed to be doing was perceiving the prototype as the best example of the recently acquired form category, and therefore recognizing it more readily than the distorted exemplar.

OVERVIEW

About 20 years ago Salapatek argued that '... the very early perception of two-dimensional visual stimuli must be regarded as the perception of parts rather than wholes' (1975, p. 226): that is, young infants do not have form perception. The virtual impossibility of eliminating alternative, non-form interpretations of stimulus discriminations is the reason why an understanding of the origins of form perception has remained elusive. Nevertheless, the evidence presented here suggests that form perception is present very early in infant perception.

Newborn infants perceive stimulus compounds, which argues against a view that they respond to parts of stimuli separately. By 3 months of age (or maybe earlier since younger infants have not been tested) infants perceive subjective contours: this ability would not be possible without form perception, since it requires the integration of perceptual information from two or more of the subjective contour's inducing elements. Also by 3 months of age infants have been shown to exhibit prototypicality effects, in the sense of extracting a form prototype from 'distorted' exemplars of the form. As discussed in the previous section, newborn babies detect the invariant (real) shapes of stimuli that vary in slant, and the real sizes of stimuli that vary in distance, and it is difficult to imagine how it would be possible to display shape and size constancy *without* having something like form perception.

Biomechanical motion

Many aspects of perceptual organization require the integration of information over space and time, and an understanding of these requires the use of dynamic stimuli. One such aspect of organization is the ability to detect the information contained in changing point-light displays. Biomechanical motions are the motions that correspond to the movements of a person (or other biological organism) when walking or displaying some other activity, and a point-light display to depict such motion is usually produced by filming a person in the dark who has some 11 points of light attached to his or her major joints (e.g. ankles, knees, hip, shoulder, elbows and wrists) and the head. Fig. 20.5A shows a display corresponding to a single, static frame, and observers shown such a picture are usually unaware that it represents a human form. However, if the displays are moving (as depicted in Fig. 20.5B) an impressive range of discriminations is easily made: adults perceive the human form and, from displays with durations as short as 200 ms, can specify its actions (e.g. walking, running, dancing, press-ups, etc.). Adults are also capable of recognizing friends and detecting gender from such displays (Bertenthal 1993).

A variety of evidence suggests that babies are sensitive to the biomechanical motions specified by the dynamic transitions of point-light displays. Displays have been produced in which the points of light either depict an upright walker with the lights at the major joints (a 'coherent' display), or with the lights moving 'off the joint', or randomly, or in a less coherent fashion than that of a real walker: random patterns (depicted in Fig. 20.5C) often suggest a moving swarm of bees. With these sorts of displays it has been found that infants as young as 3 months (younger ones have not been tested) prefer to look at a

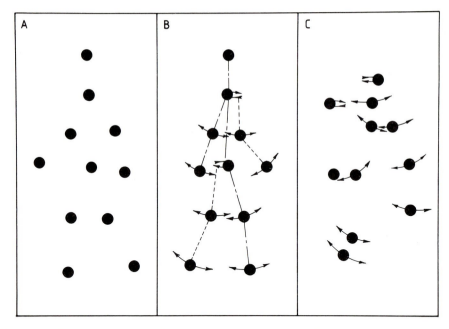

Fig. 20.5 Three possible point-light displays. (A) A static display is not usually seen as representing a human form. (B) When the display is in coherent motion, as depicted here, it is easily seen as a person walking. (C) If the point-light display moves in an incoherent or random motion perception tends to be of a swarm of bees. (Derived from Bertenthal 1993.)

coherent display in preference to a random one, and that they more readily encode 'coherent' than 'incoherent' displays, implying that they are detecting the organizational structure of the coherent one (Bertenthal *et al.* 1985; Fox and McDaniels 1982). Several processing constraints allow perception of bio-mechanical motions, as distinct from non-biomechanical forms of motion; for instance, the wrist can move back and forth and up and down relative to the position of the elbow but it is always a fixed distance from the elbow. Bertenthal (1993) discusses infants' awareness of these constraints and suggests that 'there is no clear lower-bound on the age at which they are first imple-mented. It is therefore quite reasonable to propose that these constraints are part of the intrinsic organization of the visual system' (p. 209).

There is an intriguing age change between 3 and 5 months in infants' respon-ses to these displays. Babies of 3 months discriminate between an upright and an upside down point-light walker, as do older babies. However, 3-month-olds also discriminate between an upside down point-light walker and a random pattern of lights, whereas 5- to 7-month-olds do not (Bertenthal and Davis 1988). Bertenthal and Davis's interpretation of this apparently paradoxical age change is that, by 5 months, infants are responding to the perceived familiarity of the displays, that is, as a result of experience and accumulated knowledge they recognize the upright display as a human walker, while the inverted and random displays are perceived equivalently because they are both unfamiliar. By 5 months of age, therefore, infants respond to these sorts of displays at a higher level of processing: perception interacts with prior knowledge to affect what is perceived.

Familiarity certainly affects adults' perceptions. For example, it has been known for many years that adults have great difficulty recognizing upside-down faces, most probably because of our extensive experience with upright ones. A similar 'inversion effect' is found with other stimuli: experienced dog-show judges have great difficulty matching inverted pictures of dogs (a task they can do effortlessly with upright pictures), whereas inexperienced judges do not show the inversion effect. With respect to adults' perception of point-light displays, a type of 'inversion effect' is found: an inverted display is often seen as several objects in motion, whereas the upright one is invariably seen as a moving person.

Perception of objects

As is the case with most aspects of visual development, widely different views have been expressed concerning infants' perception of objects. Piaget, who has been most influential in initiating research into object perception in infants, argued that the young infant's world is '... a world of pictures, lacking in depth or constancy, permanence or identity, which disappear or reappear capriciously' (1954, p. 3), and that 'Perception of light exists from birth (but) all the rest (perception of forms, sizes, positions, distances, prominence, etc.) is acquired through the combination of reflex activity with higher activities' (1953, p. 62). The research described earlier indicates that such an extreme constructivist view of perceptual development is unwarranted, and several authors have argued that infants perceive a much more coherent world than Piaget would have supposed. Thus, Kellman and Spelke (1983, p. 483) argued that 'perception of objects may depend on an inherent conception of what an object is', and Spelke (1985) has argued that infants begin life with an innate conception of the underlying unity, coherence and persistence of objects.

Some of the work on which Kellman and Spelke based their suggestions is from their studies (Kellman and Spelke 1983; Kellman *et al.* 1986) investigating infants' perception of partly occluded objects. Four-month-old infants were habituated to a stimulus (usually a rod) that moved back and forth behind a central occluder, so that only the top and bottom of the rod was visible (as in the upper part of Fig. 20.6). On subsequent test trials, the babies were shown two test displays without the occluder, one being a complete rod, the other being the top and bottom parts of the rod, with a gap where the occluder had been (the test trials, Fig. 20.6). Either of these test stimuli could have been the familiarized stimulus, and the question of interest was, what had the babies been seeing on the habituation trials? If they had seen the rod as being connected or complete behind the block, then the two rod pieces would be the novel of the two test stimuli. If they had seen the rod as being in two separate parts,

HABITUATION DISPLAY

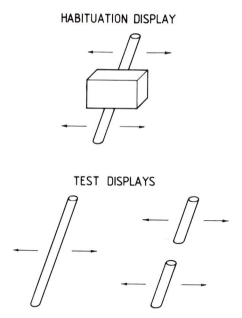

TEST DISPLAYS

Fig. 20.6 Habituation and test displays in experiments on infants' perception of partly occluded objects. During habituation the rod moved back and forth behind the occluder

the complete rod would be novel. Their results clearly supported the first of these possibilities: the babies spent more time looking at the two rod pieces on the test trials. However, when newborn babies were tested with the same arrangement they looked more on the test trials at the *complete* rod (Slater *et al.* 1990*a*).

It is possible that the newborns' limitations might result from an inability to detect the common motion *per se* of the two rod pieces, or it might be that infants' understanding of objects changes in the early months, and that, at birth, perception is dominated by that which is visible, not by that which can be inferred. Nevertheless, infants' understanding of the world of objects improves rapidly, and an experiment by Baillargeon *et al.* (1985) suggests that 5-month-olds can infer the existence of completely *invisible* objects. Their babies where shown a solid block, which was then hidden by a screen. The block was therefore no longer visible but its position was such that it should have prevented a moving drawbridge from travelling through a full 180° rotation. To make the full rotation the drawbridge would have had to pass through the block Baillargeon *et al.* found that their infants spent more time looking at an 'impossible' complete 180° rotation than at a 'possible' 120° rotation, suggesting that they were aware not only of the block's continued existence behind the screen but that they 'knew' that its presence constituted an obstacle to the drawbridge's movement.

Perception of faces

Newborn (and older) infants consistently prefer to look more at patterned than unpatterned, at moving rather than static, at three- rather than two-dimensional, at high rather than low contrast, and at low rather than high spatial frequency stimuli. These preferred stimulus characteristics are found in the human face and combine to ensure that the face will be one of the most attention-getting and attention-holding stimuli encountered by the infant. The newborn is a competent learner, as many habituation and conditioning studies have shown and, within hours from birth, learns about the specific characteristics of the mother's face. Field *et al.* (1984), and Bushnell *et al.* (1989) reported statistically reliable preferences for the mother's face, compared with that of a female stranger, at 45 hours, and 49 hours from birth, respectively. In a recent study, Walton *et al.* (1992) reported that infants aged between 12 and 36 hours of age, produced more sucking responses in order to see a videotaped image of their mother's face, as opposed to an image of a stranger's face.

Such early learning testifies to the importance of the face to the infant, and it seems that babies quickly form a prototype, or averaged version, of the face. Samuels and Ewy (1985) showed pairs of black and white slides of same-gender faces (equal numbers of female and male faces were used) to 3- and 6-month-old infants. The slides were constructed so that each of the members of a pair were as similar as possible in other respects but differing in attractiveness as rated by adults: attractive and unattractive faces were paired together. Both age groups looked longest at the more attractive face for all of the pairings. This finding of infant preferences for attractive faces was replicated and extended by Langlois *et al.* (1987; 1991), with infants as young as 2 months old, and they found that the effect generalized across faces differing in race (black and white), gender, and age (adult and infant faces). A likely interpretation of these infant preferences is the following. If faces are created by combining or averaging the features of several individual faces, these 'averaged' or prototypical faces are rated as significantly more attractive than the ones they were derived from, and such averaged faces become even more attractive as more faces are added (Langlois and Roggman 1990). Thus the babies' preferences for attractive faces can be interpreted as a prototypicality effect.

In addition to the above evidence of early learning about faces, two lines of evidence suggest that infants come into the world with some visually specified innate knowledge of the structure and organization of the face. One of these lines of evidence was first given by Goren *et al.* (1975) who reported that their subjects, who averaged only 9 *minutes* from birth at the time of testing, turned their heads and eyes more to follow (i.e. track) a two-dimensional schematic face-like pattern than either of two patterns consisting of the same facial features in different arrangements. Johnson and Morton (1991) use these, and related findings to argue for what they call a 'Conspec', which is a face-detector present at birth, and which serves to direct infants' attention to faces.

The second, and perhaps the most convincing, line of evidence that babies have an in-built knowledge of the face comes from experimental evidence for newborn infants' imitation of various facial gestures they see adults perform, the gestures including mouth opening, lip pursing, tongue protrusion, 'happy', 'sad', and 'surprised' facial expressions (Field *et al.* 1982; Meltzoff and Moore 1977). These claims of precocious imitation have been controversial, and there arose some disagreement, not only concerning which gestures newborns will imitate, but also whether they will imitate *any* facial gestures (McKenzie and Over 1983). By now, however, over 20 researchers have reported such early imitation and it is now clear that infants are innately endowed with a well-defined representational system that allows them to translate adults' facial gestures to unseen facial gestures of their own.

In a more recent paper, Meltzoff and Moore (1994), showed that 6-week-old infants can remember a facial gesture they have seen an adult produce, after a 24-hour delay. The adult produced either mouth opening or tongue protrusion on one day and, on the next day, the same adult sat in front of the babies displaying a static face: the babies then imitated yesterday's observed gesture. Meltzoff and Moore interpret this delayed recall in terms of its role in the understanding of 'persons':

Infants use imitation as a way of re-identifying and communicating with the persons they see before them ... Is this the self-same person acting differently (no facial gesture game) or a different person who merely looks the same? (1994, p. 10); and

...infants use the non-verbal behaviour of people as an identifier of who they are and use imitation as a means of verifying this identity. (1992, p. 479)

Their claim is that imitation at birth and in early infancy is an act of social cognition. Certainly, early imitation is a product of considerable innate organization of the visual system and of cross-model functioning: the claim of innate special responsiveness to and recognition of the human face is now incontestable.

Overview and conclusions

The newborn baby enters the world visually naive but with several means with which to make sense of the visual world. It is likely that rudimentary form perception is present at birth, in the sense that the infant perceives wholes rather than only separate elements, or parts, of two-dimensional visual stimuli. This conclusion results from several findings: newborns readily discriminate between different two- (and three-) dimensional shapes, and they perceive stimulus compounds in that they 'bind together' the components of a stimulus (such as colour and orientation) rather than processing these components or parts separately; infants as young as 3 months have been shown to perceive subjective contours, which is a clear indication of form perception, since such an ability requires the integration of two or more of the contour's inducing elements; infants, like adults, categorize visual stimuli and, by 3 months of age, are able to extract prototypic forms (such as a diamond or a square) from exemplars that are distorted versions of the prototypic form; infants also extract prototypes from objects encountered in their real worlds and, by 2 months, respond to a prototypic face.

Important organizational features present at birth are shape and size constancy, and an innate detection of facial structure: newborn infants detect invariant information about shape and size across changes to slant or orientation, and retinal size, indicating that size and shape constancy are present at birth; they produce imitations of a variety of facial gestures they see adults produce indicating an innate representation of the face.

As expected, learning and experience soon have an effect on perceptual organization. In the newborn period, infants learn about the visual stimuli they see, as indicated by a preference for novel stimulation after having been habituated to a now-familiar stimulus. Within hours from birth, enough has been learned about the mother's face for it to be preferred to a stranger's. The prototypicality effects mentioned earlier result from experience with exemplars of the appropriate categories; since such prototypes can be formed very quickly in an experimental setting with 3-month-olds it may be that their formation is an innate biological predisposition of the visual system. Bertenthal (1993) has argued similarly that an awareness of the processing constraints that allow perception of biomechanical motions may be part of the intrinsic organization of the visual system. However, and inevitably, some types of visual organization take time to develop. An appreciation of the underlying unity, coherence and persistence of objects is not present at birth, and a proper understanding of objects develops throughout infancy; while newborn infants imitate adult facial gestures and other body movements, it is not until around 9 months that they can copy adults' actions *on objects*. In addition, while detection of biomechanical motion from point-light displays may be present near birth, it is not until about 5 months that infants can recognize an appropriate display as being of a human walker.

These studies demonstrate that the newborn infant's visual world is, to a large extent, structured and coherent as a result of the intrinsic organization of the visual system. As development proceeds, the innate and developing organizational mechanisms are added to by experience, which furnishes the familiarity, meanings and associations that assist the infant in making sense of the perceived world.

ACKNOWLEDGEMENTS

The author's research was supported by the following grants from the Economic and Social Research Council: C00230028/2114/2278; RC00232466. Thanks are due to Liz Brown, Anne Mattock and Victoria Morison, who collected most of the data, and to the subjects' mothers and the staff of the

Maternity Unit, Royal Devon and Exeter Hospital, Heavitree, Devon, for their help and co-operation.

REFERENCES

Atkinson, J., Hood, B., Wattam-Bell, J., Anker, S., and Tricklebank, J. (1988). Development of orientation discrimination in infancy. *Perception*, **17**, 587–95.

Baillargeon, R., Spelke, E. S., and Wasserman, S. (1985). Object permanence in five-month-old infants. *Cognition*, **20**, 191–208.

Bertenthal, B. I. (1993). Infants' perception of biomechanical motions: intrinsic image and knowledge-based constraints. In *Visual perception and cognition in infancy*, (ed. C. Granrud), Erlbaum, Hillsdale, New Jersey.

Bertenthal, B. I. and Davis, P. (1988). *Dynamical pattern analysis predicts recognition and discrimination of biomechanical motions.* Paper presented at the annual meeting of the Psychonomic Society, Chicago, Illinois.

Bertenthal, B. I., Proffitt, D. R., Spetner, N. B., and Thomas, M. A. (1985). The development of infant sensitivity to biomechanical motions. *Child Development*, **56**, 531–43.

Bomba, P. C. (1984). The development of orientation categories between 2 and 4 months of age. *Journal of Experimental Child Psychology*, **37**, 609–36.

Bomba, P. C. and Siqueland, E. R. (1983). The nature and structure of infant form categories. *Journal of Experimental Child Psychology*, **35**, 294–328.

Bower, T. G. R. (1966). The visual world of infants. *Scientific American*, **215**, 80–92.

Bushnell, I. W. R., Sai, F., and Mullin, T. (1989). Neonatal recognition of the mother's face. *British Journal of Developmental Psychology*, **7**, 3–15.

Field, T. M., Woodson, R., Greenberg, R., and Cohen, D. (1982). Discrimination and imitation of facial expressions by neonates. *Science*, **218**, 179–81.

Field, T. M., Cohen, D., Garcia, R., and Greenberg, R. (1984). Mother–stranger face discrimination by the newborn. *Infant Behavior and Development*, **7**, 19–25.

Fox, R. and McDaniels, C. (1982). The perception of biological motion by human infants. *Science*, **218**, 486–7.

Ghim, H.-R. (1990). Evidence for perceptual organization in infants: perception of subjective contours by young infants. *Infant Behavior and Development*, **13**, 221–48.

Gibson, E. J. (1969). *Principles of perceptual learning and adaptation.* Appleton Century Crofts, New York.

Gibson, E. J. (1970). The development of perception as an adaptive process. *American Scientist*, **58**, 98–107.

Goren, C. C., Sarty, M., and Wu, P. Y. K. (1975). Visual following and pattern discrimination of face-like stimuli by newborn infants. *Pediatrics*, **56**, 544–9.

Johnson, M. and Morton, J. (1991). *Biology and cognitive development: the case for face recognition.* Blackwell, Oxford.

Kanizsa, G. (1979). *Organization in vision: essays on Gestalt perception.* Praeger, New York.

Kellman, P. J. and Spelke, E. S. (1983). Perception of partly occluded objects in infancy. *Cognitive Psychology*, **15**, 483–524.

Kellman, P. J., Spelke, E. S., and Short, K. R. (1986). Infant perception of object unity from translatory motion in depth and vertical translation. *Child Development*, **57**, 72–86.

Langlois, J. H. and Roggman, L. A. (1990). Attractive faces are only average. *Psychological Science*, **1**, 115–21.

Langlois, J. H., Ritter, J. M., Roggman, L. A., and Vaughn, L. S. (1991). Facial diversity and infant preferences for attractive faces. *Developmental Psychology*, **27**, 79–84.

Langlois, J. H., Roggman, L. A., Casey, R. J., Ritter, J. M., Rieser-Danner, L. A., and Jenkins, V. Y. (1987). Infant preferences for attractive faces: rudiments of a stereotype? *Developmental Psychology*, **23**, 363–9.

McKenzie, B. E. and Over, R. (1983). Young infants fail to imitate facial and manual gestures. *Infant Behavior and Development*, **6**, 85–95.

Meltzoff, A. N. and Moore, M. K. (1977). Imitation of facial and manual gestures by human neonates. *Science*, **198**, 75–8.

Meltzoff, A. N. and Moore, M. K. (1992). Early imitation within a functional framework: the importance of person identity, movement, and development. *Infant Behavior and Development*, **15**, 479–505.

Meltzoff, A. N. and Moore, M. K. (1994). Imitation, memory, and the representation of persons. *Infant Behavior and Development*, **17**, 83–99.

Piaget, J. (1953). *The origins of intelligence in the child*. Routledge and Keegan Paul, London.

Piaget, J. (1954). *The construction of reality in the child*. Basic Books, New York.

Salapatek, P. (1975). Pattern perception in infancy. In *Infant perception: from sensation to cognition*, (ed. L. B. Cohen and P. Salapatek), Vol. 1, pp. 133–248. Academic Press, New York.

Samuels, C. A. and Ewy, R. (1985). Aesthetic perception of faces during infancy. *British Journal of Developmental Psychology*, **3**, 221–8.

Slater, A. M. and Morison, V. (1985). Shape constancy and slant perception at birth. *Perception*, **14**, 337–44.

Slater, A. M., Morison, V., and Rose, D. (1983). Perception of shape by the newborn baby. *British Journal of Developmental Psychology*, **1**, 135–42.

Slater, A. M., Morison, V., and Rose, D. (1984). Habituation in the newborn. *Infant Behavior and Development*, **7**, 183–200.

Slater, A. M., Morison, V., and Somers, M. (1988). Orientation discrimination and cortical function in the human newborn. *Perception*, **17**, 597–602.

Slater, A., Morison, V., Somers, M., Mattock, A., Brown, E., and Taylor, D. (1990*a*). Newborn and older infants' perception of partly occluded objects. *Infant Behavior and Development*, **13**, 33–49.

Slater, A. M., Mattock, A., and Brown, E. (1990*b*). Size constancy at birth: newborn infants' responses to retinal and real size. *Journal of Experimental Child Psychology*, **49**, 314–22.

Slater, A. M., Mattock, A., Brown, E., and Bremner, J. G. (1991*a*). Form perception at birth: Cohen and Younger (1984) revisited. *Journal of Experimental Child Psychology*, **51**, 395–405.

Slater, A. M., Mattock, A., Brown, E., Burnham, D., and Young, A. W. (1991*b*). Visual processing of stimulus compounds in newborn babies. *Perception*, **20**, 29–33.

Spelke, E. S. (1985). Perception of object unity, persistence and identity: thoughts on infants' conceptions of objects. In *Neonate cognition: beyond the blooming, buzzing confusion*, (ed. J. Mehler and R. Fox), Erlbaum, London.

Walton, G. E., Bower, N. J. A., and Bower, T. G. R. (1992). Recognition of familiar faces by newborns. *Infant Behavior and Development*, **15**, 265–9.

Zusne, L. (1970). *Visual perception of form*. Academic Press, New York.

21

Pattern processing in infancy: hemispheric differences and brain maturation

S. de Schonen, C. Deruelle, J. Mancini, and O. Pascalis

INTRODUCTION

The various neural networks of the infant brain do not all become functional at the same rate. Investigating the relationships between emerging cognitive competences and maturational neural events can therefore be most instructive. In some respects, this approach to the neural basis of behaviour, although it involves some methodological difficulties, is similar to the neuropsychological approach to adult patients with brain lesions. The double dissociations between emerging behaviours and between neural maturational events correspond to the double dissociations that are being studied in adult patients (that is between behavioural deficits and the localization of lesions). This is not to say, however, that the emergence of a new cognitive ability in infants can be accounted for only by the functional onset of a group of neurones that has remained silent up to this point. Neural events of other kinds, which may be very similar or even identical to those underlying adult learning processes, are probably involved in the mechanisms of cognitive development. Discovering how learning mechanisms and neural maturation co-operate and are correlated with age-related behavioural changes is the main goal of this developmental approach.

Unlike the double dissociations studied in adult neuropsychology, the double dissociations observed in the changes occurring in the brain and cognitive competences during development are part of a normal functional process. The fact that specific sets of neurones are not yet functioning, or specific abilities not yet acquired, is part of the normal process of development, and may even play a decisive role in shaping and timing the course of forthcoming developmental events (Bresson and de Schonen 1979; de Schonen and Bresson 1983; de Schonen 1989; de Schonen and Mathivet 1989; Turkewitz 1988; 1989a,b), if only by simply filtering the environmental stimuli and being insensitive to some of them for example. In addition, the lack of maturity of some parts of the cortex at birth probably gives several environmental factors a non-negligible part in shaping the organization of the neuronal networks, although the role of these factors may be completely defined and anticipated in the working principles of the neuronal networks and their maturational timing (Greenough *et al.* 1987; Singer 1987).

This was the general framework within which the authors of this chapter first began to study the differences in the way the two hemispheres process visual patterns and faces in infancy and the inter-hemispheric interactions occurring at this age. The peripheral afferent pathways to the cortical areas involved in visual processing are apparently similar in the two hemispheres. Nevertheless, the contributions of the two hemispheres to some processing skills in adults, such as face processing for instance, are known to be asymmetrical. Conversely, there exists some functional plasticity between the hemispheres, as shown for example in studies on language development in infants with early unilateral brain lesions. The timing and duration of the plasticity depend on the localiza-tion of the lesion and on the subject's age at the time of the lesion. This suggests that the plasticity depends on the timetable of the maturational events, which differs from one set of networks to another. The neural organization of some portions of the two hemispheres therefore diverges at some point during de-velopment. One means of approaching these neural differences and finding our way among these populations of networks consists of looking at the develop-ment of the functional hemispheric differences, and by comparing our findings with those obtained in studies on brain maturation at other levels such as that of cellular maturation (Simonds and Scheibel 1989; Scheibel 1993).

It was only quite recently that interest began to develop in the activities in which the right hemisphere (RH) specializes and in the differences between the two hemispheres' visual modes of pattern and object processing during in-fancy. The way in which these differences develop used to be inferred simply from what was known about children (as opposed to infants) and about adults with perinatal brain damage who had been tested long after the age of a few months.

Some of the main questions dealt with in our investigations are as follows: is the adult RH advantage for some aspects of face processing (Hécaen and Albert 1978; Moscovitch 1979; Young 1983; Ellis and Young 1989; Gross and Sergent 1992) already present in infants when they begin to recognize individual faces? Or is this aspect of adult functional brain asymmetry simply the outcome of other intervening developments and neural specializations, such as the increas-ing commitment of the available left hemisphere (LH) neural space to language-related activities? If, on the contrary, the RH has an early advantage for face recognition, does this involve only the processing of faces or that of visual patterns in general? Might the functional differences between the two hemi-spheres' modes of visual pattern processing be correlated with differences between the maturational rhythms of homologous regions (the maturational lags between homologous brain regions in the two hemispheres might gener-ate differences as to how the neuronal networks are organized on both sides, as well as a differential sensitivity to pre- and post-natal environmental factors)? Are any traces of the limited visual capacities characteristic of infants during he first few months of life detectable in the adult visual processing organization? And how are the interhemispheric communication systems set up and developed?

In what follows, an attempt shall be made to answer partly a few of these questions and, where no definite answers are yet possible, a few speculations shall be made.

HEMISPHERIC SPECIALIZATION IN FACE PROCESSING

In a previous study, it was shown that, from the age of 12 weeks onwards up to the age of at least 7 months, each hemisphere is able to recognize and categorize faceness (de Schonen and Bry 1987). When tested in each visual field separately with a separate visual-field presentation technique, very short durations of presentation and an operant conditioning paradigm, infants of this age produced the same performances in the left visual field-right hemisphere (LVF-RH) and right visual field-left hemisphere (RVF-LH). However, what has been learned in one hemisphere cannot be used by the other hemisphere before the age of 19 weeks.

What about infants' ability to recognize individual faces? In a previous study, 4- to 10-month-old infants were shown colour slides of the mother's and a stranger's face. Each subject's mother's face served as the stranger's face with another subject. The photographs were taken in such a way that the discrimination between faces could be based only on physionomical features. The faces were projected, as in the faceness recognition study mentioned above, to the right or left of the central fixation point. The subjects were exposed to the stimulus for 350 ms in the case of the 4- to 6-month-old groups, and 250 ms in that of the 7- to 9-month-old group (for further details, see de Schonen *et al.* 1986). The latency between the stimulus onset and the beginning of the ocular saccade produced by the infants in response to the stimulus onset was measured. The latency of the response towards the mother's face became significantly shorter than towards the stranger's face after a few trials. The infants can therefore be said to have recognized their mothers in this situation. The decrease in the latency that occurred in response to the 'mother' stimulus took place, however, in the LVF-RH and not in the RVF-LH. Since no motor bias (de Schonen *et al.* 1978) and no difference in visual acuity or attention existed that might have accounted for this difference between the two visual fields, the RH can be said to have an advantage over the LH in recognizing—or at least in reacting spontaneously towards—a two-dimensional picture of the mother's face.

The results of another study suggested that this RH advantage is not restricted to the mother's face. The RH was again found to have an advantage when, instead of the mother's face, a photograph of a stranger's face was used with which the subjects received moderate familiarization during the experiment itself (de Schonen *et al.* 1986, experiment 2). The RH advantage for recognition of, or reactivity towards familiar faces therefore includes faces or photographs with which infants have become familiar.

In a third study, as in the previous faceness categorization study (see previous discussion) a separate visual-field presentation technique and an operant conditioning procedure were combined. The stimuli were slides of the mother's face and a stranger's face. The results again showed that in 4- to 10-month-old infants the LVF-RH had a considerable advantage for distinguishing between 'mother' and 'stranger' stimuli (de Schonen and Mathivet 1990). The boys results differed from those of the girls, not with the RH, but with the LH: none of the boys reached the learning criterion in the RVH-LH, whereas 25% of the girls reached the criterion in this visual field. A similar sex-related factor was found to operate in an earlier study on familiar face recognition (de Schonen *et al.* 1986 and unpublished data), where the male population was more strongly lateralized than the females. In the present study, the relationship between the degree of hemispheric assymmetry and the subjects' sex does not seem to vary between the age of 4 and 10 months. Therefore this was not a temporary difference such as that described by Gwiazda *et al.* (1989), for example, in their study on stereopsis (see Chapter 17 in this volume).

Contrary to what was observed in the faceness recognition study, no sign of interhemispheric transfer was observed in these infants. Although the LH is able to recognize the human face at this age, it does not score very highly with familiar face recognition and does not seem to be able to use the information learned by the RH about faces.

The above data argue against the hypothesis that the RH advantage for face recognition observed in adults might be caused by the fact that, from the age of 2 years onwards, an increasing amount of neuronal space in the LH is committed to language learning. Our data prove that if the RH lateralization of face processing has any connection with the fact that the left hemisphere is committed to language processing, the mechanism involved is present as early as the fourth month. Secondly, our data are in agreement with the idea that in adults, the RH and LH abilities to recognize individual faces do not both involve the same mechanisms.

The lack of inter-hemispheric transfer in the case of individual face recognition may contribute towards stabilizing the hemispheric specializations. Alternatively, the fact that information about faceness undergoes a transfer (after the age of 19 weeks) and also the lack of functional hemispheric asymmetry, suggest that individual face recognition and species face recognition may not involve the same neuronal networks (de Schonen 1989; de Schonen and Mathivet 1989). The latter conclusion is also supported by data from studies on neonates (Johnson and Morton 1991; Pascalis *et al.* 1995).

The fact that the degree of lateralization was found to differ between boys and girls suggests that the neuronal organization may differ between the two sexes as early as the first year of life.

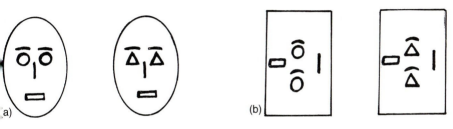

Fig. 21.1 The two pairs of stimuli: (a) symmetrical face-like patterns; (b) non-symmetrical arbitrary patterns. In each of the two pairs, the stimuli are discriminable on the basis of whether the stimulus contains a pair of small circles or a pair of triangles (from Deruelle and de Schonen 1991).

PATTERN PROCESSING BY THE RIGHT AND THE LEFT HEMISPHERES

The RH advantage for individual face recognition that emerges during the first year of life may result from a more general RH advantage for complex pattern processing, either because the neuronal networks involved in pattern processing become functional in the RH before the LH (de Schonen and Mathivet 1989), or because the RH has a general advantage for pattern processing. Another possible explanation is that, since attentional requirements are dealt with by the RH (Posner and Petersen 1990), split visual-field tasks may be performed better by the RH than by the LH when they are more difficult than simply recognizing faceness.

Deruelle and de Schonen (1991) have shown that, in infants aged 4 to 9 months, the two hemispheres both process visual patterns but not the same aspects of these patterns. In one situation, the subjects were shown two geometrical designs schematically representing a face, and differing only in the shape of the elements standing for the eyes (Fig. 21.1(a)). The second situation involved patterns composed of the same elements as previously but arranged arbitrarily and with no vertical symmetry (Fig. 21.1(b)). The stimuli were presented as in the experiments described above. It turned out that the two hemispheres were, in fact, equally able to learn to recognize the patterns in Fig. 21.1(b). The LH disadvantage in individual face processing is therefore not attributable to a general disadvantage in pattern processing.

The RH was found to score less well on learning the patterns in Fig. 21.1(a) than on the arbitrary patterns in Fig. 21.1(b), and less well than the LH on the patterns in Fig. 21.1(a). The low score obtained by the RH with the symmetrical patterns in Fig. 21.1(a) shows that this hemisphere is sensitive to the overall arrangement of the components. One might hypothesize that some configural aspects of shapes may prevent the RH from processing the components of the pattern, whereas the LH mode of processing may be better adapted to processing these local components. In Fig. 21.1(a), the relevant configural aspects

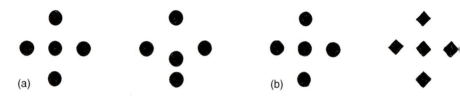

Fig. 21.2 (a) The two stimuli used in the location task, and (b) the stimuli used in th component task (see text).

that might have prevented the RH from processing the components may be either the facial ones or only the symmetrical configuration. In the situation shown in Fig. 21.1(a), the RH might have failed because the difference between the shapes of the 'eyes' did not generate any differences between the two globa configurations. The difference between the RH performances in the two situa tions suggests that the RH processing is not always blind to any local differ ences present in patterns but only when the pattern configuration is face-like or has some symmetry. In individual face recognition, the RH advantage may, therefore, stem from its propensity to process the configural aspects and differences.

CONFIGURAL AND COMPONENT PROCESSING

To investigate further the difference between the processing modes of the two hemispheres, Deruelle and de Schonen (Deruelle and de Schonen submitted de Schonen and Deruelle 1991) used a task involving recognition of sym metrical geometrical figures. Infants aged 4 to 9 months were presented, using a similar procedure to that adopted in the previous experiments (de Schonen and Mathivet 1990; Deruelle and de Schonen 1991), with either pair of the patterns shown in Fig. 21.2. Here again they had to learn to associate each o two responses with each of the two stimuli (operant conditioning). In the *component* task (Fig. 21.2(b)), the two stimuli differed by the shape of their com ponents, while in the *location* task (Fig. 21.2(a)) the two stimuli differed in the spatial position of one internal element. In the *component task* significantly more subjects were able to reach the learning criterion with the LH than with the RH in the *location task* more subjects, but not significantly so, reached the criterion with the RH than with the LH. When presented with the two symmetrical patterns in Fig. 21.2(b), the number of subjects able to learn with their LH only and not with their RH was higher than the number able to learn with the RH whereas when the patterns presented were those in Fig. 21.2(a), the number of subjects able to learn with their RH only but not with their LH tended (but not significantly) to be higher than the number able to learn with the LH (some of the subjects were able to perform the *location* task with either hemisphere)

In other words, although the RH did not perceive local differences affecting neither the overall appearance of the symmetrical pattern, the spatial relationships between the components, nor the location of a component, it perceived a change affecting the location of a component and the symmetries within the area defined by the outer contour of the figure; in contrast, the LH tended to perceive the local differences more readily than the change of location.

These data are consistent with those by Ghim and Eimas (1988) showing the contemporaneous nature of two modes of processing in early infancy (see also review by Dodwell *et al.* 1987). Our results show, however, that different neuronal networks are involved. Furthermore they argue against the hypothesis by Rothbart *et al.* (1990) that the lateralization within the LH of the processing of local aspects may be a side-product of learning to read. The LH advantage in local processing is based on a neural organization that operates long before learning to read.

The LH disadvantage for individual face recognition might be caused by the fact that local processing is not the appropriate mode for this type of recognition task. Processing the complex features of a face one by one might take too long to be efficient. The RH advantage in face recognition might be the result of the RH advantage in processing the configuration of a pattern, that is, in processing the spatial relationships between the components, or at least some of the information relating to the location of the components.

In order to determine whether this difference between the hemispheres' pattern processing modes also applies to face processing, Deruelle and de Schonen (submitted; de Schonen and Deruelle 1991) compared two situations. As in previous experiments, 4–9-month old infants had to associate each of two photographs of a face presented for a short duration in one visual field at a time, with two different responses. The stimuli were as follows. The eyes of the original photograph (O) of a woman's face (frontal view, with a scarf on her hair) were transformed in three ways. In one case (Oo) the eyes on the photograph were cut out and repasted onto the original photograph so that their orientation was more oblique. In the second case (Os), the eyes of the photograph were cut out and repasted onto the photograph after being reduced in size. These two transformations, changing the orientation of the long axis of the eyes and changing the size of the eyes, affect the overall configuration of the spatial relationships between the components of the face but not the shape of the components. In the third case (Oc), the eyes (but not the eyebrows) of another woman were pasted onto the original photograph. The outer contour of the new orbital cavities was similar in size to that of the original ones but the shape of the eyelid contour relative to the pupil and the size of the visible corneal part differed from the original eyes. This change in the shape of a local component involves minimal changes in the overall spatial relationships between the components of the face. The infants were presented with a pair of photographs (the original and one of the transformed ones). The technique was identical to that used in the experiments already described (de Schonen and Mathivet 1990; Deruelle and de Schonen 1991).

The results show that the RH had a significant advantage over the LH in recognizing and discriminating between the photographs of the configural pairs (O–Oo and O–Os) and the LH a significant advantage over the RH in performing the *component* task (O–Oc). The RH performances in the *configural* tasks were significantly higher than in the *component* task and the LH performances in the *component* task were significantly higher than in the *configural* task. Here again, the male and female populations were found to differ. Part of the female population was able to perform the configural task not only with the RH but also with the LH. This was not so in the case of the male population.

In summary, it seems likely that the RH processes faces with a configural mode. The ability of part of the female population in the previous experiments (see previous discussion) to recognize the mother's face and to discriminate it from the stranger's face with the LH might have been caused by the ability to use a configural mode of processing with the LH. This argues in favour of the hypothesis that efficient face recognition in infancy depends closely on the ability to process faces with a configural mode. The inability of the LH to recognize faces might be caused by its local mode of processing. It is worth noting that the LH is unable to recognize and discriminate between two different faces but is able to perform the task when the two faces differ in only one component (the eyes).

BRAIN MATURATION AND HEMISPHERIC SPECIALIZATION

What then are the possible factors that lead to the two hemispheres developing different visual perceptual abilities? Or in other words, what developmental mechanisms may contribute to implementing the specialization programmes?

According to a scenario developed by de Schonen (1989), de Schonen and Mathivet (1989), (see also Turkewitz 1989*a*,*b*; 1993), the RH system for processing individual faces and complex patterns might become functional before the LH system. There exist several arguments supporting the idea that, at some times *in utero* and also during the first few months of life, some parts of the RH cortex develop faster than their LH counterparts (for a review, see Geschwind and Galaburda 1985; Crowell *et al.* 1973; Rosen *et al.* 1987; Simons and Scheibel 1989; Scheibel 1993). Even quite small time lags between the two maturational rates can lead to different patterns of synaptic organizations being selected and subsequently stabilized. A neuronal network can apparently take anything from a few minutes to a few days to become stabilized (Fifkova and van Harreveld 1977; Buisseret *et al.* 1978; Fifkova 1985; Schechter and Murphy 1976; Singer 1987). The other possibility, which is compatible with the first one, is that the infant's arousal system during the first 2–3 months of life may act primarily in the RH.

During this 2–3-month period when the RH system becomes functional (or is more strongly activated by the arousal system), infants' visual capacities are still rather restricted, partly because they involve pathways that are sensitive only to the low spatial frequencies (for a review, see Banks and Dannemiller 1987; Banks *et al.* 1985; Held 1989; Atkinson and Braddick 1989). The individual face recognition system may become stabilized on the basis of this coarse visual information. Scheibel (1993; Simons and Scheibel 1989) has shown that the growth of the dendritic arborization of neurones in the human infant's left Broca cortex is slower than in the homologous part of the RH. If differences of this kind between the RH and LH cortex were also present in the extrastriate visual cortices, they would be compatible with the idea that pattern processing might develop and become stabilized earlier in the RH than in the LH, sometimes during the first 2–3 months of life, when visual information is conveyed mainly by low spatial frequencies and therefore, when configural information rather than local information is processed and memorized. The conjunction of those two series of maturational events (the time gap between right and left maturation, and the various rates of maturation of the elementary visual capacities) may give rise to two separate hemispheric modes of pattern processing. This scenario might lead one to expect that the adult RH might have an advantage for dealing, for instance, with faces when these consist of low frequencies or are presented off-centre in relation to the fovea. Sergent (1983; 1985; 1987) has suggested that the adult RH advantage in face processing may be based on its capacity to process low spatial frequencies. When tested in adults, this hypothesis has sometimes been confirmed and sometimes ruled out (Christman 1990; Fiorentini and Berardi 1984; Kitterle *et al.* 1990; Michimata and Hellige 1987; Sergent 1987; 1989; Szelag *et al.* 1987). The present authors do not believe that all the visual processing carried out by the RH is based on low spatial frequencies but that some of the visual processing systems might be fed by low spatial frequencies. Conversely, some aspects of configural processing seem to involve specifically low spatial frequency processing: Hughes *et al.* (1990) have shown that, if the low spatial frequencies are removed from a pattern, the global precedence effect disappears.

This scenario is a set of assumptions as to why face processing is more efficient in the RH than in the LH, and why the adult RH face processing system, or at least one of the RH processing systems, relies on global information more than the LH system does. However, our scenario does not tell us anything at all about how a face-processing system or a pattern-processing system may develop. Some of the constraints leading to this functional specialization of cortical networks probably operate very early, before visual experience begins. Mancini *et al.* (1994) observed face recognition or emotional expression recognition deficits in children aged 6–10 years of age who had sustained neonatal unilateral cortical damage but who were nevertheless able to learn to read and write. These data suggest that the general outline of a modular organization of the processing of the various kinds of information available on a face is prepared before the occurrence of visual experience.

Since more information is needed about functional brain maturation in human infants, a Positon Emission Tomography (PET) scan study with [15]oxygen-labelled water on alert infants aged 2 and 4 months was carried out (Tzourio *et al.* 1993 de Schonen *et al.* 1993). The aim of this study was to investigate cognitive development and brain dysfunction in infants born at risk. Among the various reasons for comparing 2- and 4-month-old infants was the fact that visual processing (including face processing) changes in many respects between the age of 2 and 4 months (see Slater 1993; Morton and Johnson 1991; Johnson 1990; Pascalis *et al.* 1995). The study involved comparing the regional activations associated with face processing with those associated with complex non-face pattern processing, and speech processing with music processing, in 2- and in 4-month-olds. Only two injections could be performed with each subject: one for the control situation and the other for one of the cognitive situations under study. The activation associated with each of these cognitive situations minus the activation associated with the control situation had therefore to be studied in different groups of subjects. The results of one group of subjects only are available so far: this group received face stimuli situation and a control situation.

The results reported here concern six 2-month-old infants who had suffered from acute fetal stress, birth asphyxia or neonatal convulsions. At the time of the study they showed only moderate neurological symptoms (minor hypotonia) and were free of neurological drugs (for the methodological background to studies of this kind see Mazoyer and Tzourio 1993).

Normalized cerebral blood flow (NrCBF) levels were recorded twice during the same session. In the first trial, which constituted the control condition, the subjects fixated a small circle consisting of red and green diodes. The red diodes were lit successively, giving the impression of a circular path moving at a speed that was varied during the whole trial. In the second trial, the subjects visually fixated photographs of female faces (borrowed from the experiments on mother's face recognition described above), which were presented every 4 s for 4 s each. Five different faces were presented repeatedly. The diode circle was chosen because three conditions had to be fulfilled: first, the control situation had to be interesting enough for the infant to remain motionless while fixating the stimulus; second, the control situation had to involve visual processing but not complex pattern processing (since knowing where pattern and face processing occur at this age was required); and last, a change in a visual aspect (but not in the shape of the pattern) had to occur parallel to the change in face stimuli—a small circular movement of the red and green diodes at a variable speed was chosen because it provided the most suitable control stimulations with which to compare the other possible patterned stimuli.

Since the results of only one age group with only one comparison are available at present, the scope of these preliminary results is necessarily limited. The first main finding to emerge from this study is that it was possible to carry it out at all. The lowest NrCBF values were obtained in pre-frontal regions and the highest in the sensory–motor and visual cortex, confirming the data obtained by Chugani and Phelps (1986) using 2-deoxy-2[^{18}F]fluoro-D-glucose (FDG). The NrCBF value was higher in the RH than in the LH during both trials in the external temporal cortex and the inferior frontal cortex (F3) (the values recorded in the medial temporal cortex, which is one of the sites specifically involved in famous-face recognition in human adults, are not yet available). The right orbitofrontal cortex was significantly more active than the left in the *circle* trial but not in the *face* trial. No significant asymmetry was detected in the sensory–motor cortex, internal occipital cortex, external occipital cortex, parietal, or superior medial frontal cortex. The right hemispheric dominance observed in both situations is compatible with our conjectures that the maturation rate in the RH may be faster than in the LH during the first 2–3 months of life. The existence of greater activity in the RH may, however, also have been caused by a differential sensitivity to visual stimulation or to a differential long-term reactivity to the fetal stress induced by asphyxia, for example.

The differences in the NrCBF levels between the two situations (*face* minus *circle*) were computed in the case of each of the regions mentioned above. Face stimuli were associated with a significant increase (relative to the circle stimulus) in the NrCBF values in both the right and left external temporal cortices (superior and middle temporal gyri), in the left inferofrontal (F3, including the Broca area) and orbitofrontal cortices. No significant differences were observed in the other regions. The increase in neural activity from circle to face stimuli therefore occurs in associative regions and not in the primary visual areas.

Some of these regional activations are similar to those recorded in PET studies on adult subjects processing faces, objects or shapes. Haxby *et al.* (1991) compared the results of two matching tasks, one with faces and the other with configurations of three dots; in the control task used in both situations, the subjects had to detect the onset of three squares. These authors observed that a lateral occipital extrastriate region was involved in both tasks. The areas activated more by face matching than by dot location were in the occipitotemporal cortex, while the areas activated more by dot-location matching than by face matching were located in the superior parietal cortex. No difference was found between RH and LH. Our data are congruent with those of Haxby *et al.* (1991) so far as they show the occurrence of rCBF increases in lateral posterior temporal regions in the *face* condition. Corbetta *et al.* (1990) used a task requiring selective attention to one of three possible kinds of near threshold changes in a display: change in shape, speed or velocity. These tasks were compared with two control tasks: in one, the subject was presented with the same display without being required to perform any task, while, in the other, the subject had to report whether any change had occurred in the display but was not informed about the kind of change (e.g. shape, speed or colour) that would occur. In fact comparisons with each of the control conditions yielded the same results. Besides activations in several medial parts of the hemisphere for which we have no equivalent data available in our study, attending to changes in shape activated a region on the lateral surface, midway along the superior temporal sulcus between areas 21 and 22. This activation was bilateral but stronger in the RH than in the LH as was the case in our study. These regions were not activated by detecting changes of either colour or velocity. The left middle external temporal region (area 21) has been described as being involved in both face and object processing in adults (Sergent *et al.* 1992). Sergent *et al.* have noted that the external temporal (area 21) activity on the left side is probably associated with object and face naming rather than with the visual type of recognition processes with which the right side deals. In our subjects, the occurrence of a right lateral temporal activity might be associated with visual pattern processing. Does the occurrence of a left activity pattern mean that some neural pathway between the networks involved in object recognition and those that will become involved later on in lexical categorization competence is already present at this age?

Sergent *et al.* (1992), as in our study, observed an activation of the orbitofrontal region (the gyrus rectus, area 11) in tasks involving object and famous face recognition. In our face task, the rCBF increases also extended to area 47. This increase might be associated with a working memory component. In our face task, five photographs of faces were presented repeatedly, providing an opportunity for some working memory processes to operate. Several authors have reported that lesions in the dorsolateral or inferior convexity of the prefrontal cortex in the monkey produced deficits in tasks requiring memory for objects (Stamm 1973; Passingham 1975), despite the fact that such regions are neither a functional nor an anatomical part of the limbo-diencephalic memory system (Kowalska *et al.* 1991). Wilson *et al.* (1993) reported more recently that in the prefrontal cortex of monkeys performing a working memory task, the neurones involved in pattern recognition were more numerous in the inferior convexity of the pre-frontal cortex, whereas neurones involved in the location recognition were more numerous in the dorsolateral pre-frontal cortex. In a PET scan study on human adults, Jonides *et al.* (1993) used a working memory task where the subject had to watch a configuration of three dots and to remember the location of one of the dots. An increase in neuronal activity in the right pre-frontal cortex centred on area 47 was associated with this task. The increase in activity observed in our subjects around area 47 may have been caused by a working memory process operating on face patterns. In our study, however, an increase in the pre-frontal cortex was significant in the LH but not in the RH, whereas the increase in the activity observed in the temporal area, which we have attributed to visual shape processing, occurred not only on the left but also on the right side, and resulted in a higher activity on the right side than on the left.

Some of the areas specifically activated in response to the *face* stimuli were different from those described in adult studies in response to faces or objects. No activation of the superior temporal gyrus was observed in the face task of Haxby *et al.* (1991) (apart from the region along the STS), or in the study on object and famous face recognition by Sergent *et al.* (1992). Ojemann *et al.* (1992), however, in a study on humans (before surgery for medically intractable epilepsy), performing a face-matching task, recorded extracellular responses in the superior and middle temporal gyri. So far as the left inferior frontal cortex (F3) including the Broca area is concerned, no specific neuronal activations were observed in adult studies in response to faces or objects. Might the greater activation of the Broca area observed here in 2-month-old infants be caused by the existence of a relationship between the visually presented faces and the tendency observed in infants to imitate mouth movements (Meltzoff and Moore 1983)? It is worth noting, however, that no visible mouth movements by the subjects were observed during the PET scanning.

CONCLUSION

There are at least three interesting outcomes of this preliminary study:

(1) The results suggest that in agreement with our predictions, some portions or some neural nets of the RH temporal cortex might mature faster than their left counterparts.

(2) The results show that, even at this early age, different regional activations of associative cortices were associated with different classes of visual events. The activations triggered by the more complex patterned stimuli, the *face* stimuli, but not by the *circle* stimuli, involved several regions of the cortex but were not spread over the whole cortex. Moreover, some of the regions activated by these face presentations are among those that are activated in the adult brain by tasks that involve attending to similar stimuli (e.g. faces, objects and shapes). Of course it is unclear as yet whether the neural activity observed is face-specific or more generally related to complex pattern and object processing.

(3) The metabolic activity associated with *face* stimuli but not with the *circle* stimuli occurs in cortical regions that still have a relatively low level of metabolic activity at this age and in which the synaptic density is still increasing (Huttenlocher 1993). This supports the notion that cerebral functional maturation proceeds network by network rather than area by area. Similar conclusions can be drawn about infant monkeys. In 5–7-week old infant monkeys Rodman *et al.* (1993) recorded cells responding specifically to faces in the IT (infero-temporal) cortex (1993). At this age, the cortical synaptic density is still increasing sharply in the monkey cortex, and the cells responded significantly more weakly than those of adults.

(4) Lastly, the fact that some of the regions activated in the infant brain by the face presentations were also activated in adults by tasks involving not only face but also object and shape processing, is in agreement with the conjecture that it is only after the age of 2 months that a system more specifically involved in face processing and more able to deal with faces emerges in infants. It has been established that neonates' mother's face recognition ability is abolished when the mother wears a scarf hiding the hair contour and the outer contour of the head (Pascalis *et al.* 1995). Morton (1993) has reported that at about 40 days of age, the infant recognizes

his/her mother even when the hair is covered with a scarf. At the age of 4 months onwards, the infant is able to recognize his/her mother's face when she is wearing a scarf, and does so better with the RH than with the LH (de Schonen *et al.* 1986; de Schonen and Mathivet 1990). These data suggest that it is between the second and fourth months that infants begin to process actual face information. This is why it is predicted that cerebral imaging data on the 4-month-old infants will show the existence of a similar pattern of activation to the adult pattern in response to our face task.

ACKNOWLEDGEMENTS

The present research was supported by the CNRS and by a grant of the Ministère de la Recherche et de la Technologie (Action Sciences de la Cognition, N°90 C 0723) to the first author.

REFERENCES

Atkinson, J. and Braddick, O. (1989). Development of basic visual functions. In *Infant Development*, (ed. A. Slater and G. Bremner), pp. 7–41. Lawrence Erlbaum, London.

Banks, M. S. and Dannemiller, J. L. (1987). Infant visual psychophysics. In *Handbook of infant perception*, Vol. 1, (ed. P. Salapatek and L. Cohen), pp. 115–84. Academic Press, Orlando.

Banks, M. S., Stephens, B. R., and Hartmann, E. E. (1985). The development of basic mechanisms of pattern vision. Spatial frequency channels. *Journal of Experimental Child Psychology*, **40**, 501–27.

Bresson, F. and de Schonen, S. (1979). Le développement cognitif. Les problèmes que pose aujourd'hui son étude. *Revue de Psychologie Appliquée*, **29**, 119–27.

Buisseret, P., Gary-Bobo, E., and Imbert, M. (1979). Ocular motility and recovery of orientational properties of visual cortical neurons in dark-reared kittens. *Nature*, **272**, 816–17.

Chugani, H. T. and Phelps, M. E. (1986). Maturational changes in cerebral function in infants determined by [18]FDG Positron Emission Tomography. *Science*, **231**, 840–2.

Christman, S. (1990). Effects of luminance and blur on hemispheric asymmetries in temporal integration. *Neuropsychologia*, **28**, 361–74.

Corbetta, M., Miezin, F. M., Dobmeyer, S., Shulman, G. L., and Petersen, S. E. (1990). Attentional modulation of neural processing of shape, color, and velocity in humans. *Science*, **248**, 1556–9.

Crowell, D. H., Jones, R. H., Kapunai, L. E., and Nakagawa, J. K. (1973). Unilateral cortical activity in newborn humans: an early index of cerebral dominance? *Science*, **180**, 205–8.

Deruelle, C. and de Schonen, S. (1991). Hemispheric asymmetries in visual pattern processing in infancy. *Brain and Cognition*, **16**, 151–79.

Deruelle, C. and de Schonen, S. (1995). Pattern processing in infancy: hemispheric differences in the processing of shape and location of visual components. *Infant Behavior and Development*, **18**, 123–32.

de Schonen, S. (1989). Some reflections on brain specialization in faceness and physiognomy processing. In *Handbook of research on face processing*, (ed. A. Young and H. D. Ellis), pp. 379–89. North Holland, Amsterdam.

de Schonen, S. and Bresson, F. (1983). Données et perspectives nouvelles sur les débuts du développement. In *Le développement dans la première année*, (ed. S. de Schonen), pp. 13–26. PUF, Paris.

de Schonen, S. and Bry, I. (1987). Interhemispheric communication of visual learning: a developmental study in 3–6-month old infants. *Neuropsychologia*, **25**, 601–12.

de Schonen, S. and Deruelle, C. (1991). Configurational and componential visual pattern processing in infancy. Poster presented at the 14th European Conference on Visual Perception, Vilnius, 26–30 August 1991. *Perception*, **20**, 123 (Abstract).

de Schonen, S. and Mathivet, E. (1989). First come first served. A scenario about development of hemispheric specialization in face recognition during infancy. *European Bulletin of Cognitive Psychology (CPC)*, **9**, 3–44.

de Schonen, S. and Mathivet, E. (1990). Hemispheric asymmetry in a face discrimination task in infants. *Child Development*, **61**, 1192–205.

de Schonen, S., MacKenzie, B., Maury, L., and Bresson, F. (1978). Central and peripheral objects distances as determinants of the effective visual field in early infancy. *Perception*, **7**, 499–506.

de Schonen, S., Gil de Diaz, M., and Mathivet, E. (1986). Hemispheric asymmetry in face processing in infancy. In *Aspects of face processing*, (ed. H. D. Ellis, M. A. Jeeves, F. Newcomber, and A. Young), pp. 199–208. Martinus Nijhoff, Dordrecht.

de Schonen, S., Tzourio, N., Mazoyer, B., Boré, A., Pietrzyk, U., Bruck, B., Aujard, Y., and Deruelle, C. (1993). Regional cerebral blood flow during visual stimuli processing in two-month-old alert infants. *16th Annual Meeting of the European Neurosciences Association*, 1993, Madrid, p. 151 (Abstract).

Dodwell, P. C., Humphrey, G. K., and Muir, D. W. (1987). Shape and pattern perception. In *Handbook of infant perception*, Vol. 2, (ed. P. Salapatek and L. Cohen), pp. 1–79. Academic Press, Orlando.

Ellis, H. D. and Young, A. W. (1989). Are faces special? In *Handbook of Research on Face Processing*, (ed. A. W. Young and H. D. Ellis), pp. 1–26. North Holland, Oxford.

Fifkova, E. (1985). A possible mechanism of morphometric changes in dendritic spines induced by stimulation. *Cellular and Molecular Neurobiology*, **5**, 47–63.

Fifkova, E. and van Harreveld, A. (1977). Long-lasting morphological changes in dendritic spines of granular cells following stimulation of the enthorinal area. *Journal of Neurocytology*, **6**, 211–30.

Fiorentini, A. and Berardi, N. (1984). Right-hemisphere superiority in the discrimination of spatial phase. *Perception*, **13**, 695–708.

Geschwind, N. and Galaburda, A. M. (1985). Cerebral lateralization. Biological mechanisms, associations, and pathology. I. A hypothesis and a program for research. *Archives of Neurology*, **42**, 428–59.

Ghim, H. D. and Eimas, P. D. (1988). Global and local processing by 3- and 4-month-old infants. *Perception and Psychophysics*, **43**, 165–71.

Greenough, W. T., Black, J. E., and Wallace, C. S. (1987). Experience and brain development. *Child Development*, **58**, 539–59.

Gross, C. G. and Sergent, J. (1992). Face recognition. *Current Opinion in Neurobiology*, **2**(2), 156–61.

Gwiazda, J., Bauer, J., and Held, R. (1989). From visual acuity to hyperacuity: A 10-year update. *Canadian Journal of Psychology*, **43**, 109–20.

Haxby, J. V., Grady, C. L., Horwitz, B., Ungerleider, L. G., Mishkin, M., Carson, R. E., Herscovitch, P., Schapiro, M. B., and Rapoport, S. I. (1991). Dissociation of object and spatial visual processing pathways in human extrastriate cortex. *Proceedings of the National Academy of Sciences, USA*, **88**, 1621–5.

Hécaen, H. and Albert, M. (1978). *Human neuropsychology*. Wiley, New York.

Held, R. (1989). Development of cortically mediated visual processes in human infants. In *Neurobiology of early infant behaviour*, (ed. C. Von Euler, H. Forssberg, and H. Lagerctantz), pp. 155–72. International Wallenberg Symposium. Macmillan, London.

Hughes, H. C., Fendrich, R., and Reuter-Lorenz, P. A. (1990). Global *versus* local processing in the absence of low spatial frequencies. *Journal of Cognitive Neuroscience*, **2**, 272–82.

Huttenlocher, P. R. (1993). Synaptogenesis, synapse elimination and neural plasticity in human cerebral cortex. In *Threats to optimal development: integrating biological, psychological, and social risk factors*. Minnesota Symposium on Child Psychology, Vol. 27, (ed. C. A. Nelson), Lawrence Erlbaum Associates, New Jersey.

Johnson, M. M. (1990). Cortical maturation and the development of visual attention in early infancy. *Journal of Cognitive Neuroscience*, **2**, 81–95.

Johnson, M. H. and Morton, J. (1991). *Biology and cognitive development: the case of face recognition*. Blackwells, Oxford.

Jonides, J., Smith, E. E., Koeppe, R. A., Awh, E., and Minoshima, S. (1993). Spatial working memory in humans as revealed by PET. *Nature*, **363**, 623–5.

Kitterle, F. L., Christman, S., and Hellige, J. B. (1990). Hemispheric differences are found in the identification, but not the detection, of low *versus* high spatial frequencies. *Perception and Psychophysics*, **48**, 297–306.

Kowalska, D. M., Bachevalier, J., and Mishkin, M. (1991). The role of the inferior prefrontal convexity in performance of delayed nonmatching-to-sample. *Neuropsychologia*, **29**, 583–600.

Mancini, J., de Schonen, S., Deruelle, C., and Massoulier, A. (1994). Face recognition in children with early right or left brain damage. *Developmental Medicine and Child Neurology*, **36**, 156–66.

Mazoyer, B. M. and Tzourio, N. (1993). Functional mapping of the human brain. In *Developmental neurocognition: speech and face processing in the first year of life*, (ed. B. de Boysson-Bardies, S. de Schonen, P. Jusczyk, P. McNeilage, and J. Morton), pp. 77–92. Kluwer, Dordrecht.

Meltzoff, A. N. and Moore, M. K. (1983). Newborn infants imitate adult facial gestures. *Child Development*, **54**, 702–9.

Michimata, C. and Hellige, J. B. (1987). Effects of blurring and stimulus size on the lateralized processing of nonverbal stimuli. *Neuropsychologia*, **25**, 397–407.

Morton, J. (1993). Mechanism in infant face processing. In *Developmental neurocognition: speech and face processing in the first year of life*, (ed. B. de Boysson-Bardies, S. de Schonen, P. Jusczyk, P. McNeilage, and J. Morton), pp. 93–102. Kluwer, Dordrecht.

Morton, J. and Johnson, M. H. (1991). Conspec and conlern: a two-process theory of infant face recognition. *Psychological Review*, **98**, 164–81.

Moscovitch, M. (1979). Information processing and the cerebral hemispheres. In *Handbook of neurobiology: neuropsychology*, (ed. M. S. Gazzaniga), pp. 379–446. Plenum Press, New York.

Ojemann, J. G., Ojemann, G. A., and Lettich, E. (1992). Neuronal activity related to faces and matching in human right non-dominant temporal cortex. *Brain*, **115**, 1–13.

Pascalis, O. and de Schonen, S. (1994). Visual recognition memory in human infants. *24th Annual Meeting of the Society for Neuroscience*, Miami Beach, USA. *Society for Neuroscience Abstracts*, **20**, part 2, 1424.

Pascalis, O. and de Schonen, S. (1995). Face recognition in 3- and 6-month-old infants. *Second Annual Meeting of the Cognitive Neuroscience Society*, San Francisco, USA. *Proceedings of the Second Meeting of the Cognitive Neuroscience Society.*

Pascalis, O., de Schonen, S., Morton, J., Deruelle, C., and Fabre-Grenet, M. (1995). Mother's face recognition in neonates: a replication and an extension. *Infant Behavior and Development*, **18**, 79–86.

Passingham, R. (1975). Delayed matching after selective prefrontal lesions in monkeys. *Brain Research*, **92**, 89–102.

Posner, M. I. and Petersen, S. E. (1990). The atttention system of the human brain. *Annual Review of Neuroscience*, **13**, 25–42.

Rakic, P., Bourgeois, J. P., Eckenhoff, M. F., Zecevic, N., and Goldman-Rakic, P. S. (1986). Concurrent overproduction of synapses in diverse regions of the primate cerebral cortex. *Science*, **232**, 232–5.

Rodman, H. R., Gross, C. G., and Scalaidhe, S. P. (1993). Development of brain substrates for pattern recognition in primates: physiological and connectional studies of inferior temporal cortex in infant monkeys. In *Developmental neurocognition: speech and face processing in the first year of life*, (ed. B. de Boysson-Bardies, S. de Schonen, P. Jusczyk, P. McNeilage, and J. Morton), pp. 63–76. Kluwer, Dordrecht.

Rosen, G. D., Galaburda, A. M., and Sherman, G. F. (1987). Mechanisms of brain asymmetry: new evidence and hypothesis. In *Duality and unity of the brain*, (ed. D. Ottoson), pp. 29–36. Plenum Press, New York.

Rothbart, M. K., Posner, M. I., and Boylan, A. (1990). Regulatory mechanisms in infant development. In *The development of attention. Research and theory*, (ed. J. T. Enns), pp. 47–66. North Holland, Oxford.

Schechter, P. B. and Murphy, E. H. (1976). Brief monocular visual experience and kitten cortical binocularity. *Brain Research*, **109**, 165–8.

Scheibel, A. B. (1993). Dendritic structure and language development. In *Developmental neurocognition: speech and face processing in the first year of life*, (ed. B. de Boysson-Bardies, S. de Schonen, P. Jusczyk, P. McNeilage, and J. Morton), pp. 51–62. Kluwer, Dordrecht.

Sergent, J. (1983). The role of the input in visual hemispheric processing. *Psychological Bulletin*, **93**, 481–512.

Sergent, J. (1985). Influence of task and input factors on hemispheric involvement in face processing. *Journal of Experimental Psychology: Human Perception and Performance*, **11**, 846–61.

Sergent, J. (1987). Failures to confirm the spatial-frequency hypothesis: Fatal blow or healthy complication? *Canadian Journal of Psychology*, **41**, 412–28.

Sergent, J. (1989). Structural processing of faces. In *Handbook of research on face processing*, (ed. A. W. Young and H. D. Ellis), pp. 57–91. North Holland, Oxford.

Sergent, J., Ohta, S., and Macdonald, B. (1992). Functional neuroanatomy of face and object processing. A positron emission tomography study. *Brain*, **115**, 15–36.

Simons, R. J. and Scheibel, A. B. (1989).The postnatal development of the motor speech area: a preliminary study. *Brain and Language*, **37**, 42–58.

Singer, W. (1987). Activity dependent self-organization of synaptic connections as a substrate of learning. In *The neural and molecular bases of learning*, (ed. J. Changeux and M. Konishi), pp. 301–36. Wiley, New York.

Slater, A. M. (1993). Visual perceptual abilities at birth: implications for face perception. In *Developmental neurocognition: speech and face processing in the first year of life*, (ed. B. de Boysson-Bardies, S. de Schonen, P. Jusczyk, P. McNeilage, and J. Morton), pp. 125–34. Kluwer, Dordrecht.

Stamm, J. S. (1973). Functional dissociation between the inferior and arcuate segments of dorsolateral prefrontal cortex in the monkey. *Neuropsychologia*, **11**, 181–90.

Szelag, W., Budohoska, W., and Koltuska, B. (1987). Hemispheric differences in the perception of gratings. *Bulletin of the Psychonomic Society*, **25**, 95–8.

Turkewitz, G. (1988). A prenatal source for the development of hemispheric specialization. In *Brain lateralization in children*, (ed. D. L. Molfese and J. Segalowitz), pp. 73–81. Guilford Press, New York.

Turkewitz, G. (1989a). Face processing as a fundamental feature of development. In *Handbook of research on face processing*, (ed. A. W. Young and H. D. Ellis), pp. 401–4. North Holland, Amsterdam.

Turkewitz, G. (1989b). A prologue to the scenario of the development of hemispheric specialization: prenatal influences. *European Bulletin of Cognitive Psychology (CPC)*, **9**, 135–40.

Turkewitz, G. (1993). The origins of differential hemispheric strategies for information processing in the relationships between voice and face perception. In *Developmental neurocognition: speech and face processing in the first year of life*, (ed. B. de Boysson-Bardies, S. de Schonen, P. Jusczyk, P. McNeilage, and J. Morton), pp. 165–70. Kluwer, Dordrecht.

Tzourio, N., de Schonen, S., Mazoyer, B., Boré, A., Pietrzyk, U., Bruck, B., Aujard, Y., and Deruelle, C. (1992). Regional cerebral blood flow in two-month-old alert infants. *Society for Neuroscience Abstracts*, **18**(2), 1121.

Wilson, F. A. W., Scalaidhe, S. P. O., and Goldman-Rakic, P. S. (1993). Dissociation of object and spatial processing domains in primate prefrontal cortex. *Science*, **260**, 1955–8.

Young, A. W. (1983). *Functions of the right cerebral hemisphere*. Academic Press, New York.

22

Practical application of the visual evoked potential in paediatric neuro-ophthalmology

Patricia Apkarian

INTRODUCTION

Within the last few decades, the impetus to study visual ontogenesis and the corresponding plethora of developmental studies have resulted in major advances in our knowledge of the relationship between various aspects of visual perception and maturation of the corresponding anatomical and physiological substrates. The basic requisite in this area of study is to understand normal visual function and its development to optimum visual capacity, as well as to understand the aetiology of abnormal visual development and its detrimental consequences. Normal maturation of the visual pathway is dependent not only upon intrinsic biological factors but upon the infant's ability to sustain normal visual experience.

While the importance of addressing developmental questions is well understood, the accurate assessment of visual capacity in the newborn, older infant and toddler is a formidable task. Vision testing that bypasses the standard, verbal responses of the more mature, more co-operative patient typically requires elaborate test methods, sophisticated data analysis procedures, considerable time and last, but not least, patience. Significant advances in our ability to test vision function in the pre-verbal infant and non-verbal child also have been made, although the majority of clinically applicable (as opposed to research) infant vision test procedures are based on preferential looking methods (Fantz *et al.* 1962). While the behavioural approach has led to reliable growth functions of spatial vision (Fantz *et al.* 1962; Teller *et al.* 1974; Fulton *et al.* 1979; Dobson 1983; Courage and Adams 1990), a major disadvantage of behavioural testing and one that is inherent to the procedure is that preferential looking estimates of visual function in the infant are 'second order'. That is, an observer subjectively judges the non-verbal behavioural response of the infant. Possible psychomotor disturbances, ocular motor instabilities and fixation instability and variability contribute to the infant's orienting behaviour. From the behavioural responses, the observer's task is to decide which of two targets has captured the child's visual preference; unreliable visual acuity assessment under these conditions may result (Katz and Sireteanu 1990). Furthermore behavioural testing is typically limited to the perceptual task at hand.

An alternative to the behavioural approach is non-invasive electrophysiology, namely visual evoked potentials (VEPs). An advantage of evoked potential assessment is that, in addition to the ability to test performance for various visual tasks (e.g. spatial acuity, temporal resolution or motion), VEPs can measure visual capacity and maturation at varying stages of processing along the visual pathway from the retina to cortex. For example, VEPs can measure retinal receptive field maturation (via optimum pattern onset responses), global organization of temporal and nasoretinal cortical projections (via potential distributions across the scalp) and cortical maturation (via age-related changes in response latency and waveform).

While there is the suggestion that VEPs, while reflecting sensory processing, do not necessarily reflect visual perception, appropriate stimulus and recording conditions result in a direct match between what is recorded and what is perceived (i.e. 'what you get is what you see'). As a caveat, however, it is important to appreciate that while the VEP is a sensitive and powerful non-invasive tool of sensory capacity and functional integrity along the visual pathway, 'short-cut' approaches with this electrodiagnostic probe also generally preclude obtaining results that are reliable and clinically useful.

In the present overview, application of the VEPs in paediatric neuro-ophthalmology is described, together with the various stimulus and recording techniques designed to optimize VEP testing in infants and young children.

PAEDIATRIC STIMULUS AND RECORDING STRATEGY

For clinical purposes, the three most common modes of stimulation for recording evoked cortical responses are: (i) the luminance flash; (ii) the pattern reversal; and (iii) the pattern onset/offset. At a slow rate of stimulus presentation, as depicted in Fig. 22.1, each of these stimulus conditions has its own response signature in terms of number, latencies and sign (negativity or positivity) of various peaks and troughs. If the stimulus rate is sufficiently slow to allow the relevant brain responses to recover prior to the next stimulus presentation, the VEP is classified as transient.

However, as depicted in the luminance VEPs from a normal infant tested at 7 days of age and again at 201 days (Fig. 22.2), with higher and higher rates of stimulation, waveshape specificity deteriorates and the responses begin to resemble a sine wave, with the fundamental frequency or harmonics of the stimulus frequency. At 7 days, the highest temporal frequency yielding a reliable response was 12 Hz, recorded during wakefulness. By 201 days, the highest temporal frequency yielding a reliable response increased to 56 Hz, also recorded during wakefulness. During quiet sleep for either age, flicker responses show considerable lower frequency cut-offs. While changes in the response profiles of pattern responses may be expected to alter with state from

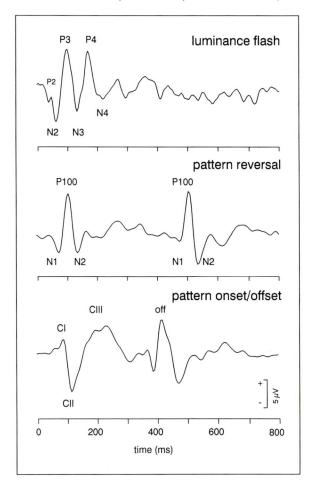

Fig. 22.1 Three classic VEP types recorded from an adult to luminance flash (upper trace), pattern reversal (centre trace) and pattern onset/offset (lower trace) stimulation. The luminance flash (recorded with 0.6 J light intensity) is a complicated waveform consisting of several major and minor positive and negative response deflections. The pattern reversal response (recorded with a 96′ check size and with each reversal presented once every 400 ms) consists of a negative–positive–negative waveform complex. The pattern onset/offset response (recorded with an 18′ check size) consists of a triphasic onset featuring a positive–negative–positive waveform complex and an offset consisting primarily of a single positive peak. In this example, the pattern was presented for 300 ms and was replaced with a homogeneous field of the same mean luminance for 500 ms. Mean luminance and contrast for both pattern responses was 95 cd/m² and 80%, respectively. (Adapted from Apkarian 1994.)

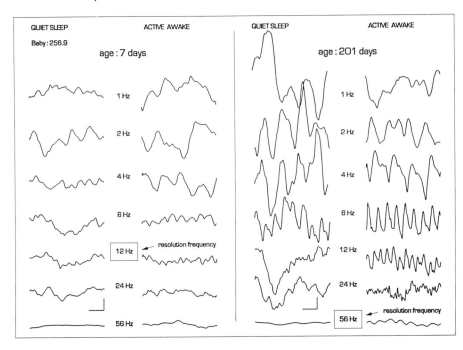

Fig. 22.2 Transition from transient to steady-state VEP with increasing stimulus frequency. The time averaged luminance VEPs depicted were recorded from a full-term normal infant tested at 7 days and 201 days during sleep and wakefulness. In response to sinusoidal homogeneous light stimulation, the resolution frequency varies with state and with age. In addition, as the frequency rate increases, the response develops a sine-wave appearance with a fundamental frequency equal to that of the stimulus frequency. (From Apkarian 1993.)

visual inattentiveness alone, resulting for example in poor fixation or defocus, the responses depicted for the luminance VEP indicate that additional state-dependent factors are involved. That is, defocus and/or poor fixation do not alter the VEP response to large-field, high-intensity, homogeneous luminance flicker. In general, the luminance response profiles depicted emphasize that if neonates and younger infants are tested, it is important to record the visual evoked responses only under behavioural state defined conditions (Apkarian *et al.* 1991; Apkarian 1993).

If the rate of stimulation is sufficiently high to preclude response recovery, the VEP is termed 'steady state'. Both the so-called higher frequency steady-state VEP and the transient VEP are important for clinical application and frequently yield complementary information. The latter, however, also yields waveform information, which, as seen in Figs 22.3 and 22.4, is particularly useful in assessing response maturation. As illustrated for both the luminance flash and the pattern onset, the response profiles, including waveform,

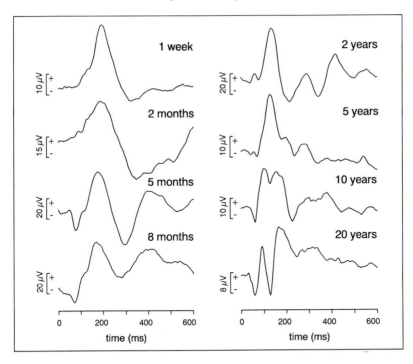

Fig. 22.3 Maturation of the luminance flash VEP from one week of age to 20 years. Within the first months of life the luminance flash response is simpler in waveform and is characterized by a major positive peak with latency of about 200 ms. During development, the luminance flash response increases in complexity and the latency of the major deflections decreases. In the adult, the first major positive peak has a latency around 100 ms. Very early latency deflections appear less sensitive to maturational changes. Note also the trend towards an inverted U-shaped function of response amplitude as a function of age. (Adapted from Apkarian 1994.)

amplitude and latency are age sensitive. The development of characteristic adult-like responses, particularly in waveform, requires a rather lengthy maturational course.

Visual stimulation

The two stimulus configurations most frequently referred to in this overview are the checkerboard/draught board (primarily pattern onset), and homogeneous luminance field (primarily luminance flash). Checkerboards, typically generated on a computer-driven monitor, are the pattern configuration of choice over more simple patterns such as horizontal or vertical stripes. The rational behind this choice is two-fold. First, because of greater contour (edge) information, checkerboards typically yield larger amplitude responses than corresponding bar patterns (Tweel van der 1979). Second, the checkerboard, with its

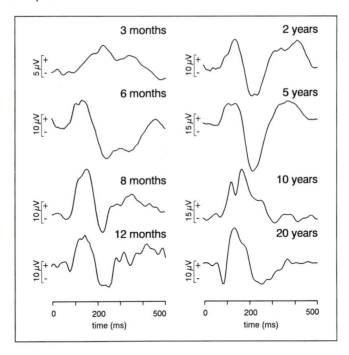

Fig. 22.4 Maturation of the pattern onset VEP from 3 months of age to 20 years. The immature pattern onset response consists primarily of a single, slightly sluggish, positive waveform deflection with a latency, after about 3 months, of about 150 ms. The major maturational improvements occur primarily in response waveform, which reaches the adult-like positive (CI), negative (CII), positive (CIII) waveform complex around puberty. Note that at around 10 years of age, identification of response components is difficult as the response begins to reflect a transitional stage. Pattern onset was 40 ms, offset 460 ms, pattern size 12′, mean luminance 90 cd/m² and contrast 80%. (Adapted from Apkarian 1994.)

multiple contour orientations is less affected by orientation-specific degradation of the stimulus from nystagmus and/or refractive errors such as astigmatism (Apkarian 1994; Rosenberg and Jabbari 1987). It should be pointed out that some experts in the field (Tyler 1991) prefer bar stimuli for VEP acuity estimates in infants, suggesting that a grating is a 'purer' stimulus configuration than Snellen chart elements or check patterns with respect to fundamental frequencies and orientation. However, as Snellen acuity and check acuity match quite well, in addition to the advantages cited above, the checkerboard remains an optimum VEP stimulus configuration.

In terms of mode of pattern stimulation, the pattern onset is the method of choice. The rational behind this preference is also two-fold. First, the pattern onset, particularly the first negative deflection, denoted CII (see also Fig. 22.1), reflects primarily spatial contrast responses compared with the stimulus reversal mode, which, in addition, also reflects stimulus motion responses (Dagnelie *et al.* 1986; Estévez and Spekreijse 1974). Pattern reversal contamination of a pattern specific response with a movement response is most likely the reason that the pattern onset (unlike the pattern reversal) correlates more directly with behavioural estimates of spatial vision. Second, the pattern onset stimulus is more appropriate for patients with ocular motor instabilities and/or misalignments, and also for younger patients, since the lengthy and highly accurate fixation demands of the pattern reversal are not required for pattern onset (Apkarian 1994; Arlt and Zangemeister 1990; Rosenberg and Jabbari 1987). During pattern reversal stimulation, it is necessary to maintain steady fixation to avoid tracking the stimulus elements, which, with poor fixation, appear to drift to the left or right. If tracking occurs, response amplitude decreases and variability increases. The compelling tendency to track the pattern elements is avoided with the pattern onset offset paradigm.

Unless otherwise noted, for data presented herein, the contrast of the check elements was 80%; mean luminance of the stimulus field was around 100 cd/m^2.

Luminance flash stimulation was typically generated with a commercially available light flasher, which allows high-intensity pulses of light (herein 1 Hz rate and 0.6 J intensity were employed). However, a homogeneous luminance stimulus, sine-wave modulated, is an appropriate stimulus configuration for assessing temporal vision (i.e. temporal responsivity). Growth functions of VEP temporal responsivity are now available (Apkarian 1993).

VEP recording

To record pattern or luminance responses, an appropriate recording montage is important. For the data presented, the electrode montage consisted of five 'active' electrodes positioned across the occiput, 1 cm above the inion and linked to a high forehead reference (or linked ear lobes). An additional ground was placed at the vertex. Filtering and amplification followed standard VEP recording procedures. For more details on stimulus and recording procedures in paediatric populations, see Apkarian (1994).

FOUR-PARAMETER VEP ASSESSMENT

In addition to emphasizing maturational changes in the VEP response profile, the approach adopted in this overview of electrodiagnosis in paediatric neuro-ophthalmology is straightforward.

Response analysis concentrates upon four simple response parameters: (i) amplitude (μV); (ii) latency (ms); (iii) waveform (component specificity); and (iv) topography (potential distribution across electrode array). The four-parameter subdivision of the evoked response is purely descriptive in that these response variables are largely interdependent.

VEP AMPLITUDE

Amplitude of the evoked potential, a stimulus time-locked average of electrical signals, reflects the summed ionic current generated from thousands of synchronously activated neurones. Voltage fluctuations from populations of neurones translate into the electrical envelopes of neuronal activity recorded at the surface of the scalp. The measurement scale for VEP amplitude is in microvolts (μV). The contributing cellular activities upon which the VEP recording procedures 'eavesdrop' are sensitive to spatial and temporal manipulations of the time-locked stimuli, recording procedures and, most importantly, the anatomical substrates in the visual pathway generating the massed electrical responses. While there is no shortage of analysis methods for calculating the amplitude of the evoked response, the relevant goal of various analysis procedures is to distinguish the evoked potential signal from the uncorrelated background activity, termed 'noise'. In its most simple form, the basic VEP amplitude question concerns whether or not a response is present. The basic amplitude query can be addressed readily by reproducing the response under the same stimulus and recording conditions. Absence or presence of a reproducible response, that is, one that can be distinguished from random fluctuations of background activity, is the most fundamental clinical application of the VEP amplitude parameter. However, if more specific questions are posed, then relative amplitude measures are required and amplitude, in a simple fashion for clinical application, can be quantified. For steady-state evoked potentials, simple Fourier analysis is applied. Amplitude of the fundamental frequency and second harmonics of the response are the most common measures. For transient-evoked responses, the two most common approaches for measuring amplitude include: (i) measurement of the voltage difference between successive waveform deflections (peak-to-peak method); and (ii) measurement of the voltage difference between a given response deflection or time window and baseline (peak-to-baseline method). The former requires identification of the designated positive and negative response deflections, which, in a poorly differentiated response, may prove difficult. The latter, peak-to-baseline method, is typically measured from the averaged amplitude of the electrical activity within a narrow time window of the VEP trace preceding the response. Advantages and disadvantages of one method over another, as well as optional measures of baseline are described in more detail elsewhere (Apkarian 1994).

Quantification of VEP amplitude emphasizes not only the high degree of response sensitivity to stimulus parameters but also the substantial intra- and intersubject amplitude variability. While for a given individual, the amplitude range remains fairly constant over time, smaller fluctuations in absolute amplitude may occur with repeated measures. The main source of intra-subject variability, apart from disease process and longer-term developmental and ageing changes, is the electrode montage and recording conditions. For example, amplitude variability may be induced by slight differences in electrode derivations from repositioning. By far, however, the greatest absolute amplitude variability is observed between individuals. While age changes play an important role in amplitude fluctuations, individual variance, including differences in cortical neuroanatomy and in the locations of response generating sources, can yield absolute interindividual differences as great as 10-fold, albeit background activity has been implicated as a major source of the variability (Apkarian 1993; Cigánek 1969).

In the case examples presented in this section, the role played by both absolute as well as relative amplitude measures is illustrated.

Dandy Walker syndrome

To address the query regarding presence or absence of a response, the luminance VEP profile from an infant with Dandy Walker syndrome is described (Fig. 22.5). Dandy Walker syndrome is characterized by posterior fossa cystic malformations (Maria *et al.* 1987; Golden *et al.* 1987; Asai *et al.* 1989). Common findings in this serious brain anomaly are: (i) partial agenesis of the inferior lobules; (ii) hypoplasia of the cerebral hemispheres; and (iii) marked dilatation of the fourth ventricle, which forms a posterior cyst and accompanying hydrocephaly. Associated central nervous system and visceral anomalies may also be present including polymicrogyria, retinal dystrophy, facial malformations, cardiac malformations, polydactyly, and syringomyelia. The pathogenesis of the disorder is not yet fully understood but early embryological maldevelopment is apparent. Outcome in children afflicted with the Dandy Walker syndrome varies from early infantile death, longer-term survival with severe intellectual retardation and cerebral palsy to longer-term survival with normal intelligence. Infants with the most severe conditions are reported to have the poorest prognosis (Maria *et al.* 1987). Intervention typically includes various forms of shunting.

Clinical history, herein, includes a male infant (Fig. 22.5), born at 42 weeks gestation without complication by spontaneous delivery. Post-natal weight was 3400 g. Within the first week post-partum, a blood transfusion was necessary for hypoglycaemia and high-level bilirubin. A CT scan within this period revealed agenesis of the vermis (inferior lobules) and marked dilatation of the fourth ventricle, with an accompanying large cyst (subarachnoid). Within the first weeks post-natally, neurological evaluation described the infant as dystrophic, presenting with low-frequency tremor, enlarged fontanelle, a sutura lamdoidea 'two fingers wide', and hypertelorism. Electroencephalogram (EEG) evaluation indicated posterior low-voltage activity and primarily right-hemisphere paroxysmal activity. Electroretinogram (ERG) showed low-amplitude a and b potentials. Ophthalmic examination revealed iris heterochromia but no outspoken fundus anomalies. The patient was referred for VEP testing to determine whether or not a light response could be evoked. VEP testing at 29 days of age revealed robust and reliable luminance flash responses and higher temporal-frequency responses to 8 Hz. Owing to severe skull malformation,

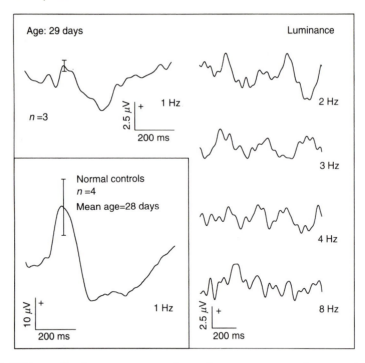

Fig. 22.5 VEP amplitude measures to determine presence or absence of a visual response from a 29-day-old infant with Dandy Walker syndrome. The luminance flash response, though reduced in amplitude compared with normal age-matched controls (insert) is clearly present and reproducible. The 1 Hz luminance flash response from the patient is the mean of three averaged responses; for the normal controls the mean luminance response depicted is the average from four age-matched infants. Error bars indicate standard error of the means. While amplitude is the relevant measure, for the patient the mean peak latency of the major positive peak was 216.7 ms ± 11.5 ms (SD); for the normal controls the mean was 192 ms ± 13.5 ms (SD). Higher frequency responses from the patient could also be elicited to 8 Hz. Note the amplitude calibration of the patient compared with the controls.

evaluation of waveform and, most notably topography, was not applicable. In this case, absolute amplitude measures clearly indicated the infant's ability to see light and to process higher temporal frequency information, facilitating decisions regarding life-support surgery. However, as a result of the severity of the malformations, the infant survived only 2 months post-partum.

VEP acuity

VEP amplitude varies with pattern size. If the smallest pattern size yielding a reliable pattern onset response is plotted as a function of age, a VEP growth function is obtained that mirrors directly maturation of spatial acuity. For the pattern onset, individual amplitude response profiles from large to small elements typically yield two useful indices of spatial function: (i) the optimum pattern size yielding a response; and (ii) the minimum pattern size yielding a response. The former emphasizes visual system processing at more distal stages, for example receptive field organization at the retina (Vries-Khoe and Spekreisje 1982), while the latter yields an estimate of acuity or spatial resolving power. Assessment of vision capacity, in general, is typically defined by the line on a Snellen acuity chart or comparable chart, for which accurate letter identification or symbol orientation can be made. The power of VEP acuity estimates is that they can be performed readily in the pre-verbal or non-verbal patient. Unlike behavioural methods for assessing acuity in infants and young children or those with mental or physical handicaps, VEP estimates based on the pattern onset paradigm do not require accurate head and ocular motor control nor lengthy fixation. Moreover, the acuity estimates obtained with the pattern onset bear a direct relation to Snellen acuity estimates as shown in Fig. 22.6, where VEP acuity is plotted against Snellen acuity. These data were from verbally co-operative subjects and patients (mean age 23 years; age range 4–66 years) from whom a reliable Snellen acuity could be obtained. The patient group consisted largely of albinos whose best corrected Snellen acuities spanned a considerable range from as low as about 0.03 (20/600) to as high as about 0.66 (20/30). The correlation diagram of Fig. 22.6 illustrates that, with appropriate stimulus and recording conditions, there is a significant and linear correlation between VEP acuity and the more traditional Snellen acuity. Under specific test conditions (Apkarian 1994), reliable pattern onset VEPs recorded to a 3' (minute) pattern size yielded a Snellen equivalent of 1 (20/20) and, as such, the minimum pattern size recorded was divided by the constant, $K = 3$; the reciprocal of the quotient yielded the Snellen equivalent. Application of this simple, yet reliable, means of determining visual acuity is depicted in the response profiles from a normal control infant tested at 26 days of age and again at 36 weeks (Fig. 22.7). Also emphasized is the application of the relative VEP amplitude measure in which acuity estimates are used to determine, among other variables, level of spatial vision, interocular comparisons, and maturational improvements. At 26 days, the optimum response was recorded with a pattern size of 110'; the minimum response was obtained with pattern size between about 55' and 36', yielding an acuity estimate of about 0.05 (20/370) to 0.08 (20/250). By 36 weeks, optimum pattern size reduced to 12' and VEP acuity estimates improved reaching from about 0.3 (20/66) to 0.5 (20/40) with corresponding minimum pattern sizes of 9' to 6'. These findings are in accord with published norms for age (for summary see Courage and Adams 1990 and Vries-Khoe and Spekreijse 1982). To the right of Fig. 22.7, response amplitude (amplitude to baseline, P1 and peak-to-peak, P1–N1) and latency (first major positive peak, P1) have been quantified in relation to pattern size. For practical purposes, VEP acuity can be estimated simply by determining the smallest pattern size yielding a reliable response. However, the amplitude *versus* pattern size functions clearly show the maturation shift towards higher-resolution

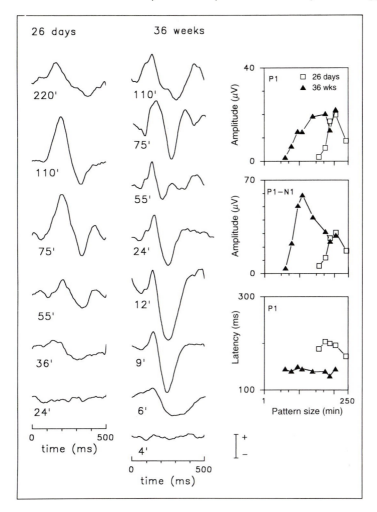

Fig. 22.7 Application of VEP relative amplitude measures illustrated with the pattern onset responses to varying pattern sizes recorded in a normal infant tested at 26 days (left traces) and again at 36 weeks (right traces). The immature pattern onset response consists of primarily a single positive peak (denoted P1), which increases in amplitude in response to the optimum pattern size and then decreases in amplitude as pattern size decreases. The relationship is shown quantitatively in the amplitude *versus* pattern size functions plotted for an occipital electrode positioned 1 cm above the inion on the midline. Peak amplitude values were measured peak to baseline (P1) or peak to peak (P1–N1; N1 = adjacent negative deflection to the right). The smallest pattern size yielding a response, shown here to decrease with age, yields the VEP acuity estimate. In addition, from the first to second session, overall response amplitude has increased markedly. VEP latency of the P1 deflection depicted in the latency *versus* pattern size function plot (lower right) also decreases with age. Calibration bar equals 10 µV at 26 days and 20 µV at 36 weeks.

maturation and increases in the elderly with ageing. In addition, latency shows a direct relationship with stimulus intensity; as stimulus intensity increases, latency (below response saturation) decreases. As a measure of neuronal conduction, decreases in latency can reflect visual pathway maturation, mirroring age-related changes in underlying functional and anatomical substrates (e.g. myelinogenesis and synaptogenesis). In contrast, latency delays inappropriate for either stimulus or age can reflect visual pathway pathology (e.g. retarded visual pathway growth, pathway obstruction or myelination anomalies). For particularly the latter, inter-peak latency measures also yield information about temporal response dispersion. An important aspect concerning the latency variable is that, unlike evoked response amplitude, absolute latency is highly stable both within and between individuals. Thus the latency measure renders reliable intra- and inter-subject comparisons, given that stimulus, recording conditions and age are comparable. While a sensitive measure of visual pathway integrity, the reliability of the latency measure is dependent upon and limited by accurate peak identification. However, owing to normal growth and ageing factors or pathological conditions, identification of specific positive and negative waveform deflections may prove ambiguous. Although this remains a problem, recording the responses under stimulus conditions that enhance or attenuate one peak over another, may facilitate peak identification. Moreover, normative VEP latency values, across the age range and under various stimulus conditions as the luminance flash, pattern reversal and pattern onset, are readily available (Blom *et al.* 1980; Chabot and John 1986; Vries-Khoe and Spekreijse 1982).

For higher temporal frequency responses, that is, steady-state VEPs, neuronal conduction velocities are described by the VEP phase. An apparent response latency can be calculated from a corresponding amplitude *versus* temporal frequency function given that a sufficient number of responses are recorded. Formulas for calculating phase from steady-state VEP responses are described by Regan (1989). One advantage of obtaining apparent latency values from steady-state VEPs is that peak identification is not required. However, such simplicity is not without disadvantage. Phase measures *per se* are more ambiguous and more variable with respect to actual response delay. In addition, it should be borne in mind that phase calculations are an indirect measure of conduction velocity and are based on several assumptions in the analysis that are not necessarily valid when applied to the visual system, or are only applicable within a limited range of conditions. In this overview, data presentation and discussion are restricted to latency measures of the transient evoked potential.

While an ultimate goal of VEP latency measures is early detection of subclinical pathology, more often than not, by the time significant response delays are observed, considerable pathway involvement has already occurred. However, latency values are invaluable for facilitating diagnosis and for the objective assessment of disease progression. In the developing visual system, an additional advantage of the latency parameter is that it can readily signal maturational interruptions and delays.

Pelizaeus-Merzbacher disease

Clinical application of both absolute latency measures compared with age-matched norms, as well as relative latency from repeated measures over time is illustrated in Fig. 22.8 and Table 22.1, by the VEP response profile of an infant with a rare leukodystrophy, Pelizaeus-Merzbacher disease (PMD). In general, leukodystrophies form a group of inherited neurological conditions reflecting inborn errors of myelin metabolism and are characterized by progressive, symmetrical, non-inflammatory demyelination or dysmyelination. Clinical features of the various leukodystrophies include loss of sensory, motor and intellectual functions and eventual death. Although the precise biochemical basis of the metabolic disorder in Pelizaeus-Merzbacher disease is yet to be determined, Gencic and colleagues (1989), as well as studies of genetic linkage and DNA analyses (Bridge *et al.* 1991), biochemical and pathological analyses (Koeppen *et al.* 1987) suggest that the condition of PMD should be restricted to genetic mutations of the proteolipid proteins. This mutation causes the failure to form myelin (i.e. dysmyelination). PMD is typically described as X-linked but sporadic cases of PMD with an autosomal recessive inheritance, as depicted in Fig. 22.8, have also been reported. Patients with the latter genotype, usually without a positive family history, are particularly difficult to diagnose and it is not unusual for patients with PMD to be incorrectly diagnosed as having cerebral palsy or other unrelated neuropathies. Electrophysiological sensory testing is reported to facilitate early PMD diagnosis in infants (Garg *et al.* 1983). In a recent VEP study of an infant with X-linked PMD (Apkarian *et al.* 1993), pattern onset, luminance flash and high temporal frequency luminance flicker evoked potentials facilitated both the PMD diagnosis and the objective assessment of visual maturation. VEP testing in the young female infant described in Fig. 22.8 proved not only useful for early detection, differential diagnosis and visual maturation assessment but also provided an accurate description of visual pathway involvement and disease progression.

Clinical history includes a female infant (Fig. 22.8, Table 22.1) born at 38.5 weeks gestation without complication by spontaneous delivery. Birth weight was 3040 g and Apgar scores were 7 and 8 at 5 and 10 min, respectively. Medical evaluation at 2 weeks was normal. However, at about 6 weeks postpartum, nystagmoid eye movements, head tremor, and excessive crying were documented. By 10 weeks, it was clear that psychomotor maturation was delayed; the presence of cramps and seizures was also documented. At 14 weeks, CT scans revealed white matter anomaly. Fixation and following were abnormal and the infant was referred for VEP evaluation. The results of the first VEP test are summarized in Table 22.1 and Fig. 22.8. By 14 weeks, the VEP showed well defined pattern onset and luminance flash responses. However, the response latencies were delayed for age compared with controls. In contrast, response waveforms were normal and estimated VEP acuity was relatively high. VEP acuity was estimated at about 0.05; the single positive peak of the pattern onset response was well differentiated, as were the multiple peaks of

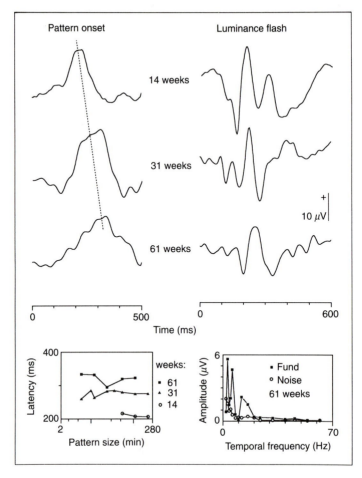

Fig. 22.8 Delayed latency for the binocular pattern onset (left) and luminance flash (right) VEPs from an infant with an autosomal recessive form of Pelizaeus-Merzbacher disease. Latency in this progressive dysmyelinating disorder is delayed for both pattern and luminance flash responses. Pattern size of the waveforms depicted was 55′. At the lower left, latency as a function of pattern size shows that, compared with normal values for age (see Table 22.1), latency is compromised severely and continues to show progressive deterioration during follow-up sessions. The major positive peak of the luminance flash response tested from 14 weeks to 61 weeks also shows an increasing latency delay, though not as dramatic as the pattern response. Despite significant latency delays, the infant's ability to respond to smaller pattern elements as depicted by the latency *versus* pattern size function (lower left) remained high, suggesting a sparing of central vision function. However, by 61 weeks the pattern response waveform, as well as the luminance waveform, began to show serious deterioration. In addition, the luminance flicker response at 61 weeks (lower right) is far below normal limits for age. (Fund, fundamental.)

Table 22.1 Latency measures compared with age-matched normals.

Study	Age (weeks)	Latency (ms) flash (P3)	Latency (ms) pattern (55′)
Present controls (*n* = 9)	14	146 ± 28	153 ± 7 (*n* = 3)
Chabot and John (1986)	≈14	135 ± 23	
Blom *et al.* (1980)	8–16	147–153	
Present PMD patient	14	209.2	217
Present controls (*n* = 6)	31	127.5 ± 24	136 ± 3 (*n* = 4)
Chabot and John (1986)	≈31	109 ± 14	
Blom *et al.* (1980)	16–32	149–154	
Present PMD patient	31	228	280
Present controls (*n* = 4)	61	120 ± 17	
Chabot and John (1986)	≈61	105 ± 21	
Blom *et al.* (1980)	52–104	126–135	
Present PMD patient	61	252	320

the luminance flash. By about 30 weeks of age, cramping was reported to increase in frequency and general hypotonia was noted. Ophthalmic examination documented the presence of an esotropia; however, the fundus was normal. EEG and ERG were also reported to be normal. MRI testing at this time was unsuccessful. However, at 31 weeks of age, VEP testing showed dramatic latency delays, which were even longer than the values obtained about 4 months earlier. Despite the significant VEP latency delays, acuity estimates improved and remained high, approximating 0.4 (20/50). At this time, the infant also showed fixation and following behaviour. However, the severely delayed response profiles confirmed the condition of a neurodegenerative disorder. By about 47 weeks of age, MRI under anaesthesia confirmed the condition of dysmyelination. A third VEP follow-up session at 61 weeks of age documented further disease progression. Central spatial vision, as assessed with VEP acuity estimates continued to show maturational improvements. The response waveforms, however, began to deteriorate, along with continued increases in response latency. Temporal frequency flicker studies at this time revealed critical fusion estimates at only between 16–20 Hz, severely below normal limits for age (Apkarian 1993). Intervention in this case was limited to medication and continued evaluation.

VEP WAVEFORM

For the transient VEP, response waveform is dependent primarily upon the stimulus configuration, stimulus mode and observer age. Examples of the three classic transient VEP waveforms are presented in Fig. 22.1 along with age-related alterations in the response profiles in Figs 22.3 and 22.4. The various positive and negative response deflections have been attributed to specific visual pathway generators and/or to specific visual processing functions. Very often, however, the purported source(s) of the so-called response components undergo alteration as analysis techniques become more sophisticated. For example, the high-frequency early wavelets of the luminance flash response were once considered to reflect subcortical sources, that is, processing at the optic tract (Siegfried 1981) or lateral geniculate body (Harding and Rubinstein 1980). More recent studies, however, suggest that the early wavelets are, in fact, cortical in origin (Ducati *et al.* 1988; Sjöström *et al.* 1991). A second example of the difficulties concerning source localization and identification of precise anatomical substrates of a particular VEP response deflection can be appreciated also with the pattern onset response. There is general consensus regarding the sensitivity of the negative CII deflection to pattern size and defocus. As such, the CII deflections are most likely to reflect contrast mechanisms. This conclusion is supported by the absence or attenuation of the CII response in the developing visual system or in patients with impaired spatial vision. However, despite the fact that the CII response most probably reflects contrast mechanisms, the exact source of this response deflection remains ambiguous. Early studies proposed that the origin of the CII component was extrastriate, that is, from cortical area 18 (Jeffreys and Axford 1972), while more recent dipole source localization studies suggest that the CII peak contains response contributions from both extrastriate and striate cortical areas (Maier *et al.* 1987). Perhaps the exact source(s) of the various response deflections that are actually recorded will have to await the introduction of more direct source localization techniques such as functional MRI. In the interim, for practical purposes it is important to appreciate that a given response deflection most probably reflects the upper envelope of multiple cortical generating sources, which overlap in space and time. Fortunately for clinical application, the global shape of a given 'upper envelope' or VEP waveform demonstrates a high degree of stability across age-matched observers and stimulus conditions. Rather than defining precisely the source(s) of a given response deflection, for practical purposes qualitative template matching is, to date, the most efficient means of assessing response waveform. For the transient pattern reversal response, which remains stable with age and stimulus conditions, template matching is quite simple. One need only identify the major positive peak. However, it is interesting to note that in the guise of a more simple waveform configuration, the pattern reversal response is actually rather complex, reflecting both motion and contrast mechanisms. In comparison, the pattern onset stimulus generates a less-contaminated contrast response but is more complicated in waveform. Regardless of which of the three classic transient responses are under analysis, template matching in the evaluation of the transient response involves two basic questions: (i) is the waveform normal for age and (ii) is the waveform appropriate for the specific stimulus and recording conditions?

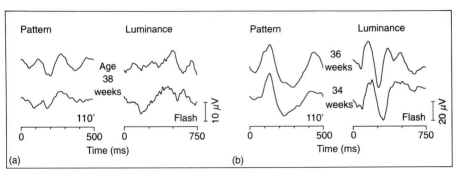

Fig. 22.9 Poorly differentiated pattern onset and luminance flash VEPs from a 38-week-old infant with a peroxisomal disorder, Zellweger syndrome (a). Repeated measures show response reliability. The abnormal responses are compared to two age-matched normal controls (b) tested with identical stimulus and recording conditions. Note the well-defined peaks and troughs of both the pattern and luminance responses for the normal controls. Note also that the responses from the normal infants are depicted at about half the amplitude (calibration for normal controls equals 20 μV; for the patient's responses, 10 μV).

Peroxisomal disorder

An attempt to address the two queries concerning waveform evaluation is described in Fig. 22.9 depicting the response profile of a 38-week-old male infant diagnosed with probable mild Zellweger syndrome. Zellweger disease, also referred to as cerebro-hepato-renal syndrome, belongs to a group of peroxisome-deficiency disorders, the primary biogenesis defect of which includes defective peroxisomal β-oxidation (Wanders *et al.* 1990). The inheritance mode for this inborn error of metabolism is autosomal recessive. Peroxisomes are organelles occurring in all mammalian cells with the exception of mature erythrocytes. These organelles house many different enzymes involved in a variety of catabolic and anabolic cellular reactions, the most significant of which are β-oxidations of very long-chain fatty acids and the synthesis of bile acids and plasmalogens. In Zellweger disease, peroxisomes are absent or greatly deficient, resulting in a wide range of serious phenotypic defects that involve nearly all organs and tissues (Schutgens *et al.* 1986; Moser 1988). Characteristic features of Zellweger syndrome include typical craniofacial dysmorphia (e.g. high forehead); neurological manifestations (e.g. hearing impairment and white matter degeneration); ophthalmic abnormalities (e.g. retinopathy); liver abnormalities, renal and adrenal pathology. Extinguished ERGs and abnormal VEPs, which are abnormal particularly in waveform (Garner *et al.* 1982) but also in amplitude and latency (Hittner *et al.* 1981; Stanescu-Segal and Evrard 1989), are typical visual electrophysiology findings in Zellweger syndrome and reflect the concomitant tapetoretinal degeneration, and visual pathway pathology, including optic nerve, optic tract and cortical pathology.

Clinical history includes a male infant (Fig. 22.9) born at 40.7 weeks gestation without complication by spontaneous delivery; the parents were not consanguine. Birthweight was 3300 g and Apgar scores were 9 and 10 at 5 and 10 minutes, respectively. Post-partum, Down's syndrome was initially suspected because of craniofacial abnormalities and a bilateral Simian crease but subsequent chromosome analysis proved negative. By 5 weeks post-partum, the infant weighed only 3490 g; heart murmur at this time was also documented. At 15 weeks of age the infant was admitted to hospital for full neurological and laboratory evaluation. For the latter, emphasis was placed on peroxisomal evaluation, which proved abnormal. Coincident with the clinical features, the patient was diagnosed as having Zellweger syndrome and possible infantile Refsum syndrome. Craniofacial involvement included high forehead, broad nasal bridge and external ear deformity. The EEG was abnormal, the ERG extinguished, and the brainstem evoked response (BAER) delayed. Ophthalmic evaluation revealed a pale optic disc and pigment anomalies; tapetal retinal degeneration was diagnosed. Subsequent ophthalmic evaluation also documented an esotropia. MRI results revealed cerebral dysmorphia characteristic of Zellweger syndrome. A few months later, deafness was also documented. At about 38 weeks of age, the infant was referred for VEP testing. The infant was to undergo dietary treatment (docosahexaenoic supplement) and VEP assessment was requested as an objective evaluation of neurological status following treatment. The response profile depicted in Fig. 22.9 was obtained prior to treatment and used as a reliable baseline with which to evaluate visual function and visual pathway maturation or delay. Fig. 22.9 depicts the binocular pattern onset responses and the luminance flash responses for the patient at 38 weeks of age. The pattern responses represent the pattern size yielding the optimum response (based on relative amplitude measures). Repeated measures under the same conditions showed that the abnormal waveforms are consistent. These responses could be compared with pattern onset (also at 110') and luminance flash for two age-matched normal controls, one tested at 36 weeks of age and the other at 34 weeks. The single positive peak of the immature pattern response and the major positive peak of the luminance flash response are clearly discernible in the responses from the two normal controls. Neither waveform deflection can be accurately identified in the patient's responses, which were, however, sufficiently reliable to yield the necessary pre-treatment baseline reference. In this case, the smallest test pattern size yielding a reliable response provided an acuity estimate of 0.08. This estimate, acceptable for infants around 12 weeks, is well below normal for the patient test age of 38 weeks. Note that the poorly differentiated responses render peak identification for latency estimation rather difficult. If anything, however, the major response deflections are definitely delayed. Follow-up on this child is underway.

VEP TOPOGRAPHY

The spatial distribution of the electrical activity (amplitude) across the electrode array at a specified time epoch (latency), and/or waveform deflection, defines VEP topography. As with absolute amplitude measures, absolute VEP topography measures, arising primarily from wide intersubject variability and recording variables, must be implemented and interpreted with caution. Anatomical aspects of retinal cortical mapping are straightforward, that is, primary foveal projection is represented posteriorly at the occipital pole, while peripheral retinal projections are represented at the medial sides of the left and right occiput. In addition, the lower visual field (upper retinal projections) is represented above the calcarine fissure; the upper visual field (lower retinal projections) is represented below the calcarine fissure. While knowledge of retinal-to-cortical mapping facilitates the practical issue of electrode positioning across the occiput, the contributing areas of cortical activity, number of sources, and their dipole positions and strengths are more complicated. Indeed, full-field stimulation of the pattern reversal response will yield a greater amplitude P100 component ipsilateral to the eye of stimulation, while a longer latency P135 component is reflected contralaterally (Barrett *et al.* 1976). If field size is reduced, the P100 deflection shows a primarily contralateral projection. In contrast, the pattern onset response and the luminance flash, independent of field size, show the expected contralateral and ipsilateral cortical representation as based on underlying retinal cortical projections. It is also of interest to note that interocular differences have been described in the topography of the pattern reversal VEP elicited by monocular hemifield stimulation in normal observers (Victor *et al.* 1991).

Despite the so-called paradoxical occipital representation and the inherent interocular half-field asymmetries, the pattern reversal stimulus mode (particularly half-field conditions) has found widespread clinical application in the investigation of chiasmal and retrochiasmal lesions (Arruga *et al.* 1980; Brecelj 1992; Haimovic and Pedley 1982). However, notwithstanding wide intersubject variability of occipital lobe morphology, the contributing factors of age, sex and stimulus and recording conditions, reliable recording of pattern reversal responses *per se* requires substantial subjective co-operation with regard to fixation (see previous discussion). For paediatric patients, and also patients with ocular motor instability appropriate fixation for the pattern reversal paradigm in general, and for partial-field stimulation in particular, is difficult and correspondingly inaccurate. Luminance flash and pattern onset are not only more straightforward in terms of expected occipital response lateralization but, with the exception of half-field stimulation, are also a more applicable stimulus mode for paediatric populations.

Regardless of stimulus mode or age of patient, if the topographical distribution across the scalp is an important variable in addressing the clinical question at hand, it is generally agreed (Blumhardt *et al.* 1977; Apkarian *et al.*

1986*b*; Apkarian and Tijssen 1992; Brecelj 1992) that multiple 'active' electrode sites, at minimum three and preferably five, are necessary for accurate estimates of the spatial distribution of electrical activity across the occiput and the corresponding determinants of response presence and lateralization. Furthermore, in general, owing to the high degree of individual response variability in cortical topography as well as the substantial influence of stimulus mode, the VEP topography measure of hemispheric response lateralization does not necessarily indicate a concomitant absence or presence of underlying visual pathway pathology. Thus absolute VEP topography measures have restricted clinical application and are best limited to the confirmation of suspected pathway lesions and as an adjunct to visual acuity, visual field, and clinical imaging techniques. Conversely, relative topography measures such as interocular hemispheric lateralization comparisons have proven invaluable, particularly for paediatric populations, in identifying the presence of misrouted pathway projections found in albinism or in patients with achiasmatic syndrome (Apkarian *et al.* 1986*a*; Apkarian and Tijssen 1992; Apkarian *et al.* 1994).

Albinism

The 'white-skinned', 'white-haired', 'dancing, pink-eyed' individual constitutes the classic percept of albinism. However, it is now appreciated that, while albinism is an inborn error of metabolism effecting abnormal melanogenesis, it is the presence of foveal hypoplasia and abnormal retinal cortical projections in the form of a preponderance of contralaterally projecting temporal retinal fibres that defines the albino condition. Extreme hypopigmentation of the hair and skin are associated with the specific albino genotype, tyrosinase-negative oculocutaneous albinism. The range of hair, skin and iris colour with other albino genotypes and/or phenotypes is widely variable, with the opposite extreme being the dark-haired, brown-eyed, heavily skin-pigmented (readily able to tan), no nystagmus, albino. While the preponderance of misguided temporal retinal fibres is a landmark albino feature, the exact aetiology of the abnormal distribution of crossed and uncrossed retinal-fugal axons is unknown. Actually, the mechanisms of retinal axon pathfinding and the corresponding divergence of crossed and uncrossed fibres is not yet fully understood in the normal vertebrate, although the albino model has assisted in this endeavour, and significant advances are now in progress (Dodd and Jessell 1988; Reese *et al.* 1992; Colello and Guillery 1990; Jeffery 1990). What is known, however, is that concomitant with abnormal melanogenesis, the albino mutation results in a strikingly abnormal patterning of retinal-fugal projections and organization. Although the effects of melanin deficiencies and abnormalities, either as transient local guidance mechanisms deposited along the developing optic stalk or as axon-labelling mechanisms, have recently been called into question (Colello and Jeffery 1991), the lack of a precise understanding of the albino pathway does not hinder application of the VEP topography parameter in detecting the misrouted optic pathway projections. With appropriate stimulus conditions that exclude pattern reversal, albino misrouting can be readily recorded from the surface of the scalp in the form of contralateral hemispheric response asymmetry following *full-field* monocular stimulation. That is, following full-field left-eye stimulation, the peak of the potential distribution shifts to the right occiput, while following full-field right-eye stimulation the peak of the potential distribution lateralizes to the left occiput. The VEP interocular asymmetry described is pathognomonic to albinism and, with age-appropriate stimulus and recording procedures, can detect the condition of albinism with virtually 100% accuracy. The albino test paradigm is dependent upon age (Apkarian *et al.* 1986*a*; Apkarian and Tijssen 1992) and an abbreviated 'misrouting test recipe' includes the luminance flash response for infants about 3 years of age and younger, both the pattern onset and luminance flash for children from about 3–6 years and the pattern onset for patients older than 6 years. The checkerboard pattern is particularly optimum for patients with nystagmus; pattern size should subtend about 1° of visual angle. Application of the VEP albino test in an albino infant and age-matched normal control is described below.

Clinical history, restricted to family pedigree and ophthalmic findings, includes a female infant (Fig. 22.10) diagnosed with autosomal recessive oculocutaneous albinism. The child is the second of two children; the family history across three generations is negative for ophthalmic anomalies. The infant was first seen for VEP evaluation at the age of 21.4 weeks. Electrophysiological assessment was requested to assess visual function and corroborate the clinical diagnosis of albinism. Hair colour was white and skin was pale. Ophthalmic examination at the same date as VEP testing revealed alternating esotropia, nystagmus, iris diaphany, photophobia, fundus hypopigmentation and foveal and macula hypoplasia, as determined by the absence of foveal or macular reflex. In addition to the classic ophthalmic, cutaneous and hair symptoms associated with oculocutaneous albinism, the infant was also diagnosed with an Axenfield anomaly; a posterior embryotoxin was present. VEP evaluation estimated binocular acuity at 0.12 (≈20/160). Luminance flash and pattern onset latencies were normal for age; waveform differentiation for either stimulus conditions was also normal for age. Abnormal was the presence of contralateral hemispheric response lateralization following full-field monocular luminance flash stimulation (Fig. 22.10). A similar trend of contralateral asymmetry with pattern onset was also observed but was less robust and more variable as expected for age. Both qualitative and quantitative evaluation of VEP contralateral asymmetry evinced the albino VEP signature. Amplitude measures of the left eye appeared greater than for the right; this is, in part, because of noisier peak amplitude to first 40 ms of the response baseline for the right-eye responses. Despite the interocular difference in absolute amplitude, relative amplitude measures across the electrode array reveal the interocular asymmetry. The albino response profile can be compared with the luminance VEP responses from an age-matched normal control. Left-eye and right-eye

368 *Patricia Apkarian*

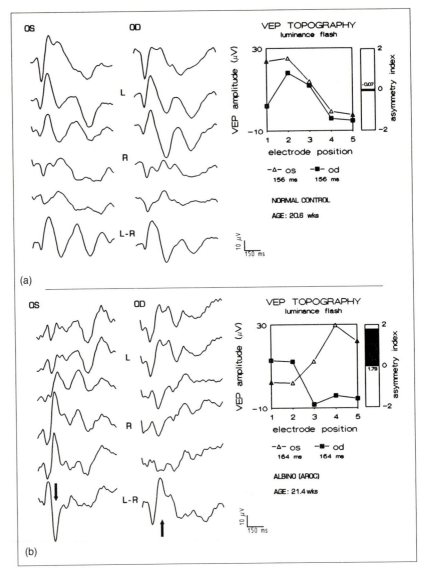

Fig. 22.10 Left occipital response lateralization in the monocular, full-field, luminance flash responses from a normal 20.6-week-old infant (a) compared with interocular contralateral asymmetry in full-field response topography from a 21.4-week-old autosomal recessive oculocutaneous albino infant (b). The upper five traces for each data set are derived from electrodes positioned from the left (L) to right (R) occiput. The bottom trace is a difference potential obtained by subtracting trace 4 (R) from trace 2 (L). For the normal control, regardless of the eye of stimulation, a major positive peak of the immature luminance flash VEP lateralizes to the left hemisphere. For the albino, however, following left-eye (OS) stimulation, the peak response lateralizes to the right

continued

luminance flash responses for the age-matched normal control infant show distinct left-hemispheric response lateralization. The left-hemispheric response dominance for either left- or right-eye full-field stimulation re-emphasizes the fact that VEP asymmetry or hemispheric lateralization can be observed readily in normal subjects and can vary from midline dominance or midline attenuation, to left- (as seen in the present example) or right-hemispheric response dominance. Thus, absolute response asymmetry may not be indicative of underlying visual pathway pathology. However, relative VEP topography measures as shown here are invaluable for disease detection and differential diagnosis.

CONCLUSION

In this overview, a practical approach to electrodiagnostic assessment of visual function in paediatric neuro-ophthalmology has been presented. Stimulus and recording techniques were outlined and substantial attention was paid to the 'four-parameter approach' to VEP assessment for clinical application. The four basic VEP parameters, amplitude, latency, waveform, and topography, were described in detail, together with unique paediatric neuro-ophthalmology case studies, including Dandy Walker syndrome, Zellweger syndrome, Pelizaeus-Merzbacher disease, and albinism with Axenfield anomaly.

The purpose for a non-invasive and accurate method of paediatric evoked potential testing arises from the acute need

(1) to assesss the integrity of visual function during various stages of ontogeny; and

(2) to detect at an early stage, visual system anomalies that can lead to serious and irreversible visual impairment.

Early detection and diagnosis in the developing visual pathway facilitate effective and timely patient care.

Fig. 22.10 *continued.*

hemisphere; with right-eye stimulation the response lateralizes to the left hemisphere. Note also for the albino, the polarity reversal of the difference potentials (see arrows), the crossover of the monocular response amplitudes plotted across the electrode array, and the high asymmetry index (maximum contralateral albino asymmetry equals 2). Compare these resutls with those of the age-matched normal control. The asymmetry index (hemispheric response lateralization of OS minus OD) for the control is near zero. Topography plots are derived from amplitude values across the electrode array at the latencies denoted. (For further details regarding asymmetry calculations see Apkarian and Tijssen 1992.)

REFERENCES

Apkarian, P. (1993). Temporal frequency responsivity shows multiple maturational phases: state-dependent visual evoked potential luminance flicker fusion from birth to 9 months. *Visual Neuroscience*, **10**, 1007–18.

Apkarian, P. (1994). Visual evoked potential assessment of visual function in pediatric neuroophthalmology. In *Principles and practice of ophthalmology: basic sciences*, (ed. D. M. Albert and F. A. Jakobiec), pp. 622–47. W. B. Saunders Co., Philadelphia.

Apkarian, P. and Tijssen, R. (1992). Detection and maturation of VEP albino asymmetry: an overview and a longitudinal study from birth to 54 weeks. *Behavioural Brain Research*, **49**, 57–67.

Apkarian, P., Veenendaal van, W., and Spekreijse, H. (1986a). Albinism: an anomaly of maturation of the visual pathway. *Documenta Ophthalmologica*, **45**, 271–84.

Apkarian, P., Veenendaal van, W., and Spekreijse, H. (1986b). Measurement of visual acuity in infants and young children by visual evoked potentials. *Documenta Ophthalmologica*, **45**, 168–89.

Apkarian, P., Mirmiran, M., and Tijssen, R. (1991). Effects of behavioural state on visual processing in neonates. *Neuropediatrics*, **22**, 85–91.

Apkarian, P., Koetsveld-Baart, J. C., and Barth, P. G. (1993). Visual evoked potential characteristics and early diagnosis of Pelizaeus-Merzbacher Disease. *Archives of Neurology*, **50**, 981–5.

Apkarian, P., Bour, L., and Barth, P. G. (1994). A unique achiasmatic anomaly detected in non-albinos with misrouted retinal-fugal projections. *European Journal of Neuroscience*, **6**, 501–7.

Arlt, A. and Zangemeister, W. H. (1990). Influence of slow eye movements and nystagmus on pattern induced visual evoked potentials. *Neuro-ophthalmology*, **10**, 241–51.

Arruga, J., Feldon, S. E., Hoyt, W. F., and Aminoff, M. J. (1980). Monocularly and binocularly evoked visual responses to patterned half-field stimulation. *Journal of Neurological Sciences*, **46**, 281–90.

Asai, A., Hoffman, H. J., Hendrick, E. B., and Humphreys, R. P. (1989). Dandy-Walker syndrome: experience at the hospital for sick children, Toronto. *Pediatric Neuroscience*, **15**, 66–73.

Barrett, G., Blumhardt, L., Halliday, A. M., Halliday, E., and Kriss, A. (1976). A paradox in the lateralisation of the visual evoked response. *Nature*, **261**, 253–5.

Blom, J. L., Barth, P. G., and Visser, S. L. (1980). The visual evoked potential in the first six years of life. *Electroencephalography and Clinical Neurophysiology*, **48**, 395–405.

Blumhardt, L. D., Barrett, G., and Halliday, A. M. (1977). The asymmetrical visual evoked potential to pattern reversal in one half field and its significance for the analysis of visual field defects. *British Journal of Ophthalmology*, **61**, 454–61.

Brecelj, J. (1992). A VEP study of the visual pathway function in compressive lesions of the optic chiasm. Full-field versus half-field stimulation. *Electroencephalography and Clinical Neurophysiology*, **84**, 209–18.

Bridge, P. J., MacLeod, P. M., and Lillicrap, D. P. (1991). Carrier detection and prenatal diagnosis of Pelizaeus-Merzbacher disease using a combination of anonymous DNA polymorphisms and the proteolipid protein (PLP) gene cDNA. *American Journal of Medical Genetics*, **38**, 616–21.

Chabot, R. J. and John, E. R. (1986). Normative evoked potential data. In *Handbook of electroencephalography and clinical neurophysiology*, Vol. 2. Clinical applications of computer analysis of EEG and other neurophysiological signals, (ed. F. H. Lopes da Silva, W. Storm van Leeuwen, and A. Rémond), pp. 263–309. Elsevier, Amsterdam.

Cigánek, L. (1969). Variability of the human visual evoked potential: normative data. *Electroencephalography and Clinical Neurophysiology*, **27**, 35–42.

Colello, R. J. and Jeffery, G. (1991). Evaluation of the influence of optic stalk melanin on the chiasmatic pathways in the developing rodent visual system. *Journal of Comparative Neurology*, **305**, 304–12.

Colello, J. and Guillery, R. W. (1990). The early development of retinal ganglion cells with uncrossed axons in the mouse: retinal position and axonal course. *Development*, **108**, 515–23.

Courage, M. L. and Adams, R. J. (1990). Visual acuity assessment from birth to three years using the acuity card procedure: cross-sectional and longitudinal samples. *Optometry and Vision Science*, **67**, 713–18.

Dagnelie, G., Vries de, M. J., Maier, J., and Spekreijse, H. (1986). Pattern reversal stimuli: motion or contrast? *Documenta Ophthalmologica*, **61**, 343–9.

Dobson, V. (1983). Clinical applications of preferential looking measures of visual acuity. *Behavioural Brain Research*, **10**, 25–38.

Dodd, J. and Jessell, T. M. (1988). Axon guidance and the patterning of neuronal projections in vertebrates. *Science*, **242**, 692–9.

Ducati, A., Fava, E., and Motti, E. D. F. (1988). Neuronal generators of the visual-evoked potentials: intracerebral recording in awake humans. *Electroencephalography and Clinical Neurophysiology*, **71**, 89–99.

Estévez, O. and Spekreijse, H. (1974). Relationship between pattern appearance–disappearance and pattern reversal responses. *Experimental Brain Research*, **19**, 233–8.

Fantz, R. L., Ordy, J. M., and Udelf, M. S. (1962). Maturation of pattern vision in infants during the first six months. *Journal of Comparative and Physiological Psychology*, **55**, 907–17.

Fulton, A. B., Manning, K. A., and Dobson, V. (1979). Infant vision testing by a behavioral method. *Ophthalmology*, **86**, 431–9.

Garg, B. P., Markand, O. N., and DeMyer, W. E. (1983). Usefulness of BAER studies in the early diagnosis of Pelizaeus-Merzbacher disease. *Neurology*, **33**, 955–6.

Garner, A., Fielder, A. R., Primavesi, R., and Stevens, A. (1982). Tapetoretinal degeneration in the cerebro-hepato-renal (Zellweger's) syndrome. *British Journal of Ophthalmology*, **66**, 422–31.

Gencic, S., Abuelo, D., Ambler, M., and Hudson, L. D. (1989). Pelizaeus-Merzbacher disease: an X-linked neurologic disorder of myelin metabolism with a novel mutation in the gene encoding proteolipid protein. *American Journal of Human Genetics*, **45**, 435–42.

Golden, J. A., Rorke, L. B., and Bruce, D. A. (1987). Dandy-Walker syndrome and associated anomalies. *Pediatric Neuroscience*, **13**, 38–44.

Haimovic, I. C. and Pedley, T. A. (1982). Hemi-field pattern reversal visual-evoked potentials. II. Lesions of the chiasm and posterior visual pathways. *Electroencephalography and Clinical Neurophysiology*, **54**, 121–31.

Harding, G. F. A. and Rubinstein, M. P. (1980). The scalp topography of the human visually evoked subcortical potential. *Investigative Ophthalmology and Visual Science*, **19**, 318–21.

Hittner, H. M., Kretzer, F. L., and Mehta, R. S. (1981). Zellweger syndrome. Lenticular opacities indicating carrier status and lens abnormalities characteristic of homozygotes. *Ophthalmology*, **99**, 1977–82.

Jeffery, G. (1990). Distribution of uncrossed and crossed retinofugal axons in the cat optic nerve and their relationship to patterns of fasciculation. *Visual Neuroscience*, **5**, 99–104.

Jeffreys, D. A. and Axford, J. G. (1972). Source locations of pattern-specific components of human visual evoked potentials II. Component of extrastriate cortical origin. *Experimental Brain Research*, **16**, 22–40.

Katz, B. and Sireteanu, R. (1990). The Teller acuity card test: a useful method for the clinical routine? *Clinical Vision Sciences*, **5**, 307–23.

Koeppen, A. H., Ronca, N. A., Greenfield, E. A., and Hans, M. B. (1987). Defective biosynthesis of proteolipid protein in Pelizeus-Merzbacher disease. *Annals of Neurology*, **21**, 159–70.

Maier, J., Dagnelie, G., Spekreijse, H., and Dijk van, B. W. (1987). Principal components analysis for source localization of VEPs in man. *Vision Research*, **27**, 165–77.

Maria, B. L., Zinreich, S. J., Carson, B. C., Rosenbaum, A. E., and Freeman, J. M. (1987). Dandy-Walker syndrome revisited. *Pediatric Neuroscience*, **13**, 45–51.

Moser, H. W. (1988). The peroxisome: nervous system role of a previously underrated organelle. *Neurology*, **38**, 1617–27.

Reese, B. E., Guillery, R. W., and Mallarino, C. (1992). Time of ganglion cell genesis in relation to the chiasmatic pathway choice of retinofugal axons. *Journal of Comparative Neurology*, **324**, 336–42.

Regan, D. (1989). *Human brain electrophysiology*. Elsevier, Amsterdam.

Rosenberg, M. L. and Jabbari, B. (1987). Nystagmus and visual evoked potentials. *Neuro-ophthalmology*, **7**, 133–8.

Schutgens, R. B. H., Heymans, H. S. A., Wanders, R. J. A., Bosch vd, H., and Tager, J. M. (1986). Peroxisomal disorders: a newly recognised group of genetic diseases. *European Journal of Pediatrics*, **144**, 430–40.

Siegfried, J. B. (1981). Early potentials evoked by macular stimulation: optic nerve potentials? *Documenta Ophthalmologica*, **23**, 201–7.

Sjöström, A., Abrahamsson, M., Norrsell, K., Helgason, G., and Roos, A. (1991). Flashed pattern-induced activity in the visual system: I. The short latency evoked response recorded from the cat visual cortex. *Acta Physiologica Scandinavica*, **143**, 1–9.

Stanescu-Segal, B. and Evrard, P. H. (1989). Zellweger's syndrome and retinal involvement. *Neuro-ophthalmology*, **9**, 111–14.

Teller, D.Y., Morse, R., Borton, R., and Regal, D. (1974). Visual acuity for vertical and diagonal gratings in human infants. *Vision Research*, **14**, 1433–9.

Tweel van der, L. H. (1979). Pattern evoked potentials: facts and considerations. In *Proceedings of the 16th International Society for Clinical Electrophysiology of Vision Symposium*, pp. 27–46, Morioka, Japan.

Tyler, C. W. (1991). Visual acuity estimation in infants by visual evoked cortical potentials. In *Principles and practice of clinical electrophysiology of vision*, (ed. J. R. Heckenlively and G. B. Arden), pp. 408–16. Mosby, St Louis.

Victor, J. D., Conte, M. M., and Iadecola, C. (1991). Ocular dependence of hemifield visual evoked potentials: relevance to bilateral cortical representation of central vision. *Clinical Vision Sciences*, **6**, 261–76.

Vries-Khoe de, L. H. and Spekreijse, H. (1982). Maturation of luminance and pattern EPs in man. *Documenta Ophthalmologica*, **31**, 461–75.

Wanders, R. J. A., Roermund van, C. W. T., Schutgens, R. B. H., Barth, P. G., Heymans, H. S. A., Bosch van den, H., and Tager, J. M. (1990). The inborn errors of peroxisomal β-oxidation: a review. *Journal of Inherited Metabolic Disease*, **13**, 4–36.

23

MRI findings in children with cerebral visual impairment

G. Cioni, A. E. Ipata, R. Canapicchi, B. Fazzi,
and J. van Hof-van Duin

INTRODUCTION

The classical definition of cortical blindness in both adults and children refers to complete loss of vision, including appreciation of light and dark, loss of OKN with preservation of pupillary responses, normal eye motility and normal retina on examination (Marquis 1934).

Cerebral visual impairment (CVI) is now recommended as a better term by many authors (Wong 1991; Flodmark *et al.* 1990; Hertz *et al.* 1988) for several reasons. Complete blindness is rare in these patients. Most of them have some residual vision, which it is often difficult to test because they show inattention and variability in their visual performance (Foley 1987; Jan *et al.* 1987). Secondly, 'cerebral' seems to be a more appropriate term than 'cortical'. Visual impairment is secondary to a cerebral disease from multiple causes (e.g. infection, trauma, cerebrovascular disease, etc.), involving retrochiasmatic visual pathways but not necessarily the visual cortex.

According to the timing of the cerebral injury, CVI in children can be classified as congenital or acquired (Foley 1987). The latter can be caused by meningitis, encephalitis, head trauma, hydrocephalus, or metabolic derangements. Occipital infarctions are often observed in these cases.

Congenital CVI includes visual loss caused by malformations, intrauterine infections or perinatal hypoxic ischaemic encephalopathy (HIE). HIE is the most common cause of CVI, and is often accompanied by other motor and cognitive impairment owing to the diffuse nature of this pathology.

Ischaemic lesions in term infants occur in different parts of the brain in comparison with pre-term ones. This is for complex vascular and metabolic reasons (Volpe 1987; Hill 1991). In pre-term infants the necrotic processes are often located in the white matter of the periventricular zone at the level of the trigona (periventricular leukomalacia), involving the optic radiations. In full-term infants, however, more diffuse damage, including diffuse atrophy, occipital infarctions or multicystic encephalopathy is often correlated with a visual impairment (De Vries *et al.* 1989).

Neuroimaging techniques such as cranial ultrasounds (US), computed tomography (CT) and magnetic resonance imaging (MRI) (for recent reviews in this field see Cioni *et al.* 1992 and De Vries *et al.* 1992) allow us to identify *in vivo*, from the first days or weeks of life, the parts of the brain (posterior visual pathways and visual cortex) that are mainly involved in CVI.

Some authors have tried to correlate imaging findings with the severity and the duration of CVI in children (Whiting *et al.* 1985; Lambert *et al.* 1987; van Nieuwenhuizen and Willemse 1988; Koeda and Takeshita 1992; Ipata *et al.* 1992; Weisglas-Kuperus *et al.* 1993). The results reported by these researchers are not unanimous. This may be because of the different techniques of visual testing applied (e.g. flash VEPs, acuity card procedure, visuomotor responses to toys, visuoperceptual responses). Also, in these studies imaging findings were often obtained by means of US or CT scans, whose value in detecting brain lesions is inferior to that of MRI. Finally, the ages of the patients at which images and visual testing were performed and the cause of the encephalopathy determining the CVI were often variable.

The authors of this chapter decided to carry out a study in which the results of MRI investigation were evaluated in a group of small children suffering from perinatal HIE, and presenting a CVI identified by means of visual testing including the acuity card procedure. This technique has already shown its value in assessing visual acuity both in normal (even very young) infants and in patients with different neurological disorders (Mohn *et al.* 1988).

SUBJECTS AND METHOD

From the patients admitted to the Infant Section of the Institute of Developmental Neurology, Psychiatry and Educational Psychology of the University of Pisa, all the cases fulfilling the following criteria were selected:

(1) perinatal HIE as confirmed by medical history, neonatal US and EEG;
(2) no evidence of prenatal neurological damage or other congenital disease;
(3) cranial MRI carried out in our institute;
(4) complete visual assessment (see discussion following) with reliable results;
(5) no ophthalmological abnormalities or minimal disorders, such as minor refraction problems.

Magnetic resonance imaging

MRI scans were evaluated by a paediatric neuroradiologist (RC) who was unaware of patient history or the results of visual assessment. MRI studies were carried out by means of a system operating at 0.5 Tesla (MR MAX, GE CGR) with sections of 5 mm in sequence spin-echo. T1, proton density, and T2-weighted images were obtained in the axial, coronal, and sagittal planes.

The MRIs were generally carried out at around 1 year of age. When multiple scans were available, only the most recent scan was used for this study. In all scans various abnormalities of the signal, characteristic of perinatal HIE (Cioni *et al.* 1992) were found.

For the aims of this study three degrees of impairment were scored for optic radiations: I 'no impairment'; II 'moderate impairment'; III 'severe impairment'. The area of the visual cortex (striate and parastriate areas) was graded as: I 'normal'; or II 'impaired'. Right and left hemispheres were assessed separately and, when differences in the scoring were obtained, the most severe scores were taken. Examples of normal and abnormal MR appearance of optic radiations and visual cortex are given in Figs 23.1, 23.2 and 23.3.

Visual assessment

Binocular grating acuity was tested by means of Teller Acuity Card procedure (McDonald *et al.* 1985), which sometimes had to be adapted when comparing norms because of the severe neurological problems of our patients. In many cases, more trials than usually recommended were required to obtain the visual threshold. The grey screen surrounding the cards was often not used and testing distances were varied. In cases of severe strabismus, visual acuity was also tested monocularly.

Ophthalmological examination, including retinoscopy, ocular motility and ocular alignment was carried out for all infants.

The visual assessment protocol also included visual field, binocular OKN, visual, and tactile threat response (Mohn and van Hof-van Duin 1986; van Hof-van Duin and Mohn 1986) and flash-VEPs. These results will not be discussed in this book.

Spontaneous visual behaviour (e.g. reponses to the light, to mother's face and to moving and stationary objects) was also observed and videorecorded for all cases.

From the patients fulfilling the selection criteria, the records of all infants for whom visual assessment indicated a CVI, defined as visual acuity values below the 5th percentile of normative data were selected as reported by Mohn *et al.* (1988) and Heersema and van Hof-van Duin (1990).

Forty subjects were included in this group (18 males, 22 females); their mean age at the last (or only) visual assessment was 22 months (range 4–87 months). Thirty-one of these infants showed a severe loss of vision, whereas nine infants were considered as totally blind, because they did not show any response either to the cards or to their mother's face or to objects.

Nine of these 40 infants were tested twice and 15 of them for three times or more, and they were all consistently visually impaired.

The second group of neuropaediatric children also included in this study was randomly selected from subjects responding to the abovementioned criteria but showing normal acuity values obtained by means of the acuity card procedure.

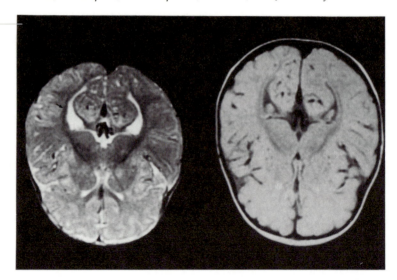

Fig. 23.1 Axial MR proton density (left) and T$_2$-weighed (right) images of a 12-month-old infant. Symmetrical low-intensity areas in the region of the optic radiations, consistent with normal myelination (arrow). There is normal white and grey matter in both visual areas.

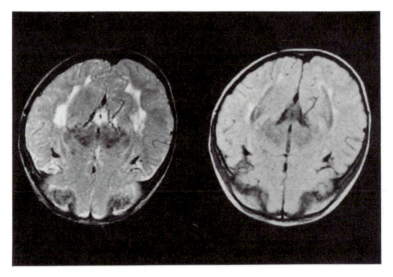

Fig. 23.2 Axial MR proton density (left) and T$_2$-weighed (right) images of a 13-month-old infant. Symmetrical hyperintensity is seen in the optic radiations. The visual areas are normal.

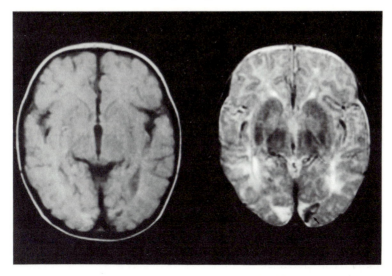

Fig. 22.3 Axial MR proton density (left) and T_2-weighed (right) images of a 9-month-old infant. Cortical–subcortical areas of hyperintensity are seen in both visual regions. The hypointensity is consistent with hemosiderin deposition (arrow).

Twenty-two subjects were included in this group (12 males, 10 females); their mean age at the last (or only) visual assessment was 18 months (range 8–60 months). Eleven of them were tested at least twice.

RESULTS

The results of visual assessment in relation to MRI findings for optic radiations and for visual cortex are reported in Tables 23.1 and 23.2, respectively.

In seven cases (three with normal and four with impaired vision), optic radiations could not been scored by the images. This was because the MRI were taken at too young an age (less than 6–7 months), when the optic radiations are scarcely myelinated and therefore they can hardly be differentiated from the surrounding white matter. In the remaining 55 cases, a significant correlation was found between lesions, mild or severe, of the optic radiations and CVI (Fisher exact test $p < 0.00001$).

Only four infants with normal visual outcome showed some degree of impairment of the optic radiations. In these cases, repeated visual assessments were available; they showed some visual impairment at one or more observations, especially at the younger ages. Of the visually impaired infants, normal optic radiations were observed only in five infants, whereas they were mildly impaired in 15 cases and severely impaired in the other 16. Interestingly, seven

Table 23.1 Visual acuity in relation to MRI findings for optic radiations in 62 neuropaediatric patients.

Optic radiations	Visual acuity		
	Normal	Impaired	Total
Normal	15	5	20
Mildly impaired	1	15	16
Severely impaired	3	16	19
Unscorable	3	4	7
Total	22	40	62

Table 23.2 Visual acuity in relation to MRI findings for visual cortex in 62 neuropaediatric patients.

Visual cortex	Visual acuity		
	Normal	Impaired	Total
Normal	21	23	44
Impaired	1	17	18
Total	22	40	62

out of the nine totally blind infants had a severe impairment of the optic radiations.

Sensitivity of MRI appearance of the optic radiations for a visual impairment (i.e. number of infants with CVI presenting MRI abnormalities) was 77.5%, whereas specificity of this technique was 68.2%, which gives an accuracy value (i.e. all correct predictions made from MRI findings) of 72.8%.

Lesions of the visual cortex (striate and parastriate areas) were rarer. They related to visual impairment, although not so closely as the optic radiations (Fisher exact test $p < 0.002$).

Only one infant with normal vision had some cortical impairment on the MRI, and that was unilateral. Out of the 40 infants with CVI, 17, including seven of the cerebrally blind, showed lesions of the visual cortex.

Accuracy of MRI evaluation of the visual cortex with respect to visual impairment was quite good (68.9%): this was because of high specificity (95.45%), whereas sensitivity was low (42.5%).

By looking at the two MRI scores together, it was found that lesions of the visual cortex were often combined with lesions of the optic radiations, especially in cerebrally blind children.

Only four infants in the group with CVI showed normal MRI scoring for both parameters.

DISCUSSION

Cerebral visual impairment in children is being recognized with increasing frequency, especially in association with other neurological deficits. Schenk-Rootlieb *et al.* (1992) recently reported impaired visual acuity in 71% of children with cerebral palsy.

Improvement in neonatal care has led to an increasing number of very low birthweight infants surviving. Unfortunately, some of them show brain lesions and consequent motor, cognitive and perceptual deficit. Newer visual assessment techniques, behavioural (e.g. visual acuity cards) and electrophysiological (VEPs) allow us to identify visual disturbances even in very young or uncooperative patients.

Identification of CVI in the first months of life is crucial, in order to establish an early intervention programme to stimulate the visual and cognitive development of these children (Sonksen *et al.* 1991).

Neuroimaging studies of these children could, on the one hand, help to identify the anatomical structures involved in CVI and, on the other, could also be very useful for evaluating the visual potential of infants with brain lesions.

Our results indicate a strong correlation between lesions of posterior visual pathways, as shown by MRI, and visual impairment in patients with peri-natal HIE. This correlation is higher for abnormalities in the area of the optic radiations than for those in the striate and parastriate areas.

This latter finding contrasts with those for adults and older children (McAuley and Ross Russell 1979; Aldrich *et al.* 1987), in which occipital infarctions are the most common cause of CVI. So far as studies on children are concerned, our findings are in full agreement with those of Lambert *et al.* (1987), whereas they are partially in contrast with other reports.

In a group of 50 patients with permanent CVI, Whiting *et al.* (1985) reported that CT scanning was helpful in determining the extent and the pathophysiology of the brain damage but was unrelated to the type and degree of visual loss and recovery. This study was carried out using CT and not MRI; moreover, the age range of the patients was very wide, aetiology of CVI varied and no standardized tests were used to test the patients' vision.

Ipata *et al.* (1992) more recently reported that MRI findings were not highly correlated with acuity deficit, testing with visual acuity cards, unless the lesions were very severe. The different results obtained in the present study may be because of a more precise MRI scoring of visual pathways applied and to different patient selection procedure.

Koeda and Takeshita (1992) indicated that lesions of the optic radiations, evaluated at MRI by means of a quantitative computer-aided method, correlated with visuoperceptual impairments but not with visual impairment. Ages at testing of their subjects (between 5 and 9 years) were different to those in the present study, and no details were provided of the methods applied to test visual acuity.

Although MRI abnormalities and visual assessment correlated nicely in most of our patients, there were some exceptions. Normal MRI was found in four patients with CVI; this may be explained by oculomotor disturbances of these patients, by errors in their acuity estimate from their neurological problems, or by the presence of lesions in the visual system not observable by MRI.

The discovery of infants with lesions in visual pathways at the MRI and normal vision is interesting. Longitudinal data suggest a visual recovery of these patients from an initial visual loss.

Visual improvement after peri-natal asphyxia is a well-known phenomenon, occurring not only in young children but also in patients up to 16 years of age (Groenendaal and van Hof-van Duin 1992). The use of extra-geniculate visual pathways (Atkinson 1992), the recruitment of adjacent neurones and restoration of normal excitability of the surviving neurones (Lambert *et al.* 1987) have been indicated as possible explanations of visual recovery after lesions.

Our patients were still quite young at the age of their last visual assessment. Further studies will provide more information about their long-term visual outcome and its relationship with early MRI findings.

ACKNOWLEDGEMENTS

This work was supported by grants from the Italian Ministry of Health (Current Research Projects 1991). The authors thank C. Romano MD for ophthalmological advice, and P. Morse for reviewing the English of the manuscript.

REFERENCES

Aldrich, M. S., Alessi, A. G., Bech, R. W., and Gilman, S. (1987). Cortical blindness: etiology, diagnosis and prognosis. *Annals of Neurology*, **21**, 149–58.

Atkinson, J. (1992). Early visual development: differential functioning of parvocellular and magnocellular pathways. *Eye*, **6**, 129–35.

Cioni, G., Bartalena, L., Biagioni, E., Boldrini, A., and Canapicchi, R. (1992). Neuroimaging and functional outcome of neonatal leukomalacia. *Behavioural Brain Research*, **49**, 7–19.

De Vries, L. S., Dubowitz, L. M. S., Pennock, J. M., and Bydder, G. M. (1989). Extensive cystic leukomalacia: correlation of cranial ultrasound, magnetic resonance imaging and clinical findings in sequential studies. *Clinical Radiology*, **40**, 158–66.

De Vries, L. S., Eken, P., and Dubowitz, L. M. S. (1992). The spectrum of leukomalacia using cranial ultrasound. *Behavioural Brain Research*, **49**, 1–6.

Flodmark, O., Jan, J. E., and Wong, P. K. H. (1990). Computed tomography of the brains of children with cortical visual impairment. *Developmental Medicine and Child Neurology*, **32**, 611–20.

Foley, J. (1987). Central visual disturbances. *Developmental Medicine and Child Neurology*, **29**, 110–20.

Groenendaal, F. and van Hof-van Duin, J. (1992). Visual deficits and improvements in children after perinatal hypoxia. *Journal of Visual Impairment and Blindness*, 215–18.

Heersema, D. J. and van Hof-van Duin, J. (1990). Age norms for visual acuity in toddlers using the acuity cards procedure. *Clinical Vision Science*, **5**, 167–74.

Hertz, B. G., Rosenberg, J., Sjo, O., and Warburg, M. (1988). Acuity card testing of patients with cerebral visual impairment. *Developmental Medicine and Child Neurology*, **30**, 632–7.

Hill, A. (1991). Current concepts of hypoxic-ischemic cerebral injury in the term newborn. *Pediatric Neurology*, **7**, 317–25.

Ipata, A. E., Bottai, P., Salvadori, P., and Cioni, G. (1992). Magnetic resonance imaging and cerebral visual impairment in infants between 6 and 18 months (in Italian). *Giornale di Neuropsichiatria dell'Eta' Evolutiva*, **12**, 73–9.

Jan, J. E., Groenveld, M., Sykanda, A. M., and Hoyt, C. S. (1987) Behavioral characteristics of children with permanent cortical visual impairment. *Developmental Medicine and Child Neurology*, **29**, 571–6.

Koeda, T. and Takeshita, K. (1992). Visuo-perceptual impairment and cerebral lesions in spastic diplegia with preterm birth. *Brain and Development*, **14**, 239–44.

Lambert, S. R., Hoyt, C. S., Jan, J. E., Barkovich, J., and Flodmark, O. (1987). Visual recovery from hypoxic cortical blindness during childhood. Computed tomographic and magnetic resonance imaging predictors. *Archives of Ophthalmology*, **105**, 1371–7.

McAuley, D. L. and Ross Russell, R. W. (1979). Correlation of CAT scan and visual field defects in vascular lesions of the posterior visual pathways. *Journal of Neurology, Neurosurgery and Psychiatry*, **42**, 298–311.

McDonald, M. A., Dobson, V., Sebris, S. L., Baitch, L., Varner, D., and Teller, D. Y. (1985). The acuity card procedure: a rapid test of infant acuity. *Investigative Ophthalmology and Visual Science*, **26**, 1158–62.

Marquis, D. G. (1934). Effects of removal of visual cortex in mammals with observations on the retention of light discrimination in dogs. *Proceedings of the Association of Research into Nervous and Mental Disease*, **13**, 588–92.

Mohn, G. and van Hof-van Duin, J. (1986). Development of the binocular and monocular visual field during the first year of life. *Clinical Vision Science*, **1**, 51–64.

Mohn, G., van Hof-van Duin, J., Fetter, W. P. G., de Groot, L., and Hage, M. (1988). Acuity assessment of non-verbal infants and children: clinical experience with the acuity cards procedure. *Developmental Medicine and Child Neurology*, **30**, 232–44.

Schenk-Rootlieb, A. J., van Nieuwenhuizen, O., van der Graaf, Y., Witteboi-Post, D., and Willemse, J. (1992). The prevalence of cerebral visual disturbance in children with cerebral palsy. *Developmental Medicine and Child Neurology*, **34**, 473–80.

Sonksen, P. M., Petrie, A., and Drew, K. J. (1991). Promotion of visual development of severely visually impaired babies: evaluation of a developmentally based program. *Developmental Medicine and Child Neurology*, **22**, 320–35.

van Hof-van Duin, J. and Mohn, G. (1986). Visual field measurement, optokinetic nystagmus and the visual threatening response: normal and abnormal development. *Documenta Ophthalmologica Proceding Series*, **45**, 305–16.

van Nieuwenhuizen, O. and Willemse, J. (1988). Neuro-imaging of cerebral visual disturbances in children. *Neuropediatrics*, **19**, 3–6.

Volpe, J. J. (1987). *Neurology of the newborn*. (2nd edn). W. B. Saunders, Philadelphia.

Weiglas-Kuperus, N., Heersema, D. J., Baerts, W., Fetter, W. P. F., Smrkovsky, M., van Hof-van Duin, J., and Sauer, P. J. J. (1993). Visual functions in relation with neonatal cerebral ultrasound, neurology and cognitive development in very-low-birthweight children. *Neuropediatrics*, **24**, 149–54.

Whiting, S., Jan, J. E., Wong, P. K. H., Flodmark, O., Farreil, K., and McCormick, A. Q. (1985). Permanent cortical visual impairment in children. *Developmental Medicine and Child Neurology*, **27**, 730–9.

Wong, V. C. N. (1991). Cortical blindness in children: a study of etiology and prognosis. *Pediatric Neurology*, **7**, 178–85.

24

Occlusion therapy for childhood amblyopia: current concepts in treatment evaluation

The burden remains on the vision research community to assess more completely the impact of various occlusion regimens on long-term gains in visual performance.

Fulton and Mayer, 1988

Merrick J. Moseley and Alistair R. Fielder

INTRODUCTION

This chapter, as its title suggests, is concerned primarily with practical issues surrounding amblyopia therapy. It is our thesis that imprecise or inappropriate measurement techniques have limited our understanding of occlusion therapy as alluded to by Fulton and Mayer above. To examine these issues we draw upon observations made in the literature and on some techniques recently developed in our own laboratory. Finally, experimental data that indicate how our proposals work in practice are presented. Our discussions are necessarily restricted in scope[1] and do not address the many neuroscientific contributions that have increased our understanding of this curious condition. To readers wishing to familiarize themselves with these basic topics and other clinical aspects of amblyopia, the excellent monograph by Ciuffreda *et al.* (1991) is recommended.

The history of amblyopia therapy provides rich pickings for medical historians seeking exotic anecdotes to illustrate the pseudoscience which to this day underpins much medical practice (Smith 1991). Indeed, a review of past therapies reveals a truly eclectic range including diet, massage, hypnosis and

---

[1] Throughout this chapter our attention is focused on the amblyopic child as opposed to infant and we define the former as being of an age at which a visual task involving 'linear' optotypes can be performed, either by the elicitation of a verbal response or by the child indicating the target seen at distance on a hand-held key card. Also, we make no specific reference to the taxonomy of amblyopia although we acknowledge this to be an obvious factor likely to influence treatment outcome (Hiscox *et al.* 1992). Rather, we address measurement issues applicable to treatment evaluation independent of the category of amblyopia to which therapy is directed.

electrical stimulation (Unwin 1991). Perhaps of some significance, however, is that, while the above have their origins in the 20th century they are seldom if ever practised today. In contrast, occlusion therapy, which remains the mainstay of amblyopia therapy, was first described by Saint Yves in the early 18th century. This suggests that more than two centuries of accumulated clinical wisdom have led to a consensus as to its effectiveness—yet there have been few, if any, rigorously conducted clinical trials that would satisfy the criteria of, for example, the evaluation of a new drug. This is a timely observation as new medicinal remedies for amblyopia are now under evaluation (Levi 1994). One is left to conclude that there is little understanding of the relationship between the factors that define the nature of the occlusion (e.g. duration and regimen) and the change (improvement?) in the patient's visual status. This notion may be supported by quoting from among the many diverse opinions as to the regimen of choice. In one of the most frequently cited studies, Watson and co-workers (1985) conclude that '... minimal (20–30) minutes occlusion should be the first method of treatment'. This statement may be contrasted with the opinion expressed by von Noorden (1990), 'Occlusion of the sound eye for an hour or so a day rarely is beneficial'. Borrowing loosely from terminology more often associated with drug remedies, it can be stated unequivocally that there is no known dose–effect relationship for occlusion therapy. How we might eventually achieve such an understanding is the aim of this chapter.

TREATMENT AND OUTCOME

While it is accepted that the 'amount' of occlusion prescribed will bear upon the visual improvement, this notion has not been defined clearly. The term 'regimen' is used to indicate the duration of occlusion prescribed on a *per day* basis and numerous regimens have been promoted, broadly categorized thus: 'minimal' (20–60 min/day), 'part-time' (>1–4 h/day) and 'full-time' (most of the waking day). An alternative approach, although not to our knowledge adopted in practice, would be to define a specific duration of occlusion, for example 100 h, and to evaluate treatment progress as a function of accumulated time. For the purposes of the arguments presented here, the term 'dose rate' is substituted for regimen (occlusion/24 h) and dose[2] for accumulated duration. Although this may appear merely a semantic distinction, the authors believe these expressions not only clarify our perceptions of the treatment but prompt us to inquire how one might actually attain greater precision in the measurement of occlusion (i.e. dose and dose rate). Clinicians will be well aware, however, of the practical difficulties involved in achieving this laudable goal—lack of compliance routinely hinders our ability to determine either the dose or

---

[2] Doran and co-workers (1990) we believe were the first to adopt the term 'dose' in referring to the amount of occlusion.

dose rate of occlusion the patient actually receives. This is of particular consequence for the clinical investigator who, being effectively unable to quantify the treatment, is greatly limited in the conclusions they can draw as to the efficacy of any particular dose or dose rate.

For those unfamiliar with the practice of occlusion therapy, it is worth elaborating upon the issue of non-compliance of which at least three factors come into play. First, and most obviously, by limiting the visual input to the amblyopic eye one is imposing upon the child an abnormal visual percept that is unpleasant in its own right or may functionally inhibit the child in his or her activities. Second, even the best designed occlusor provides a degree of physical irritation that should not be underestimated, as even a brief period of self-occlusion will readily demonstrate. Third, in common with other paediatric medical regimens, the overall compliance achieved will arise from a combination of parental and child factors. Taken together it is hardly surprising that compliance is a recurring topic in the literature; indeed, quite drastic measures to ensure effective occlusion have been adopted in the relatively recent past, including plaster-cast arm restraints (Hiles and Galket 1974) and even eyelid suture (Weckert 1932). Such extreme methods excepted, it has been said that, beyond parental report and a positive record of clinic attendance, there are no methods with which compliance can be established with certainty (Nucci *et al.* 1992). This view, as we shall see later, may need to be modified in the light of some recent technical developments.

Intuitively one might predict that compliance would be negatively correlated with prescribed occlusion dose rate and while, no doubt, this describes the overall situation, wide individual differences limit the usefulness of this observation.

The implications for evaluating treatment in view of non-compliance are clearly spelled out in the literature—it is one of the most significant predictors of visual outcome independent of regimen (Lithander and Sjöstrand 1991; Fulton and Mayer 1988; Oliver *et al.* 1986). Thus it would appear crucial to gain precise measurements of compliance, that is, dose and dose rate, actually administered.

Turning our attention from the factors that define or influence occlusion, the variables with which treatment outcome is quantified shall now be addressed. One of the defining characteristics of amblyopia is the absence of any lesion visible upon ophthalmoscopy or indeed located by other means at any point in the visual pathway. Thus, from its earliest descriptions, amblyopia has been quantified solely by the measured loss in visual performance and, specifically, that of spatial resolving power (acuity) measured using recognition (optotype) targets. Emphasis in the literature on this single measure should not mislead us into believing that the loss of recognition acuity characterizes perfectly the visual deficit. It is generally agreed that a reduction of contrast sensitivity may accompany the loss of spatial resolution and, on theoretical grounds alone, provides a better indication of spatial visual discrimination for targets of varying size. Yet another anomaly of spatial visual processing characteristic of amblyopia is that of a loss of position acuity on, for example, vernier tasks. Although such losses may be quite profound, vernier acuity testing, perhaps due to the unavailability of simple tests, has not made the transition from laboratory to clinic. Finally, it is worth recalling that the amblyopic visual system may demonstrate several subtle abnormalities in temporal processing, eye movements and accommodation, and pupillomoter function, although since none of these can, in themselves, account for the deficits of spatial processing they remain of secondary consideration.

Measurement of occlusion: subjective and objective methods

There are four methods capable of measuring compliance: (i) parental interview; (ii) occlusion diary; (iii) clinic attendance; and (iv) occlusion dose monitor.

Parental interview

This is the simplest subjective method but information so obtained is likely to overestimate compliance. Patients tend to tell clinicians what they believe they wish to hear (Cramer 1991). In addition, unless specific instructions have been given, it is unfair to expect of a parent anything other than a purely qualitative description of compliance. As such, this technique does not meet the precise requirements necessary for the accurate determination of dose or dose rate. Despite these obvious limitations, parental interview remains almost exclusively the only means by which occlusion is monitored currently during routine therapy.

Occlusion diary

This is another subjective method, the principle of which has been previously adopted for medical (drug) regimens (Spilker 1991) but has found little favour in amblyopia therapy. Its use is subject to problems of parental literacy, although our own experience suggests that, when used in a formal clinical trial, an occlusion diary can elicit an accurate record of occlusion dose and dose rate. These were, however, somewhat artificial circumstances with considerable effort devoted to optimizing compliance. Analysis of 'free-form' diary records may be somewhat time-consuming, particularly where problems of legibility occur as, for example, in the diary entries shown in Fig. 24.1. A better approach is the use of machine-readable forms, with parents ticking a series of boxes corresponding to the periods of occlusion.

Clinic attendance

Clinic attendance is arguably the crudest measure of compliance, nonetheless it is an objective measure and has been used to differentiate compliant and non-compliant subjects in a retrospective study (Nucci *et al.* 1992).

Occlusion Dose Monitor (ODM)

This device comprises two principal components: (i) a miniature battery driven data logger; and (ii) a modified occlusor. The data logger is encapsulated within

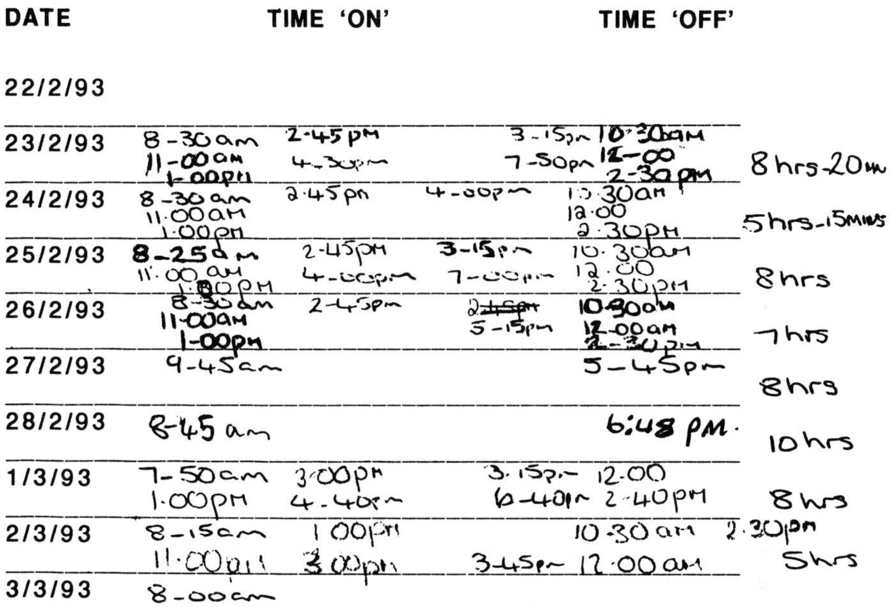

DATE	TIME 'ON'				TIME 'OFF'			
22/2/93								
23/2/93	8-30am 11-00am 1-00pm	2-45pm 4-30pm			3-15pm 10:30am 7-50pm 12-00 2-30pm			8 hrs 20m
24/2/93	8-30am 11-00am 1-00pm	2-45pm	4-00pm		10-30am 12-00 2-30pm			5hrs-15mins
25/2/93	8-25am 11-00am 1-00pm	2-45pm 4-00pm	3-15pm 7-00pm		10-30am 12-00 2-30pm			8hrs
26/2/93	8-30am 11-00am 1-00pm	2-45pm	2-15pm 5-15pm		10-300m 12-00am 2-30pm			7hrs
27/2/93	9-45am				5-45pm			8hrs
28/2/93	8-45 am				6:48 pm			10 hrs
1/3/93	7-50am 1-00pm	3-00pm 4-40pm			3-15pm 12-00 6-40pm 2-40pm			8 hrs
2/3/93	8-15am 11-00am	1-00pm 3-00pm			10-30am 2-30pm 3-45pm 12-00am			5hrs
3/3/93	8-00am							

Fig. 24.1 'Freeform' occlusion diary. Problems of legibility may cause difficulties in eliciting an accurate occlusion time history.

a small plastic case and placed within a shoulder bag (Fig. 24.2). The occlusor is a standard eye patch modified by the addition of two miniature skin electrodes to its undersurface. It is connected to the data logger by a 'flying lead', which can be readily concealed under clothing. The occlusor is a disposable item and is connected distally to the lead by an in-line connector. The data logger monitors the resistance across the skin electrodes and stores within its memory (as a function of time) whether this is at a level indicative of occlusor-skin contact. The ODM can operate continuously for a period of several weeks and, on eventual return to clinic, is interrogated by a personal computer to provide an 'occlusion time-history' an example of which is shown in Fig. 24.3. From such data a variety of statistics can be derived as described later. In contrast to interview and diary methods, the ODM has the significant advantage that it provides an *objective* occlusion record and offers the first precise means of defining dose and dose rate.

Measurement of visual performance: specifying appropriate tests

Visual acuity
The Snellen chart (Fig. 24.4) and its associated scale resolutely remain the most commonly employed means of recording visual recognition acuity. However, in recent years, strenuous attempts to improve upon this system

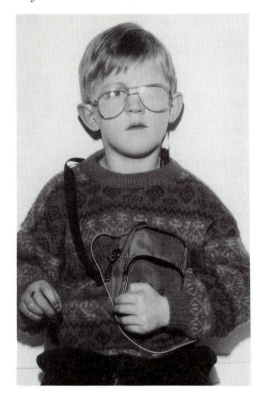

Fig. 24.2 Occlusion dose monitor in use.

Total time on = 23 hours 11 minutes
Total time off = 552 hours 49 minutes

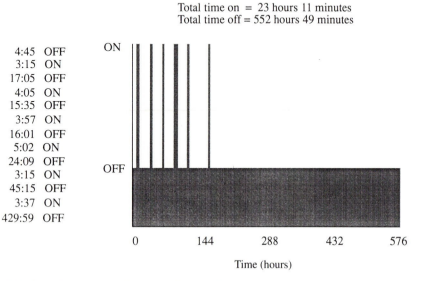

4:45	OFF
3:15	ON
17:05	OFF
4:05	ON
15:35	OFF
3:57	ON
16:01	OFF
5:02	ON
24:09	OFF
3:15	ON
45:15	OFF
3:37	ON
429:59	OFF

Fig. 24.3 Time history recorded by occlusion dose monitor.

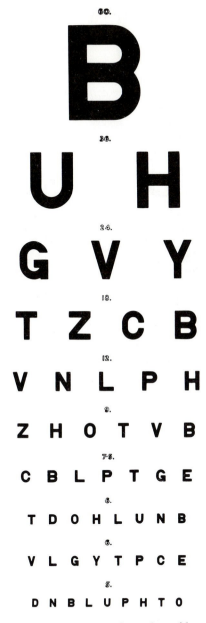

Fig. 24.4 Typical Snellen chart. Note unequal number of letters per line and arbitrary increments in line size.

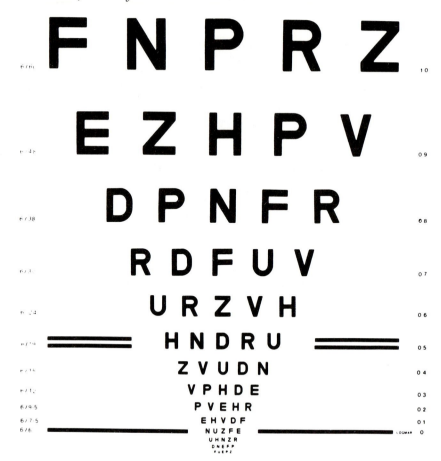

Fig. 24.5 Typical logMAR chart (Bailey and Lovie 1976). Note equal number of letters per line (5) and constant geometric scaling of lines sizes (0.1 log units).

have been made and, at least in North America, are beginning to make inroads into clinical research (Waring *et al.* 1983; Blackhurst *et al.* 1989). Specifically, there is evidence that charts scaled according to the logarithm of the minimum angle of resolution (logMAR) approximate more faithfully to the underlying properties of human visual discrimination (Westheimer 1979) and provide significantly better test–retest reliability (Lovie-Kitchin 1988). The design criteria of these charts specify an equal number of letters per line with spacing between optotypes held constant as a function of their dimensions (Fig. 24.5). Thus task difficulty varies only upon the dimension of optotype size. In addition, such charts are amenable to scoring on a letter-by-letter basis (Kitchin and Bailey 1981), which may be particularly appropriate for use with amblyopic observers who show a tendency to resolve a proportion of letters spanning several line sizes (Flom 1966). LogMAR charts tend, in comparison with Snellen charts, to comprise optotypes of near equal legibility and again this may be a significant advantage when testing amblyopes whose acuities differ proprotionately more than normals as a function of differences in the legibility of the individual optotypes (Jagerman 1970). Finally, while many Snellen charts 'truncate' at 6/6 or 6/5, logMAR charts extend to the acuity limit (–0.3 logMAR, 6/3)—a typical Snellen chart will therefore be unable to detect improvements in performance much beyond the so-called normal level of acuity: 6/6.

While logMAR charts provide us with the opportunity to record acuity with a considerably enhanced precision, their use with children has yet to be reported. However, there is every reason to believe that the advantages that these charts possess would be as applicable to children as to adults as the following example indicates:

A child achieves a score of 6/60 in their amblyopic eye when tested on a standard Snellen chart (at this level of vision the patient need only correctly recognize one letter (Fig. 22.4)). Testing with a logMAR chart confirmed the Snellen score, the child reading correctly all 5 letters, which comprise the 1.0 logMAR (=6/60) line. The child is prescribed an occlusion regimen and, after an appropriate interval, returns for reassessment. On this occasion, the acuity obtained using the Snellen chart is identical to that of the previous visit, whereas that recorded using the logMAR chart is 0.9 logMAR, an improvement of 0.1 logMAR. This beneficial change was not apparent when testing with the Snellen chart as the line size below that of 6/60 is 6/36—an acuity greater than that possessed by the child.

In the absence of the logMAR score the clinician may have concluded incorrectly that the prescribed treatment had been completely ineffective but, in fact, the Snellen chart lacked the precision to document the small but perhaps significant improvement that occurred. Such a finding is necessarily of even greater significance when striving to relate treatment to outcome in some quantifiable manner.

Contrast sensitivity

Although visual acuity is the defining feature of amblyopia and therefore a primary outcome measure, it has long been appreciated that this merely quantifies the eye's ability to resolve high-contrast targets whereas 'real-world vision' requires the perception of objects of varying sizes and contrasts. This raises the following questions:

1. Do amblyopic observers suffer an impairment of contrast sensitivity?
2. If so, is there a characteristic loss of sensitivity?
3. Can the measurement of contrast sensitivity serve usefully as an outcome measure of occlusion therapy?

The answer to question 1 is a qualified yes—although it is possible to have an essentially normal contrast sensitivity function yet exhibit a defining loss of recognition acuity (Hess *et al.* 1978). There are, however, sufficient studies indicating that a loss of contrast sensitivity in amblyopia if not an absolute defining feature, is very commonly present. As to the characteristics of the loss, in a review of 12 papers cited by Leguire (1991), which include a heterogeneous case mix, the predominant loss of sensitivity occurred at high spatial frequencies—although in most instances losses could also be demonstrated at both medium (3–8 cycles/degree) and low (<3 cycles/degree) spatial frequencies.

The finding that greatest loss of contrast sensitivity occurs in the high spatial frequency region suggests initially that it is here that one should preferentially seek to measure. However, this proposition is countered by the fact that it is this region that is most closely 'associated' with (resolution) acuity. Although, as a rule, resolution acuity may underestimate recognition (optotype) acuity (Friendly *et al.* 1990) it will still be *highly correlated* with recognition acuity. Thus from the standpoint of treatment evaluation, measurement of contrast sensitivity at high spatial frequencies may be considered superfluous as one will, by necessity, be undertaking separate measurement of recognition acuity. On these grounds, the authors suggest that it may prove more useful to measure contrast sensitivity in the low-to-medium spatial frequency region, where, if a change in sensitivity occurs, it will on *a priori* grounds be less likely to be predicted by (correlated with) the measured recognition acuity.

Having reached the conclusion that an optimized test strategy will assess selectively the sensitivity in the low-to-medium spatial frequency region, one must next decide upon an appropriate test (version). Possibly the most important decision is whether to test using 'traditional' grating targets or with letter optotypes. The authors believe that, within the defined goals of this chapter, it is the latter that are most appropriate. For the relative merits of grating *versus* letter targets the reader is referred to the discussions by Leguire (1991), Regan (1991), and Pelli and Robson (1991). Here, two specific issues will be considered: (i) ease of testing; and (ii) its likely sensitivity in detecting changes in the amblyopic visual system occurring during therapy. Testing with letter little additional time in explaining to the child the nature of the test, which is, from their viewpoint, grossly similar in the demands made upon them by the acuity test. The authors also favour the use of letter targets on the somewhat more speculative reasoning that the perception of complex optotypes may be more impaired than that of grating targets (Friendly *et al.* 1990)— by adopting letter targets one is adding an extra dimension of difficulty to the task.

The most widely used letter contrast-sensitivity chart (Fig. 24.6) is that developed by Pelli and co-workers (Pelli *et al.* 1988). Age norms for its use among 6–12-year-old children have been obtained recently (Fitzgerald *et al.* 1993). The authors have successfully administered this test to even younger children by use of a 'key card'. Several other authors have proposed the use of low-contrast letter charts for paediatric use (France and France 1988; Regan 1988).

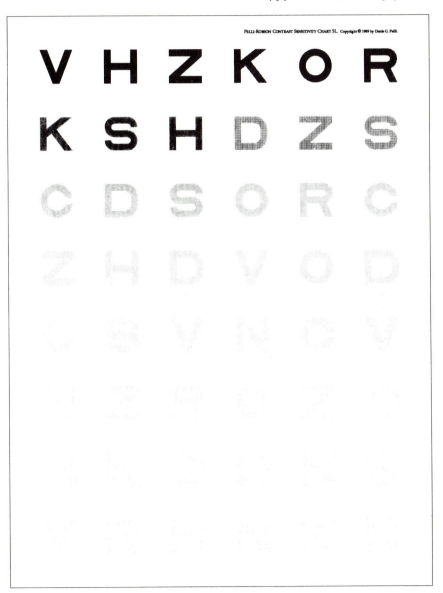

Fig. 24.6 The Pelli-Robson chart (Pelli *et al.* 1988).

TOWARDS AN EVALUATION OF OCCLUSION THERAPY

In the final section of this chapter, some objective and subjective occlusion data and corresponding visual performance data are presented. Measurements were undertaken as part of a pilot study to evaluate the measurement techniques (occlusion and visual performance) discussed here. The experimental design did not set out to mimic a controlled trial of occlusion therapy—it was conducted over a relatively short period, did not include controls and no attempt was made to draw conclusions on the efficacy of occlusion.

Methods and experimental design

The pilot study divided into three phases: preliminary assessment, 'baseline' and treatment. Preliminary assessment comprised a full ophthalmological and orthoptic examination including cycloplegic refraction and the prescription of spectacle correction if required. The nature of the study was explained to parents from whom written informed consent was obtained. Emphasis was placed on the requirement of subjects to return to clinic at regular intervals over the following weeks and that occlusion monitoring was to be undertaken.

The baseline phase comprised a series of repeat clinic visits (typically at 7–14-day intervals) during which spatial visual performance (logMAR visual acuity and letter contrast sensitivity) was measured using a LIGHTHOUSE distance visual acuity test and the Pelli-Robson chart. These visits commenced immediately in the case of children not requiring spectacles or otherwise as soon as spectacles were available. The baseline phase lasted a minimum of two visits, continuing until visual acuity in the amblyopic eye failed to improve beyond the score obtained on the previous occasion. The purpose of the baseline phase was to isolate changes in visual performance arising from adaptation to spectacle wear or that attributable to practice/familiarization effects. No attempt to occlude the subjects was made during this phase.

As soon as a subject's acuity ceased to improve, the treatment phase commenced with the prescription of occlusion with dose rates ranging from 1–8 h/day. These regimens were monitored subjectively using the diary method and objectively using the ODM. Data retrieval took place at weekly intervals for the following 4 weeks at which time visual performance measurements were repeated.

Results

Our overall qualitative impressions of the ease with which the tests could be undertaken and of occlusion monitoring were favourable. The vision tests could be completed before the child's concentration lapsed to the point at which it was likely to impair the accuracy of the test result. In particular, subjects had little difficulty in performing the letter contrast sensitivity test whose use among children has only been reported recently (Fitzgerald *et al.* 1993).

Likewise, objective occlusion monitoring did not present any problems to patients or parents. With almost a year's accumulated use of the ODM in

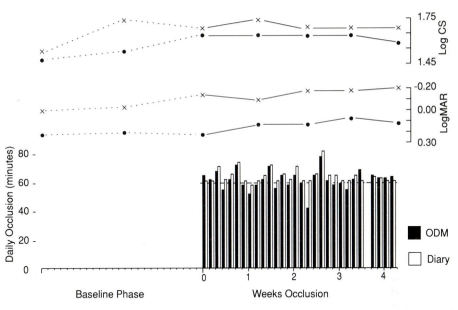

Fig. 24.7 Visual perfomance and occlusion data of subject SM. Upper line graph: visual acuity and contrast sensitivity as a function of trial duration: • = amblyopic eye, × = fellow eye. Broken line indicates performance during baseline phase, whereas solid line indicates performance during treatment. NB: The logMAR axis has been inverted such that an increment on the vertical scale indicates an improvement in acuity. Lower bar graph: daily occlusion recorded subjectively and objectively (NB: No occlusion was prescribed during baseline). Prescribed occlusion = 60 min/day indicated by the horizontal broken line.

the field, only one monitor became damaged during use (by a child who chose to ride his bike during occlusion and met with a minor accident!). Diary records were generally well kept but, as previously mentioned, problems with deciphering occurred, as did the occasional missing entry.

Performance data were recorded in log units for both tests: logMAR for acuity and log contrast sensitivity for the Pelli-Robson chart. In addition to the dose and dose rate parameters, which could be ascertained directly from both the subjective and objective records, three derived units were used: the monitor compliance ratio (MCR) calculated as the objective occlusion dose divided by the prescribed occlusion dose; (ii) the diary compliance ratio (DCR) calculated as the subjective occlusion dose divided by the prescribed occlusion dose; and (iii) the precision index (PI), the ratio of the MCR to the DCR—in other words, taking the ODM as the objective 'gold standard', the extent to which the diary record was accurately kept.

Fig. 24.7 shows the visual performance and subjective and objective occlusion records obtained from a 10-year-old child with anisometropic amblyopia prescribed 60 min/day. This subject's visual acuity at the beginning of the baseline phase was 0.24 logMAR (6/10) in the amblyopic eye and 0.0 logMAR (6/6) in the other eye. At the end of baseline (25 days later) the acuity of the amblyopic eye remained the same as at the beginning of baseline (having improved marginally by 0.02 logMAR in the intervening period) whereas the acuity of the other eye had improved to –0.16 logMAR (6/4). Corresponding improvements in contrast sensitivity also occurred during the baseline phase: both amblyopic and other eye improving by 0.15 log units. (These findings are illustrative of the obvious need to rule out, so far as possible, the influence of long-term spectacle adaptation, practice and familiarization effects when attributing an improvement in visual performance to the beneficial effects of treatment.)

During the treatment phase, visual acuity of the amblyopic eye improved to 0.14 logMAR (6/8) and in the other eye to –0.2 logMAR (>6/4). Corresponding changes in contrast sensitivity were an improvement of 0.05 log units in the amblyopic eye, while no improvement occurred in the other eye. Interestingly, the changes in acuity and contrast sensitivity only appear to be loosely correlated during treatment, for example, while the acuity of the amblyopic eye improved between the onset and the third week of occlusion, no change in contrast sensitivity occurred during this period.

The MCR, DCR and PI indices were 0.98, 1.02 and 0.96 respectively. As immediately apparent from Fig. 24.7 and the compliance indices, compliance was excellent—of a prescribed dose of 1800 min, 1763 min was recorded objectively and 1840 min recorded subjectively, indicating a very slight tendency (as indicated by the PI) for the child's parents to report longer periods of occlusion than that known objectively to have occurred. Only on 1 day during the final treatment week was no occlusion undertaken.

Although small improvements in visual performance were apparent during the treatment phase, visual acuity remained unequal at the end of occlusion. The objective (and subjective) compliance record, however, rules out non-compliance as playing a role in this outcome.

SUMMARY AND CONCLUSIONS

At the beginning of this chapter, attention was drawn to the lack of empirical (as opposed to clinical, anecdotal) support for the use of occlusion therapy. It was suggested that this arose because of inadequate or inappropriate measurement of compliance and visual outcome. The authors have proposed several ways in which this state of affairs may be improved: by using objective recording of treatment compliance and refined measurements of visual performance. Finally, in preparing to undertake a comprehensive evaluation of occlusion therapy a preliminary appraisal of some of our proposals has been performed in clinical practice.

The way forward lies in attempting to establish a relationship (the 'dose–effect relationship') between treatment and outcome using some of the techniques described in this chapter. For the first time one is able to monitor, precisely and objectively, treatment compliance in occlusion therapy.

Clearly some issues remain unaddressed, for example the use of controls. Indeed the notion of a dose-effect relationship in a strict mathematical sense may not exist or may be dependent upon some characteristic of the individual patient of which we have no knowledge—there is unlikely to be a single definitive answer to the question 'How much occlusion should I prescribe'. Doubtless the 'plot will thicken'!

ACKNOWLEDGEMENTS

We would like to thank Ken Cocker and Mary Irwin for technical support, Rosemary Auld for undertaking the vision testing, and Helen Jones for statistical help.

REFERENCES

Bailey, I. L. and Lovie, J. E. (1976). New design principles for visual acuity letter charts. *American Journal of Optometry and Physiological Optics*, **53**, 740–5.

Blackhurst, D. W., Maguire, M. G., and the Macular Photocoagulation Study Group (1989). Reproducibility of refraction and visual acuity measurement under a standard protocol. *Retina*, **9**, 163–9.

Ciuffreda, K. J., Levi, D. M., and Selenow, A. (1991). *Amblyopia: basic and clinical aspects.* Butterworth-Heinemann, Boston.

Cramer, J. A. (1991). Overview of methods to measure and enhance patient compliance. In *Patient compliance in medical practice and clinical trials*, (ed. J. A. Cramer and B. Spilker), pp. 3–10. Raven Press, New York.

Doran, R. M. L., Yarde, S., and Starbuck, A. (1990). Comparison of treatment methods in strabismic amblyopia. In *Strabismus and ocular motility disorders*, (ed. E. C. Campos), pp. 51–9. Macmillan, London.

Ferris, F. L. III, Kassoff, A., Bresnick, G. H., and Bailey, I. (1982). New visual acuity charts for clinical research. *American Journal of Ophthalmology*, **94**, 91–6.

Fitzgerald, A., Mitchell, J., and Munns, J. (1993). Pelli-Robson contrast sensitivity on 122 children aged six to twelve years. *Australian Orthoptic Journal*, **29**, 40–5.

Flom, M. C. (1966). New concepts on visual acuity. *Optometric Weekly*, **57**, 63–8.

France, T. D. and France, L. W. (1988). Low-contrast visual acuity cards in pediatric ophthalmology. *Graefe's Archive for Clinical and Experimental Ophthalmology*, **226**, 158–60.

Friendly, D. S., Jaafar, M. S., and Morillo, D. L. (1990). A comparative study of grating and recognition visual acuity testing in children with anisometropic amblyopia without strabismus. *American Journal of Ophthalmology*, **111**, 293–9.

Fulton, A. B. and Mayer, D. L. (1988). Esotropic children with amblyopia: effects of patching on acuity. *Graefe's Archive for Clinical and Experimental Ophthalmology*, **226**, 309–12.

Hess, R. F., Campbell, F. W., and Greenhalgh, T. (1978). On the nature of the neural abnormality in human amblyopia; neural aberrations and neural sensitivity loss. *Pflügers Archive*, **377**, 201–7.

Hiles, D. A. and Galket, R. J. (1974). Plaster cast arm restraints and amblyopia therapy. *Journal of Pediatric Ophthalmology*, **11**, 151–2.

Hiscox, F., Strong, N., Thompson, J. R., Minshull, C., and Woodruff, G. (1992). Occlusion for amblyopia: a comprehensive survey of outcome. *Eye*, **6**, 300–4.

Jagerman, L. S. (1970). Visual acuity measured with easy and difficult optotypes in normal and amblyopic eyes. *Journal of Pediatric Ophthalmology*, **7**, 49–54.

Kitchin, J. E. and Bailey, I. (1981). Task complexity and visual acuity in senile macular degeneration. *Australian Journal of Optometry*, **64**, 235–42.

Leguire, L. E. (1991). Do letter charts measure contrast sensitivity? *Clinical Vision Sciences*, **6**, 391–400.

Levi, D. M. (1994). Pathophysiology of binocular vision and amblyopia. *Current Opinion in Ophthalmology*, **5**, 3–10.

Lithander, J. and Sjöstrand, J. (1991). Anisometropic and strabismic amblyopia in the age group 2 years and above: a prospective study of the results of treatment. *British Journal of Ophthalmology*, **75**, 111–16.

Lovie-Kitchin, J. E. (1988). Validity and reliability of visual acuity measurements. *Ophthalmic and Physiological Optics*, **8**, 363–70.

Nucci, P., Alfarano, R., Piantanida, A., and Brancato, R. (1992). Compliance in anti-amblyopia occlusion therapy. *Acta Ophthalmologica*, **70**, 128–31.

Oliver, M., Neumann, R., Chaimovitch, Y., Gotesman, N., and Shimshoni, M. (1986). Compliance and results of treatment for amblyopia in children more than 8 years old. *American Journal of Ophthalmology*, **102**, 340–5.

Pelli, D. G., Robson, J. G., and Wilkins, A. J. (1988). The design of a new letter chart for measuring contrast sensitivity. *Clinical Vision Sciences*, **3**, 187–99.

Pelli, D. G. and Robson, J. G. (1991). Are letters better than gratings? *Clinical Vision Sciences*, **6**, 409–11.

Regan, D. (1988). Low-contrast visual acuity test for pediatric use. *Canadian Journal of Ophthalmology*, **23**, 224–7.

Regan, D. (1991). Do letter charts measure contrast sensitivity? *Clinical Vision Sciences*, **6**, 401–8.

Smith, R. (1991). Where is the wisdom …? (Editorial) *British Medical Journal*, **303**, 798–9.

Spilker, B. (1991). Methods of assessing and improving patient compliance in clinical trials. In *Patient compliance in medical practice and clinical trials*, (ed. J. A. Cramer and B. Spilker), pp. 37–56. Raven Press, New York.

Unwin, B. (1991). The treatment of amblyopia – a historical review. *British Orthoptic Journal*, **48**, 28–31.

von Noorden, G. K. (1990). *Binocular vision and ocular motility: theory and management of strabismus*. Mosby, St Louis.

Waring, G. O. III, Moffitt, S. D., Gelender, H., Laibson, P. R., Lindstrom, R. L., Myers, W. D., Obstbaum, S. A., Rowsey, J. J., Safir, A., Schanzlin, D. J., Bourque, L. B., and The PERK study group (1983). Rationale for and design of the National Eye Institute Prospective Evaluation of Radial Keratotomy (PERK) study. *Ophthalmology*, **90**, 40–58.

Watson, P. G., Sanac, A. S., and Pickering, M. S. (1985). A comparison of various methods of treatment of amblyopia: a block study. *Transactions of the Ophthalmological Societies of the United Kingdom*, **104**, 319–28.

Weckert, H. (1932). Neue Wege zur Bekämpfung der Schielamblyopie. *Zentralblatt für die gesamte Ophthalmologie und ihre grenzgebiete*, **27**, 239.

Westheimer, G. (1979). Scaling of visual acuity measurements. *Archives of Ophthalmology*, **97**, 327–30.

25

Visual development following treatment of a unilateral infantile cataract

Ronald G. Boothe

INTRODUCTION

An understanding of the ways in which vision develops following treatment of an infantile cataract is of considerable interest to a broad spectrum of basic scientists and clinicians. Devising improved methods for treatment, or ideally methods for prevention, of the amblyopia that typically develops following surgical removal of the cataract poses a significant challenge for clinicians. Psychophysicists are interested in the precise nature of the perceptual deficits that sometimes develop in these children. Neuroscientists are particularly interested in questions regarding the neuropathology in the visual pathways in the brain that correlate with reduced visual function. Developmental psychologists are intrigued by the implications this topic has for broad issues having to do with the relative importance of 'nature versus nurture' in guiding development.

Over the past several years a number of research programmes pertaining to these separate issues have been carried out and published within isolated subspecialties. However, the visual development that occurs in children following treatment for an infantile cataract will only be understood fully by bringing together the perspectives of all of these diverse research groups. This chapter attempts to summarize some of the main findings from the literatures from all of these disciplines in order to synthesize an understanding of visual development in children being treated for infantile cataracts.

Infants with a unilateral cataract are subjected to unequal inputs to the two eyes during an early sensitive period of visual development. If left untreated, this imbalance will cause vision in the deprived eye to deteriorate rapidly to very poor levels of acuity. However, a lensectomy is usually performed to remove the cataractous lens. This surgery renders the eye aphakic. Thus the name *aphakic amblyopia* is commonly used to describe the resulting functional disorder.

However, the name *aphakic amblyopia* should not be taken to imply that it is the aphakia that causes the amblyopia. The exact causal relationships between the initial deprivation conditions and the resulting amblyopia are difficult to determine in these children. The eyes are initially subjected to stimulus deprivation from the cataract until it is removed, then severe defocus until an optical correction is applied, and finally the aphakic child continues to be subjected to anisometropia and aniseikonia even after optical correction. The deprivation conditions that lead to aphakic amblyopia could be either primarily stimulus deprivation, or primarily optical defocus, or any combination of the two, depending on factors such as age at surgery, and age at which optical correction is applied. In addition, these children often develop crossed eyes so that the deprivation conditions that occur secondary to a strabismus are also likely to operate.

Aphakic amblyopia is one of the most difficult forms of amblyopia to treat because the deprivation starts at such an early age that there is little or no opportunity for normal binocular experience to get development off to a normal start. In fact, until about 20 years ago, an infant with a cataract was generally considered to be hopeless to treat except for cosmetic purposes. An early study by Frey and co-workers (1973) was one of the first to indicate that it might be possible to retain some functional vision by treating these infants with a combination of early surgical removal of the cataract, optical correction of the resulting aphakia with a contact lens, and aggressive occlusion of the fellow eye. Since then several studies have been reported of children treated along these lines. Some of the major findings of these studies will be discussed in the next section.

Even though much valuable information has been gleaned from human children, there are several limitations that always plague even the best designed studies. These include incomplete medical histories, associated ocular abnormalities, inability to directly monitor amblyopia therapy, difficulty assuring patient follow-up, absence of untreated controls, failure to assign randomly infants to treatment groups, and lack of information about underlying neuropathology.

Research with an appropriate animal model can overcome some of these limitations and provide a useful source of adjunct information about the effectiveness of established or potential new treatments. Infant macaque monkeys provide an excellent animal model for these studies. Behavioural studies have established close similarities in post-natal visual development in human and monkey infants, except that the monkey develops about four times faster (Boothe *et al.* 1985). Thus, it is possible to extrapolate age-related results from monkeys to humans by using a 1:4 ratio of ages (age in monkeys in weeks is roughly equivalent to human age in months). This accelerated development in the monkey also means that one can obtain the answer to a specfic question regarding the functional results of a particular treatment within about 3 years in a group of monkeys, compared with the more than a decade that would be required to obtain the answer from studies in human children. The close anatomical similarities of macaque monkey and human primary visual pathways facilitates extrapolation of neuroanatomical and neurophysiological results from the monkey to human neuropathology. Relative ages for many pre-natal neuroembryological events in visual-system development of the monkey and human have also been established and are summarized elsewhere (Boothe 1988).

STUDIES OF HUMAN CHILDREN

The first step in trying to treat an infant with a cataract is to improve the quality of visual stimulation received by the cataractous eye. This can be accomplished by a combination of surgery and optical correction. However, it has been found that this first step is usually insufficient to promote recovery of visual function by itself. The second step of treatment usually involves occlusion, in the form of patching therapy, that is applied to the patient's unaffected eye. The modern scientific rationale for patching therapy is usually attributed to models of binocular competition that have, in turn, been derived from animal deprivation rearing studies. This issue is discussed further later on in this chapter in conjunction with the results of the animal studies.

Studies of human children in which the aphakic eye has been corrected optically and the other eye patched for some of the time, report a wide variety of outcomes. The median Snellen acuities reported in aphakic eyes are about 1.0 logMAR (log minimum angle of resolution in minutes of arc), in other words, about 10 times poorer than in normal eyes (Catalano *et al.* 1987), although better outcomes have been reported in individual cases.

One more recent study (Drummond *et al.* 1989) was able to achieve acuities of 0.4 logMAR or better in 43% of aphakic eyes following an aggressive patching regimen. However, at least one of the patients in this study exhibited evidence of mild but persistent occlusion amblyopia in the patched eye.

A series of studies by Birch and colleagues (Birch *et al.* 1986; Birch and Stager 1988) reported prospective measures of acuity in 16 patients and a retrospective review of 38 patients. All infants developed good acuities in their aphakic eyes, as assessed by preferential looking over the first couple of years. However, recognition acuities on 19 patients conducted between 3–7 years were not so encouraging. Only about half of their patients achieved 0.6 logMAR or better. However, the most recent study from this research group reports normal or near normal acuity in a subset of infants that received very early surgery (Birch *et al.* 1993).

The Maurer and Lewis research group (Maurer *et al.* 1989; Maurer and Lewis 1993) report acuities of about 0.5 logMAR in unilateral patients in which surgery and optical correction occurred before 5 months of age and compliance with part-time patching was excellent. However, the median acuity value when surgery was performed after 5 months of age was only 1.5 logMAR. Another point emphasized by the studies performed by this research group is that children with corrected unilateral aphakia exhibit deficits in other functions besides acuity including reductions in contrast sensitivity, nasotemporal asymmetries in optokinetic nystagmus, and alterations in visual field sensitivity. These findings underscore the general conclusion from previous studies that caution is needed when using any tests based on gratings because grating acuities tend to overestimate Snellen or other recognition acuities in amblyopic eyes (Mayer *et al.* 1984).

It is sometimes presumed in the clinical literature that patching therapy needs to be full time, or nearly full time, in order to achieve good acuity in cases where the amblyopia begins very early such as in cases of unilateral infantile aphakia. However, examination of results from individual subjects in all of the studies reported to date does not provide strong support for this assumption. There are reasonably large individual differences in the outcomes from patient to patient regardless of treatment condition, and the ranges of acuity values obtained across all conditions overlap considerably. For example, patients in one study who were patched 90% of their waking hours had acuities that ranged from as good as 0.17 logMAR to as poor as 1.3 logMAR (Pratt-Johnson and Tillson 1981). A recent study with human infants attempted to use preferential looking measures of acuity as a basis for titrating the amount of patching (Catalano *et al.* 1987). Patching was allowed to vary between 25% and 100% of daily waking hours, depending on the outcomes of the PL assessments. Patients in this study achieved recognition acuities of 0.7 logMAR or better when the amount of patching was only 50–60%.

There is currently no consensus about the exact amounts or schedules of patching that should be used in order to be both effective and safe under all conditions and at all ages. The uncertainty is particularly acute when patching pre-verbal children where it is difficult to assess the effects of the treatment on visual function. Very young children are particularly susceptible to occlusion amblyopia and should be monitored carefully during periods of aggressive patching therapy. A common recommendation is to follow-up at intervals of no more than 1 week per year of age during periods of aggressive patching. The presence of an occlusion amblyopia in an eye undergoing patching therapy has now been documented in several studies (von Noorden 1981; Simon *et al.* 1987; Drummond *et al.* 1989). Catalano *et al.* (1987) reported results from one patient in whom early surgery was followed by patching without the vision being monitored. The first time this infant was assessed with preferential looking, an occlusion amblyopia was detected in the fellow eye that would have gone undiscovered if the patient had not been undergoing careful monitoring.

STUDIES OF VISUAL DEPRIVATION REARING IN MONKEYS

The historical basis for understanding amblyopia within the basic science literature comes from studies of unilateral visual deprivation rearing carried out with animals. Wiesel and Hubel (1963; 1965) proposed binocular competition as a mechanism to account for the effects of unilateral visual deprivation. The basic idea of this mechanism is that neurones carrying information from the left and right eyes must compete against one another for a limited number of neural connections in the developing brain. When one eye experiences visual deprivation during the period when the brain is still developing, its ability to compete is weakend, and thus the connections formed in the brain end up being dominated by the other eye. This failure of the deprived-eye pathways to form appropriate connections results in permanent impairments that can be assessed electrophysiologically and anatomically in the brain and are manifest behaviourally as impaired vision.

Unilateral deprivation has been studied most frequently in animals by performing a tarsorrhaphy during infancy. Monkeys raised under these conditions for extended periods have severely impaired acuity in the deprived eye and are often able to exhibit only light–dark perception. These animal studies are most directly analogous to conditions such as ptosis and dense cataracts that lead to stimulus-deprivation amblyopia in humans. The sensitive period during which stimulus deprivation can lead to amblyopia extends to about 2 years in the monkey, which is equivalent to about 8 years in the human (Harwerth *et al.* 1983). The animal studies also sometimes involve reverse deprivations. The results of these studies may be pertinent to full-time patching therapy in human children. The initial deprivation mimics the development of an amblyopia, and the reversal mimics patching therapy.

The neuropathology that results from visual deprivation rearing has received extensive study in monkeys. Following monocular deprivation, neurones in layers of the lateral geniculate nucleus (LGN) that receive input from the deprived eye have smaller somas than neurones in layers receiving input from the other eye. The amount of soma shrinkage is proportional to the duration of deprivation. The largest changes are seen for deprivation that occurs during the first 3 months after birth, although smaller changes have been reported during a sensitive period that lasts for several additional months (von Noorden and Middleditch 1975; von Noorden *et al.* 1976; Blakemore and Vital-Durand 1986; Headon *et al.* 1988). There appears to be a gradation in susceptibility to deprivation within subdivisions of the LGN, with binocular portions of the parvocellular laminae being most susceptible, followed by binocular portions of the magnocellular laminae, and finally the monocular segments (von Noorden and Middleditch 1975; von Noorden and Crawford 1978; Vital-Durand *et al.* 1978).

The anatomical ocular dominance columns in the cortex that can be revealed by histological staining procedures are also abnormal. Those columns associated with the deprived eye are shrunken in width compared with the columns associated with the fellow eye (Vital-Durand *et al.* 1978; LeVay *et al.* 1980). Throughout the layers of the visual cortex, electrophysiological recordings from neurones demonstrate a shift in the ocular dominance distribution such that there are very few binocular cells, and most of the monocularly driven cells are activated only by the non-deprived eye (Crawford 1988; Blakemore 1988; Hubel 1988). The loss of binocular cells provides a neural correlate for loss of binocular function. The anatomical losses of territory and physiological shifts in ocular dominance balance provide a neural correlate of the general functional deficits that are present in amblyopic eyes. A neural correlate that is probably related more specifically with the acuity losses that accompany amblyopia is provided in studies of spatial resolution properties of neurones in cortex. Prolonged monocular deprivation during infancy has profound detrimental effects on spatial resolution properties of neurones of the striate cortex (Blakemore 1988).

Simply removing an initial deprivation condition does not, in itself, lead to recovery of the behavioural, anatomical, or physiological effects of visual-deprivation rearing. However, reversal of the deprivation condition to the opposite eye (the formerly deprived eye now receives normal stimulation whereas the formerly untreated eye is now deprived) can lead to at least partial reversal of the deprivation effects if it is carried out within the sensitive period (Harwerth *et al.* 1989; Crawford *et al.* 1989). These results from animal studies of reverse deprivation are often used as the rationale for patching therapy in human infants that have an amblyopia. It is surmised that an amblyopic eye will be 'given a chance to win the battle' for functional connections in the brain if it is competing against the other eye that is deprived (by patching) of all visual stimulation. However, this rationale is incomplete and may even be misleading if it is applied to this situation in an uncritical manner (Jastrzebski *et al.* 1984). Reverse-deprivation studies in animals have demonstrated clearly deficits in the eye treated second, or worse, to bilateral deficits (Harwerth *et al.* 1989). Also, binocular function is almost always obliterated following reverse deprivation (Crawford *et al.* 1989).

A MONKEY MODEL OF TREATMENTS FOR INFANTILE CATARACTS

For the past several years, my laboratory has been conducting studies with infant monkeys that are designed specifically for evaluating treatments of children with infantile cataracts. Our monkey model is created by placing a diffusing contact lens onto one eye within a few hours after birth to simulate a unilateral cataract. Then, within a few days after birth, a lensectomy is conducted on the same eye of the deeply anaesthetized infant monkey using sterile procedures similar to those that would be used with human babies. Following surgery, the infant monkeys are fitted with extended-wear contact lenses. The lenses used are manufactured in our own laboratory specifically for research with infant monkeys (Gammon *et al.* 1985). Some contact lenses provide an optical correction to the eye, allowing the eye to see more clearly. Other lenses occlude light, thus forcing the animal to use its opposite eye. Animals are checked every 2 hours during the daylight hours throughout the rearing period in order to maintain accurate records of compliance (Fernandes *et al.* 1988). Missing lenses are noted and replaced immediately.

Several assessments are made on the animals during and after the rearing period. The animals receive ophthalmological examinations at regular intervals to document their clinical status and demonstrate that the monkeys provide a good clinical model of human children with aphakic amblyopia. Two behavioural methods are used to assess acuity in our monkeys. Preferential-looking procedures, similar to those sometimes used in clinical settings with human infants (Sebris *et al.* 1987), are used when testing the infant monkeys. These procedures are easy to implement and are adequate for providing us with a rough estimate of near acuity in each eye during development. However, our aim is to confirm all of our results at older ages with operant methods in which the animal is trained to respond for a food reward (Boothe 1990). Also, outcome measures are obtained which attempt to determine the underlying neuropathology. The Sweep method for obtaining visually evoked potentials (Norcia and Tyler 1985) is used for electrophysiological assessment of spatial resolution. Intracortical extracellular recordings are also obtained in some animals (Wilson *et al.* 1991). Neuroanatomical studies conducted at the termination of each study further document central nervous system changes (Tigges *et al.* 1992).

There are two important baseline conditions that need to be established before the outcomes of our various treatment groups (normal controls and untreated aphakia controls) can be evaluated. Normal control infants have an acuity of about 1.5 logMAR at birth and improve steadily to about 0.0 logMAR by 1 year of age. Acuities in the aphakic eyes of our untreated aphakia control animals are typically reduced by more than two log units from the normal adult value (2.0 logMAR), which is a deterioration from the acuity levels present at birth. In fact, many of these eyes exhibit only *light–dark perception*. These findings obtained from infant monkeys are similar to those obtained in previous studies of human infants and reassure us that our procedures have produced a valid monkey model of human infantile aphakia.

One of the questions the author has been trying to address has to do with the relative benefits and risks associated with patching therapy. As already discussed, there is no consensus in the clinical literature about the schedule of patching that should be followed in order to be both effective and safe. Recommendations range from minimal patching to aggressive full-time patching that extends for long periods. Obviously there are both benefits and risks associated with patching and detailed information about these trade-offs is needed if one wants to establish a rational basis for treatment. The author has attempted to obtain this information by conducting a parametric study with a group of aphakic monkeys in which the aphakic eyes were optically corrected to a near point (at about arm's length) and then the daily occlusion schedule of the fellow eyes systematically varied from 0–100% of the daylight hours. The results of these studies are summarized in Fig. 25.1.

One of the unexpected findings was that even our no-patching group (0%) showed some advantage compared with our untreated aphakic controls. Optically corrected aphakic eyes in which the other eye was not patched achieved median acuity values near 1.2 logMAR, which is about 1 log unit poorer than normal, but still about 1 log unit better than untreated aphakic

GRATING ACUITY FOLLOWING PATCHING

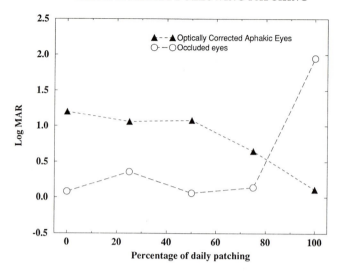

Fig. 25.1 The mean acuity values, expressed as log minimum angle of resolution in minutes (logMAR), are shown for the optically corrected aphakic eyes and the fellow eyes of monkeys in treatment groups that received varying amounts of daily patching. As a standard of reference it can be noted that normal monkeys typically have acuity values near 0.0 logMAR and untreated aphakic eyes are typically poorer than 2.0 logMAR.

eyes. This finding was somewhat surprising, because of the discussion in the clinical literature in which it is usually assumed that providing an optical correction to an aphakic eye will not provide any benefit unless it is coupled with patching. The explanation is probably that good contact lens wear compliance was maintained in the aphakic eyes. Studies in the clinical literature on humans that include children with no patching are likely to include many subjects who were initially prescribed patching but who failed to comply. Thus, the poor outcomes reported for children who do not patch, may be influenced strongly by the fact that many of these children do not comply with prescribed treatment in general. The implication of the results from our no-patching group is that children prescribed only optical correction with no patching will derive some benefit from this treatment if they can be made to comply with the prescribed lens wear. This treatment will not achieve normal vision in aphakic eyes but may be useful in cases where the primary goal is to prevent vision from further deterioration or to maintain the aphakic eye as a 'spare tire' in case there is damage to the other eye later in life.

Acuity results from our monkeys in which the aphakic eye was treated with near-point optical correction and the other eye received daily part-time occlusion ranging from 25–75% of the daylight hours fall within the same range as reported from the studies of human infants described in the previous section.

Our monkey results combined with the results in the published human clinical literature indicate that, even though excellent outcomes are sometimes reported for individual cases, it is probably not realistic to expect, in general, to obtain normal acuity, even when using relatively aggressive (75%) patching schedules.

Our results from monkeys that were patched 100% of the time demonstrate that it is, in fact, possible to obtain near-normal acuity in an aphakic eye by continuous full-time occlusion of the fellow eye. However, this was achieved at the expense of vision in the eye occluded full-time. It is not yet known what happens in the intermediate range (between 75 and 100%). Our laboratory is currently engaged in studies with monkeys that are exploring intermediate levels of patching within this range in order to establish the shape of the benefit–risk trade-off function. In the meantime, the results obtained to date underscore the clinical recommendation that caution, coupled with frequent follow-ups, should be employed whenever using full-time patching in young children.

There is relatively little information available in the human literature regarding alternative treatments that do not involve any patching. Studies have also been conducted by the author and colleagues in monkeys with an alternative treatment that involves selective defocus. The aphakic eye is provided with an optical correction for distance. Then a positive lens is placed on the other eye so that its focusing range is restricted to near vision. This treatment has the same rationale as patching therapy in the sense that it promotes forced usage. The subject will be forced to use the aphakic eye when viewing distant objects, and will be forced to use the other eye when viewing near objects. However, this selective defocus treatment differs from patching therapies in that neither eye is occluded. This treatment has several potential advantages over daily occlusion therapy. There should be less risk of damage to the other eye since it will received near-field stimulation. Also this treatment provides the potential for at least a gross level of binocular stimulation from objects that happen to fall at intermediate distances. Finally, there may be less psychosocial resistance to compliance with a treatment that involves two clear lenses as opposed to a cosmetically unappealing patch. The preliminary results obtained from monkey subjects reared with this treatment indicate that the results for both eyes are as good or better than those obtained with 75% daily occlusion.

SUMMARY AND CONCLUSIONS

A broad spectrum of basic scientists and clinicians are conducting research that has relevance to clinical treatment of infants with unilateral cataracts. The goal is to devise methods for treatment of this disorder that are based on a sound scientific rationale. In this chapter, the author has attempted to summarize some of the major findings from studies reported in the literature on humans, as well as animal-deprivation studies that have a bearing on these issues. Studies conducted in the author's own laboratory have been emphasized, using monkey models that were designed specifically for the purpose of serving as a model of aphakic amblyopia in human infants.

Neonatal monkeys that receive a lensectomy for a simulated unilateral cataract develop a profound aphakic amblyopia with characteristics similar to those found in human children suffering from this condition. Providing a good optical correction to the aphakic eye is of some benefit even in the absence of patching. This treatment appears to be able to prevent further deterioration of vision and may be able to provide at least enough functional vision to provide some insurance in case of later damage to the other eye.

Daily part-time patching can improve the vision in the aphakic eye over and above that obtained using an optical correction alone. Individual subjects sometimes have normal or near-normal acuity with this treatment. However, it does not appear to be realistic to expect this treatment to result in completely normal acuity in general. More aggressive patching schedules that approach 100% occlusion are more likely to result in normal or near-normal acuity in the aphakic eye. However, this form of treatment poses a significant risk of occlusion amblyopia.

Finally, our preliminary monkey results suggest that treatments that involve selective defocus instead of patching may be able to achieve the goal of forced usage of each eye. These forms of treatment may be as effective as patching therapy, and offer some potential advantages in terms of decreased risk of occlusion amblyopia and decreased resistance to compliance with prescribed treatment. Treatments along these lines deserve further study and they are a main focus of the current research in the author's laboratory.

ACKNOWLEDGEMENTS

All of the results described in this chapter obtained from my own laboratory involve a multidisciplinary team of basic and clinical scientists that include: D. Bradley, A. Fernandes, M. Tigges, J. Wilson, J. A. Gammon, H. Eggers, and S. Lambert. My graduate students, M. Quick, C. O'Dell, and R. Brown, also participated in many aspects of these studies. Preparation of this chapter and support of some of my own research that is described here has been supported in part by NIH grants EY-05975 and by RR-00165 from the National Center for Research Resources to the Yerkes Regional Primate Research Center. The Yerkes Center is fully accredited by the American Association for Accreditation of Laboratory Animal Care.

REFERENCES

Birch, E. E. and Stager, D. R. (1988). Prevalence of good visual acuity following surgery for congenital unilateral cataract. *Archives of Ophthalmology*, **106**, 40–3.

Birch, E. E., Stager, D. R., and Wright, W. W. (1986). Grating acuity development after early surgery for congenital unilateral cataract. *Archives of Ophthalmology*, **104**, 1783–7.

Birch, E. E., Swanson, W. H., Stager, D. R., Woody, M., and Everett, M. (1993). Outcome after very early treatment of dense congenital unilateral cataract. *Investigative Ophthalmology and Visual Science*, **34**, 3687–99.

Blakemore, C. (1988). The sensitive periods of the monkey's visual cortex. In *Strabismus and amblyopia*, Vol. 49, (ed. G. Lennerstrand, G. K. von Noorden, and E. C. Campos), pp. 219–34. Macmillan, London.

Blakemore, C. and Vital-Durand, F. (1986). Effects of visual deprivation on the development of the monkey's lateral geniculate nucleus. *Journal of Physiology* (*London*), **380**, 493–511.

Boothe, R. (1988). Visual development: central neural aspects. In *Handbook of human growth and developmental biology I*, Part 1, (ed. E. Meisami and P. Timiras), pp. 179–91. CRC Press, Boca Raton, Florida.

Boothe, R. G. (1990). Experimentally induced and naturally occurring monkey models of human amblyopia. In *Comparative perception*, Vol. I, *Basic mechanisms*, (ed. M. A. Berkley and W. C. Stebbins), pp. 461–8. John Wiley & Sons, New York.

Boothe, R. G., Dobson, V., and Teller, D. Y. (1985). Post-natal development of vision in human and nonhuman primates. *Annual Review of Neuroscience*, **8**, 495–545.

Catalano, R. A., Simon, J. W., Jenkins, P. L., and Kandel, G. L. (1987). Preferential looking as a guide for amblyopia therapy in monocular infantile cataracts. *Journal of Pediatric Ophthalmology and Strabismus*, **24**, 56–63.

Crawford, M. L. (1988). Electrophysiology of cortical neurons under different conditions of visual deprivation. In *Strabismus and amblyopia*, Vol. 49, (ed. G. Lennerstrand, G. K. von Noorden, and E. C. Campos), pp. 207–18. Macmillan, London.

Crawford, M. L. J., Defaber, J. T., Harwerth, R. S., Smith III, E. L., and von Noorden, G. K. (1989). The effects of reverse monocular deprivation in monkeys. 2. Electrophysiological and anatomical studies. *Experimental Brain Research*, **74**, 338–47.

Drummond, G. T., Scott, W. E., and Keech, R. V. (1989). Management of monocular congenital cataracts. *Archives of Ophthalmology*, **107**, 45–51.

Fernandes, A., Tigges, M., Tigges, J., Gammon, J. A., and Chandler, C. (1988). Management of extended-wear contact lenses in infant rhesus monkeys. *Behavior Research Methods, Instruments, and Computers*, **20**, 11–17.

Frey, T., Friendly, D., and Wyatt, D. (1973). Re-evaluation of monocular cataracts in children. *American Journal of Ophthalmology*, **76**, 381–8.

Gammon, J. A., Boothe, R. G., Chandler, C. V., Tigges, M., and Wilson, J. R. (1985). Extended-wear soft contact lenses for vision studies in monkeys. *Investigative Ophthalmology and Visual Science*, **26**, 1636–9.

Harwerth, R. S., Smith III, E. L., Boltz, R. L., Crawford, M. L. J., and von Noorden, G. K. (1983). Behavioral studies on the effect of abnormal early visual experience in monkeys: spatial modulation sensitivity. *Vision Research*, **23**, 1501–10.

Harwerth, R. S., Smith III, E. L., Crawford, M. L. J., and von Noorden, G. K. (1989). The effects of reverse monocular deprivation in monkeys. 1. Psychophysical experiments. *Experimental Brain Research*, **74**, 327–37.

Headon, M. P., Sloper, J. J., and Powell, T. P. S. (1988). Effects of abnormal visual experience on the morphology of lateral geniculate neurons in the infant primate.

In *Strabismus and amblyopia*, Vol. 49, (ed. G. Lennerstrand, G. K. von Noorden, and E. C. Campos), pp. 185–95. Macmillan, London.

Hubel, D. H. (1988). *Eye, brain, and vision*. Scientific American Library, New York.

Jastrzebski, G. B., Hoyt, C. S., and Marg, E. (1984). Stimulus deprivation amblyopia in children. *Archives of Ophthalmology*, **102**, 1030–4.

LeVay, S., Wiesel, T. N., and Hubel, D. H. (1980). The development of ocular dominance columns in normal and visually deprived monkeys. *Journal of Comparative Neurology*, **191**, 1–51.

Maurer, D. and Lewis, T. L. (1993). Visual outcomes after infant cataract. In *Early visual development: normal and abnormal*, (ed. K. Simons), pp. 454–84. Oxford University Press, New York.

Maurer, D., Lewis, T. L., and Brent, H. P. (1989). The effects of deprivation on human visual development: studies of children treated with cataracts. In *Applied developmental psychology*, Vol. 3, Psychological development in infancy, (ed. F. J. Morrison, C. Lord, and D. P. Keating), pp. 139–227. Academic Press, San Diego.

Mayer, D. L., Fulton, A. B., and Rodier, D. (1984). Grating and recognition acuities of pediatric patients. *Ophthalmology*, **91**, 947–53.

Norcia, A. M. and Tyler, C. W. (1985). Spatial frequency sweep VEP. Visual acuity during the first year of life. *Vision Research*, **25**, 1399–1408.

Pratt-Johnson, J. A. and Tillson, G. (1981). Visual results after removal of congenital cataracts before the age of one year. *Canadian Journal of Ophthalmology*, **16**, 19–21.

Sebris, S., Dobson, V., McDonald, M., and Teller, D. (1987). Acuity cards for visual acuity assessment of infants and children in clinical settings. *Clinical Vision Science*, **2**, 45–58.

Simon, J. W., Parks, M. M., and Price, E. C. (1987). Severe visual loss resulting from occlusion therapy for amblyopia. *Journal of Pediatric Ophthalmology and Strabismus*, **24**, 244–6.

Tigges, M., Boothe, R. G., Tigges, J., and Wilson, J. R. (1992). Competition between an aphakic and an occluded eye for territory in striate cortex of developing rhesus monkeys: cytochrome oxidase histochemistry in layer 4C. *Journal of Comparative Neurology*, **316**, 173–86.

Vital-Durand, F., Garey, L. J., and Blakemore, C. (1978). Monocular and binocular deprivation in the monkey: morphological effects and reversibility. *Brain Research*, **158**, 45–64.

von Noorden, G. K. (1981). New clinical aspects of stimulus deprivation amblyopia. *American Journal of Ophthalmology*, **92**, 416–21.

von Noorden, G. K. and Crawford, M. L. J. (1978). Morphological and physiological changes in the monkey visual system after short-term lid suture. *Investigative Ophthalmology and Visual Science*, **17**, 762–8.

von Noorden, G. K. and Middleditch, P. R. (1975). Histology of the monkey lateral geniculate nucleus after unilateral lid closure and experimental strabismus: further observations. *Investigative Ophthalmology*, **14**, 674–83.

von Noorden, G. K., Crawford, M. L. J., and Middleditch, P. R. (1976). The effects of monocular visual deprivation: disuse or binocular interaction? *Brain Research*, **111**, 277–85.

Wiesel, T. N. and Hubel, D. H. (1963). Single-cell responses in striate cortex of kittens deprived of vision in one eye. *Journal of Neurophysiology*, **26**, 1003–17.

Wiesel, T. N. and Hubel, D. H. (1965). Comparison of the effects of unilateral and bilateral eye closure on cortical unit responses in kittens. *Journal of Neurophysiology*, **28**, 1029–40.

Wilson, J. R., Tigges, M., Boothe, R. G., Tigges, J., and Gammon, J. A. (1991). Effects of aphakia on the geniculostriate system of infant rhesus monkeys. *Acta Anatomica*, **142**, 193–203.

26

Visual development in children with congenital cataract

A. Sjöström, M. Abrahamsson, E. Byhr, and J. Sjöstrand

INTRODUCTION

Visual-deprivation experiments on cats and monkeys have showed that complete unilateral eye occlusion of these animals until 12 weeks of age can produce a permanent amblyopia (Hubel and Wiesel 1965; von Noorden 1972) and a decrease in cell density along the geniculocortical pathway (Blakemore and van Sluyters 1974). Reversal of the amblyopia was possible if the occlusion was removed before 8 weeks of age in monkeys. Although this critical age is established for animals, the exact critical period has not been determined for humans, partly because of the problem with assessment of infant vision. Attempts to estimate such a critical period have, however, been performed (Ellston and Timms 1992; Vaegan and Taylor 1979).

During the last decade, preferential-looking techniques have enabled studies of visual resolution of gratings in infants and young children (Dobson and Teller 1978; Gwiazda *et al.* 1980; Atkinson and Braddick 1979) as well as in longitudinal studies of visual development of children with congenital cataract (Lorenz and Wörle 1991; Schulz *et al.* 1985).

In recent years also, estimates of visual acuity based on electrophysiological methods have been presented (Norcia and Tyler 1985; Sokol 1978). Together, these two approaches to child vision have made it possible to describe visual development during the first years of life (Cornell and McDonnell 1986). Age-related norms for visual resolution are slowly being established although the two types of methods used show somewhat divergent results (Vaegan and Taylor 1979; Sokol 1978; McDonald 1986). The acuity of children older than 3 years of age has been possible to measure by a variety of tests based on letter or picture charts (e.g. Landholt-C, Sjögrens hand test, HTOV, tumbling E) for a long time, and normative data for different age levels are well established (McDonald 1986; Simons 1983).

In this chapter, the relationship between visual development and age at surgery for patients with total congenital cataract shall be focused upon. In patients with total congenital cataract, retinal image formation is severely degraded from birth until the lens is removed by surgery and the optics is restored by a contact lens. Several studies have indicated that early surgery of congenital cataract within the first month induces favourable functional results in both bilateral and unilateral cases (Enoch and Rabinowicz 1976; Gelbart *et al.* 1982; Pratt-Johnson and Tillson 1985; Ellis 1983) while less favourable reports with respect to vision continue to appear despite early treatment (Robb *et al.* 1987; Taylor 1982).

In 1980, a project was initiated in order to develop optimized clinical routines for treatment and care of children with congenital cataract. The problem was to be studied from different developmental aspects. A cohort was formed of all children born during the 1980s (1980–1989) in the western part of Sweden with the diagnosis of congenital cataract ($n = 55$). The cataracts were then classified according to functional aspects. Four categories were used: (i) *bilateral*; (ii) *unilateral*; (iii) *total*; or (iv) *partial*. In the cohort, 16 out of the 38 children with bilateral cataract had a total cataract. In these children, the type of cataract, parents' statements and visual behaviour of the child implied that there had not been any period with partially clear media. Seven out of the 17 children with unilateral congenital cataract had a total cataract. Thus, 32 children had partial cataracts.

A family history of congenital or juvenile cataract was always obtained. Among the cases with total cataract, seven could be related to heredity. However, in two cases, owing to the family situation, it was impossible to evaluate fully the possible heredity. Counting all cases with congenital cataract, the prevalence of heredity was approximately 35%, which is in agreement with findings in other studies (Rice and Taylor 1982; Bardelli *et al.* 1989). General systemic disease, such as Mb, Down and Lowe's disease, was present in five of the children and microphthalmos in one. No cases of rubella related cataract were found in the cohort.

A total lensectomy with anterior vitrectomy was performed in the majority of cases. Initially a few extracapsular extractions were also performed, but postoperative complications seemed to be more common with this technique.

VISUAL TESTING

Visual resolution was monitored with a method based on electrophysiology during the first 2 years of life and from approximately 30 months of age a HVOT letter chart was used for estimation of visual acuity.

The method based on transient flash VEP has been described in detail previously (Sjöström *et al.* 1991). A flash light stimulus of high intensity (0.2 J) and short duration (<100 μs) was used with a temporal stimulus frequency of 0.2–0.5 Hz. Activity was recorded at Oz and A1 and A2 were used as reference and ground (10–20 international EEG system). For analysis an average of 20–30 recordings were used.

The light stimulus was flashed when the infant was looking at the flash or directing its eyes at the stimulus direction. For patterns, the retro-illuminated checkerboards of different check sizes with high contrast were used. For the non-pattern stimulus, a similar board with check size well below human resolution was used. Pattern and non-pattern stimuli were given in a quasi-random order.

A VER resolution is calculated as the inverse of the length of the side of a cheque measured in minutes of visual angle at the eye. The VER resolution can then be plotted in the same type of graph as visual acuity.

From approximately 30 months of age, visual performance was tested by HVOT letter chart. The test is based on four symbols, H, V, O and T mixed in rows on a chart. The child has a matching chart with the symbols in his or her lap. The chart is based on rows of the abovementioned letters in approximately logarithmic steps from 0.1 to 1.0 when viewed at a distance of 3 m. The visual acuity was defined as the line at which at least 70% of the optotypes were identified correctly. In cases with visual acuity below 0.2, the testing distance was decreased appropriately and values transformed. In order to avoid sudden steps in the acuity data caused by variations among different type of letter charts the HVOT letter chart was used for all children during the whole test period.

VISUAL DEVELOPMENT IN TOTAL, BILATERAL CATARACT

Visual development in children following the removal of 'congenital' cataract is influenced by such factors as whether the opacity is present at birth or develops later, the density and location of the lens opacity, the age at which the cataract is removed and the quality of the optical correction. It is often impossible to distinguish between truly congenital, neo-/post-natal and/or acquired cataract (Parks 1982) when a cataract is first recognized some time after birth. In this study, the children with a total cataract from birth were focused upon. Total cataract was defined as a lens opacity that covered the whole of the pupillary area of the eye and in which it was impossible to obtain a red fundus reflex or a focused image of the retina. Were there any evidence or suspicion of a period with at least partly clear media for daily vision, the child was classified as a partial cataract. In a recent study, Parks *et al.* (1993) compared long-term visual results and complications in children with aphakia as a function of cataract type. Comparing these two methods of classifying cataracts gave much the same visual outcome; this is because there is a good correlation between type of cataract and the way it obstructs vision.

Our study is an attempt to describe the visual development in these selected children with congenital cataract in eyes with no associated ocular or other abnormality, except microphthalmos. In monkeys, a complete occlusion of the eye for more than 8–12 weeks causes an irrevocable amblyopia. This 'critical period' for visual development has been established for cats and monkeys but it has not been determined in detail for humans. In a paper by Elston and Timms (1992) they stated that neonates with a III or VI nerve palsy or afferent visual pathway pathology at birth, which have these abnormalities removed before the sixth week of life, developed normal visual acuity, motor fusion and stereopsis. This can be interpreted either as an sensitive period for visual development that start after 6 weeks of life or that the obstruction of the vision must be longer than 6 weeks. Gelbaert and co-workers (1982) noticed that all children with total congenital cataract with surgery later than 91 days of age, that is 13 weeks, had a pre-operative nystagmus that lasted, although in some cases become less pronounced, after surgery. The children with nystagmus all developed a poor acuity.

In our study the cataracts were diagnosed at a mean age of 71 days (10 weeks). Surgery was normally performed within 4 days after diagnosis. The median interval between surgery in first and second eye was 3 days.

The visual development was monitored with an electrophysiologically based method during infancy and early childhood. When the child reached 3 years of age we started to use letter charts. In Fig. 26.1 visual acuity data for each case at three different age levels (4, 7 and 10 years of age) are presented. The acuity is presented as a function of age at surgery. In Fig. 26.1(a), data from children without nystagmus are presented. The acuity continuously increases as the child grows older. All children developed an acuity of 0.2 or better at 7 years of age and no child had an acuity less than 0.4 at 10 years of age. It should be noted that all children have not yet reached 10 years of age. In contrast, the data in Fig. 26.1(b) are acuity levels of children with pre- and/or post-surgical nystagmus. In only one case, who started to have nystagmoid movements at the time of the surgery, these disappeared after the operation. This patient was operated on at 81 days of age and developed an acuity of 0.4 at 7 years of age. In the remainder of cases with nystagmus, acuity remains poor and only a very limited age related acuity increase can be detected. One case reached 0.2 at 10 years of age. In several other studies, it is noted that nystagmus does not develop after surgery nor does a nystagmus already developed disappear with surgery. The mean acuity for the children without nystagmus was 0.22, 0.35 and 0.55 at 4, 7 and 10 years of age, respectively. In comparison the mean acuities are 0.09, 0.14 and 0.2, respectively, for the same age levels for the nystagmus group.

Our data imply that there is a 'critical period' at approximately 100 days of age. The oldest child operated on without nystagmus was 130 days of age and the youngest with nystagmus, however reversible, was 81 days of age at surgery. Our sample shows, despite few patients, indications for a 50-day interval in which the children develop a nystagmus that may be cured by surgery. One child had nystagmus before surgery, which vanished afterwards. In this child, acuity develops much better than in the rest of the children in the nystagmus group (Fig. 26.1(b)). The presence or absence of nystagmus pre-operatively seems to be a much more important indicator for a successful or poor visual outcome than age at surgery in itself.

The acuity value continuously increases for all children from the day of surgery and so long as we have been able to follow them (11–13 years of age).

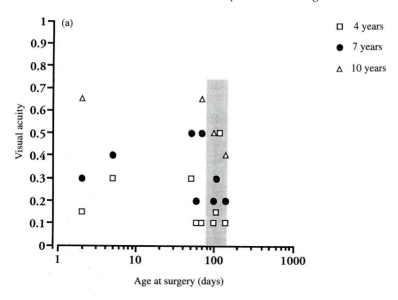

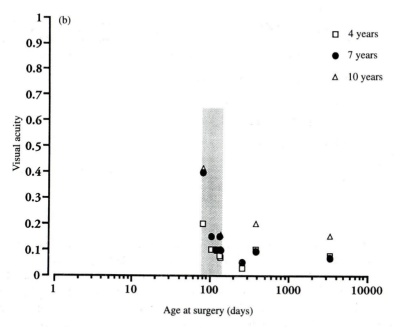

Fig. 26.1 Visual acuity as a function of age at surgery for the children with total bilateral congenital cataract. Visual acuity is determined at three age levels: 4, 7 and 10 years, respectively. Each patient can contribute to three data points. Only one eye, the best, is shown for each patient. In (a) the data from the patients without nystagmus are shown and in (b) the data from the patients with nystagmus are shown. The stippled area indicates the critical period in which nystagmus develops.

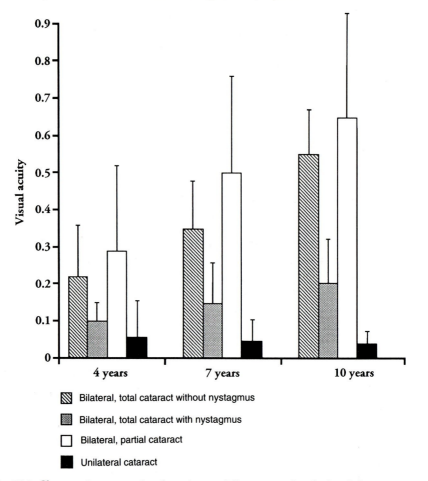

Fig. 26.2 Changes in mean visual acuity at different age levels for different types of congenital cataract.

For children without nystagmus, acuity data from different age levels indicate that visual acuity at 4 years of age does not predict the acuity level at for example 10 years of age. The final visual outcome cannot be determined before the child reaches adolescence. Three children in our study had a rapid increase in acuity after 8 years of age. In these cases, the acuity was stabilized at an acuity level of 0.1–0.15 for 4–5 years before it started to increase. In one out of the three cases, the acuity rose from 0.1 at 8 years of age to 0.65 at 11 years of age. The same acuity test was used during the whole period.

Furthermore, the mean acuity for all children with cataract in the cohort was compared at different age levels. In Fig. 26.2 the acuity change for all 55 children in the cohort is presented. All bilateral cases show an age-related increase in acuity. The partial as well as the total bilateral cataract. This is also in concordance with data from Hamburg (Schulz 1985).

Thus, the acuity data for the children without nystagmus indicate that there is a continuous increase in acuity with age. The acuity data for 4-year-olds cannot be used as an indicator for visual outcome at 10 years of age. There are no simple developmental parameters that can predict the acuity increase.

UNILATERAL CATARACT

The cases with unilateral cataract develop a very poor acuity. Even those cases that responded well to treatment initially showed a negative visual development as they grew older. However, more recent studies have shown that it is possible also to treat these children successfully (Lloyd *et al*. 1993; Bradford *et al*. 1992; Scott *et al*. 1989). The important conclusion is that these children demand very extensive occlusion therapy over a long period of time in order to have a good visual outcome. In these studies treatment periods of total daily occlusion of 50% or more of waking hours were used. A visual outcome of 0.4 or better in the aphakic eye demands surgery before 4–5 weeks of age. Another problem with unilateral congenital cataract is that these eyes often are related to other eye malformations such as microphthalmos. Isolated microphthalmos does not seem to be related closely to poor visual outcome but, in combination with other factors including development of glaucoma, optic nerve and retinal pathology, it becomes an important negative sign.

CONCLUSIONS

Total congenital cataract in a child without nystagmus can be treated successfully by surgery followed by careful amblyopia treatment. Nystagmus develops between 80 and 130 days of life. During this interval, every day's delay of surgery decreases the possibility of a good visual outcome. Unilateral cataract is a challenge to the ophthalmologist that can be successfully treated with a consistent and extensive occlusion therapy. Good methods for acuity test and experienced clinical specialists are of great necessity in this work.

REFERENCES

Atkinson, J. and Braddick O. (1979). New techniques for assessing vision in infants and young children. *Child Care, Health and Development*, **5**, 389–98.

Bardelli, A. M., Lasorella, G., and Vanni, M. (1989). Congenital and developmental cataracts and multimalformation syndromes. *Ophthalmic Paediatrics and Genetics*, **10**, 293–8.

Blakemore, C. and van Sluyters, R. (1974). Reversal of the physiological effects of monocular deprivation in kittens. *Journal of Physiology (London)*, **137**, 195–203.

Bradford, G. M., Kutschke, P. J., and Scott, W. E. (1992). Results of amblyopia therapy in eyes with unilateral structural abnormalities. *Ophthalmology*, **99**, 1616–21.

Cornell, E. and McDonnell, P. (1986). Infant acuity at twenty feet. *Investigative Ophthalmology and Visual Science*, **27**, 1417–20.

Dobson, V. and Teller, D. (1978). Visual acuity in infants: a review and comparison of behavioral and electrophysiological studies. *Vision Research*, **18**, 1469–83.

Ellis, P. (1983). Extended wear contact lenses in pediatric ophthalmology. *CLAO Journal*, **9**, 317–21.

Elston, J. and Timms, C. (1992). Clinical evidence for the onset of the sensitive period in infancy. *British Journal of Ophthalmology*, **76**, 327–9.

Enoch, J. and Rabinowicz, I. (1976). Early surgery and visual correction of an infant born with unilateral eye lens opacity. *Documenta Ophthalmologica*, **41**, 371–82.

Gelbart, S., Hoyt, S., Jastrebski, G., and Marg, E. (1982). Long-term visual results in bilateral congenital cataract. *American Journal of Ophthalmology*, **93**, 615–21.

Gwiazda, J., Brill, S., and Mohindra, I. (1980). Preferential looking acuity in infants from two to fifty-eight weeks of age. *American Journal of Optometry and Physiological Optics*, **57**, 428–34.

Hubel, D. and Wiesel, T. (1965). Comparison of the effects of unilateral and bilateral eye closure on cortical unit responses in kittens. *Journal of Neurophysiology*, **28**, 1060.

Lloyd, I. C., Dowler, J., Kriss, A., Thompson, D. A., Russel-Eggit, J., and Taylor, D. (1993). Modulation of amblyopia therapy in unilateral congenital cataract using acuity cards. *Investigative Ophthalmology and Visual Science*, **27** (suppl.), 1351.

Lorenz, B. and Wörle, J. (1991). Visual results in congenital cataract with the use of contact lenses. *Graefe's Archive for a Clinical and Experimental Ophthalmology*, **229**, 123–32.

McDonald, M. (1986). Assessment of visual acuity in toddlers. *Survey of Ophthalmology*, **31**, 189–210.

Norcia, A. and Tyler, C. W. (1985). Spatial frequency sweep VEP: visual acuity during first year of life. *Vision Research*, **25**, 1399–1408.

Parks, M. (1982). Visual results in aphakic children. *American Journal of Ophthalmology*, **94**, 441–9.

Parks, M. M., Johnson, D. A., and Reed, G. W. (1993). Long-term visual results and complications in children with aphakia. *Ophthalmology*, **100**, 826–41.

Pratt-Johnson, J. and Tillson, G. (1985). Hard contact lenses in the management of congenital cataract. *Journal of Pediatric Ophthalmology and Strabismus*, **22**, 94–6.

Rice, N. S. C. and Taylor, D. (1982). Congenital cataract: a cause of preventable blindness in children. *British Journal of Ophthalmology*, **285**, 581–2.

Robb, R., Mayer, D., and Moore, B. (1987). Results of early treatment of unilateral congenital cataract. *Journal of Pediatric Ophthalmology and Strabismus*, **24**, 178–81.

Schulz, E. (1986). Refractive changes and retarded visual development in aphakic children after operation for congenital cataract. In *Detection and measurement of visual impairment in pre-verbal children*, (ed. B. Jay), pp. 260–70. Martinus Nijhoff/Dr Junk Publishers, Dordrecht.

Schulz, E., Pabst-Hofacker, M., and von Domarus, D. (1985). Postoperative Nachsorge und visuelle Entwicklung congenitaler Katarakte. *Fortschritte der Ophthalmologie*, **82**, 370–3.

Scott, W. E., Drummond, G. T., Keech, R. V., and Karr, D. J. (1989). Management and visual acuity results of monocular congenital cataracts and persistent hyperplastic primary vitreous. *Australian and New Zealand Journal of Ophthalmology*, **17**, 143–52.

Simons, K. (1983). Visual acuity in young children. *Survey of Ophthalmology*, **28**, 84–92.

Sokol, S. (1978). Measurements of infant visual acuity from pattern-reversal evoked potentials. *Vision Research*, **18**, 33–41.

Sjöström, A., Abrahamsson, M., Norrsell, K., Helgasson, G., and Roos, A. (1991). Pattern light-flash induced activity in the visual system. I. The evoked response recorded from the primary visual cortex of cat. *Acta Physiologica Scandinavica*, **143**, 1–9.

Taylor, D. (1982). Risk and difficulties of the treatment of aphakia in infancy. *Transactions of the Ophthalmological Society of the UK*, **102**, 403–6.

Vaegan and Taylor, D. (1979). Critical period for deprivation amblyopia in children. *Transactions of the Ophthalmological Society of the UK*, **99**, 432–9.

von Noorden, G. (1973). Experimental amblyopia in monkeys: further behavioral observation and clinical evaluations. *Investigative Ophthalmology and Visual Science*, **12**, 721–6.

27

Visual instrumentation for use with visually deficient children: the Point Mobile

Serge Portalier and François Vital-Durand

INTRODUCTION

Factors affecting the development of visual capacities in infants can be categorized as biological or environmental. In the first category, maturation of sensory and motor systems allows detection and visual capture of external features. Body movements and possibly sensory stimulation itself provide the elements of a feedback loop reinforced by the interaction with adults (Favez *et al.* 1992). The development of such a sensory-cognitive signal processing system is largely dependent upon genetic and biological constraints. In the second category, cognitive information processing is generated by the infant when exploring, more or less randomly, the environment and is reinforced by social interaction (top-down process, Kosslyn *et al.* 1978; Brossard 1992). This results in complex behaviours and, ultimately, in formation of symbolic representations. This latter category is more dependent upon the social and environmental conditions in which the individual is reared. It is assumed that the individual's future performances are, at least in part, shaped by his or her interactions with the human environment.

The visual system is involved at all stages of development, initially as a feature detector and then as a channel for interactive communication with its utmost symbolic expression mediated by smile or subtle gaze games. The whole process can be considered as a unique association between a highly differentiated sensory organ and a motor organ under the control of the thinking brain (MacKenzie and Marteniuk 1985). As a consequence of this exquisite combination, in this chapter, the eye will be considered as a privileged site for intelligent interaction between the subject and his or her environment.

The development of visual capacities relies on the eye acting like a mobile limb with three pairs of muscles, transporting the retinal sense organ that 'carpets' its back surface. Organized eye movements are already present at birth and adult patterns of eye dynamics have been recorded at a very early age (Hainline *et al.* 1984; Harris *et al.* 1993). Neonatal spatial resolution allows fixation of a face and improves swiftly (Banks and Salapatek 1978; Vital-Durand

1992). An attentive infant stares at an observer and plays 'peek-a-boo' as early as 2 months of age. Inaccuracy of accommodation is not a factor limiting resolution (Cornell and McDonnell 1986). Eye fixations and movements are clinically used as early signs of normality and constitute a test of the maturation of the neural plant subserving eye position.

Psychological studies have indicated that cognitive development can be deduced from behaviours resulting from information processing abilities in young children. Finally, ecological psychology has proved the great signific-ance of the stimulation of different sensory systems by the outer world in which the face of the mother or other adult seems to be one of the most salient stimuli (Bower *et al.* 1970; Slater 1996, this volume).

In visually deficient infants, the whole system is disturbed and new land-marks of development have to be considered for each category of pathology (Fielder *et al.* 1991; Sonksen *et al.* 1991). Since a proper estimation of residual visual capacities is difficult, children have often been considered blind on the ground of their deficient eye movements or poor fixation (Aitken and Buultjens 1991). The resolution defect can be tested with acuity cards (Mohn and van Hof-van Duin 1983; Birch and Bane 1991) and evaluated by VEP to be classified as ophthalmological or central disorder with a special reference to delayed maturation syndrome (Beauvieux, see Tresidder *et al.* 1990). Most pathological eye movements fall into the following categories (Gauthier and Hofferer 1983): lack of stable fixation superimposed upon nystagmic oscillations; absence of smooth pursuit; saccadic instabilities; and increased saccadic reaction time. As a consequence of such motor disorders, Arditi *et al.* (1988) have described modi-fications in the parameters of mental imagery processing, such as topological relationships.

More specifically, fixation pathology is considered in addition to the ophthal-mological disorder and should be treated to assist partially sighted patients. Low-vision care is becoming a speciality area within optometry, orthoptics and ophthalmology. It is assumed here that training of eye movements at an early age would facilitate the capture of visual objects when the deficit is a conse-quence of ocular, muscular or neurological pathology.

Since the pioneer attempts of Baraga in 1964 (Ben-Yishay and Diller 1981), several authors have used visual stimulation for very low-vision subjects and low-vision training for mildly defective ones in order to train fixation, eye movements and functional vision in visually handicapped adult patients. Patients with hemianopsia have been reinforced to move their eyes in their blind field by Zihl (1980; 1994) and also by Ducarne de Ribaucourt and Barbeau (1993). Ron and Gur (1986), and Pommerenke and Markowitsch (1989) have trained patients with cortical damage. Lacert and Picard (1987) have trained multi-handicapped children to follow a moving target to promote pursuit eye movements. All these studies describe some degree of improvement in terms of visual exploration. Nevertheless, very few studies have succeeded in demonstrating proper improvement and even fewer examined infants (review in Tavernier 1993).

Bullinger (1984) used the term 'visual instrumentation' to describe a means for achieving an intelligent interaction of this type between the low-vision infant and his or her environment. Bullinger and Mellier showed (1988) that the use of artificial means to provide sensory flow, for example, a highly contrasted geometric pattern on a large surface, or the temporary use of an ultrasonic guide, leads to behavioural changes interpreted in terms of instrumentation that extends the body's function.

THE STUDY

In our study, described in this chapter, the concept of instrumentation is applied to the deficient visual system of visually handicapped infants to explore the extent to which the use of poor vision can be developed rather than relying exclusively upon vicarious sensory systems, such as an extensive use of auditory or tactile cues. Our study describes the use of a simple computer program designed to stimulate detection, localization and capture of visual targets by visually deficient infants. These young children, aged 2–4 years, presented some degree of residual vision. They attend a multi-disciplinary educational centre (Centre d'Action Médico-Sociale Précoce) where vision therapists, psychologists and researchers try to develop their visual instrumentation, as well as their vicarious sensory systems.

Subjects

The procedure is designed to test infants aged 2.5–5 years of age whose vision is deficient (acuity $< 20/100$ or 6 cycles/degree). Mean age at the beginning of the study 3 years and 11 months; range 2.4–4.11.

The experiment began with 15 children. Eight children were excluded from the data because they did not master the first task or were absent on too many occasions. Only seven children (three boys and four girls) performed enough sessions for data analysis. They had one session of 15 min/week for 6 weeks. In these subjects, low vision was associated with central or peripheral lesions. The following symptoms were often associated with our study population: optic atrophy; retinopathy; bilateral congenital cataract; Arnold-Chiari syndrome; spina bifida; nystagmus; strabismus; prematurity; neonatal brain damage; and cerebral atrophy. Near acuity was between 20/400 and 20/100 (1.5 and 6 cycles/degree).

Materials and methods

The experimental tool is an electronic space game played on a computer screen. The program is called 'Point Mobile'. Point Mobile is composed of four games each made up of a series of 10 trials (Fig. 27.1). For each game, the task can be

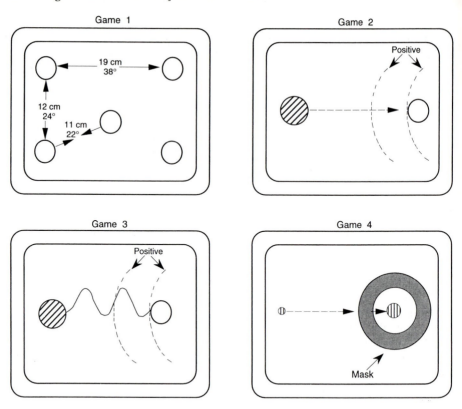

Fig. 27.1 The four games as they appear on the monitor.

made easy or difficult by altering the size of the stimulus (from 31–3.5 mm), the luminance contrast associated to a chromatic displacement (CIE coordinates were B/W 0.93, Y/B 0.70, R/G 0.50), the velocity (from 4.7–28 cm/s) and the delay of the response making the time constraints either more or less demanding.

The first game evaluated the capacity to detect a round target appearing on the screen. Each child had to shout or point with his or her hand when he or she detected a target. After the child has performed a series of 10 with a resonable score, the computer began a record of the reaction time and the score.

The second game was devoted to training the child to track a moving spot heading toward a target at one end of a rectilinear path. The child had to react sufficiently quickly to prevent the spot from striking the target.

The third task was similar to the second one except that the moving spot followed a sinusoidal path.

In the fourth task, the rectilinear moving spot is temporarily hidden by a circular mask surrounding the target at some distance from it. The mask is visible to the child who must react when the moving spot emerges from the mask but before it hits the target.

The child performs the test when seated next to an adult. A short session (10–15 min) took place each time the child came to the Special Education Center, once or twice a week, between September and December 1992. Each individual performed 20–30 sessions during this period of time. One year later, a similar procedure was performed. From each series of initial and late exposure to the test, uncompleted sessions where the child was inattentive or complied badly were discarded. Six sessions with good performances were chosen for statistical processing. Sessions representative of the best performances that the child could reach were chosen deliberately. Results from six initial and late sessions were compared.

Results

Half the infants did not master the first task or were absent on too many occasions.

Game 1

All subjects except one (six out of seven) improved their performances between the initial and late sessions. The child who did not show improvement suffered a maturational delay and later caught up with the others, to the point that she became one of the subjects who would not need Braille. Fig. 27.2(a) compares the results according to the size of the stimulus between the two sessions at an interval of 1 year. These data are based upon six sessions of 10 trials for seven children for each stimulus size (420 trials). In 1 year, the performance for detection had obviously increased. The difference in performance between small and large stimuli was attenuated by the training. Fig. 27.2(b) shows the score when chromatic composition of the stimulus was changed (constant size). There was no clear difference connected with chromatic content between the early and late performances at the 1-year interval.

The plateau was obviously reached because of a trade-off between contrast and size of the stimulus which varied with individuals. However, all subjects preferred higher contrast to larger stimulus size. Several chromatic contrasts were used and it was found that red/green was the most salient stimulus. Chromatic sensitivity was not checked in these infants.

Game 2

Two-thirds of the infants had initial difficulties in mastering movement detection and pursuit. Although velocity was low, it appeared to be a critical limiting factor of the performance, to the point that two children could not perform the test reliably. A total of 300 responses were analysed for the three velocities used. Fig. 27.3 is a comparison of the scores for a red/green stimulus. Significant improvement of the performances was only found for low and intermediate velocities but not for the higher ones. As a consequence the data are not globally significant.

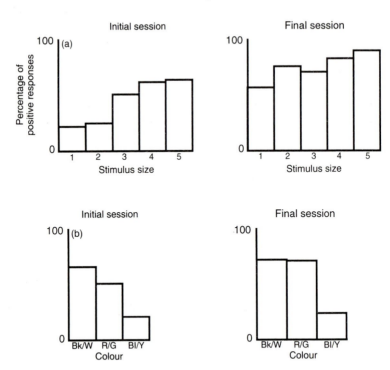

Fig. 27.2 Game 1: mean scores when: (a) size was decreased; (b) chromatic composition was changed. (a) When the size was decreased in the first session a significant difference was found ($\chi^2 = 153$; $p < 0.001$ (significant)). In the second session a significant difference was also found when the size was varied ($\chi^2 = 35$; $p < 0.01$ (significant)). A significant improvement was found between session 1 and 2, especially for size 2 ($\chi^2 = 57.8$; for size 2 $p < 0.01$ (significant)). (b) Mean scores when chromatic composition is changed from Black(Bk)/White to Red/Green and Blue(Bl)/Yellow. In the first session a significant difference was found ($\chi^2 = 95$; $p < 0.001$ (significant)). In the second session a significant difference was found when the colour was varied Bk/W $> =$ R/G $>$ Bl/Y ($\chi^2 = 35$; $p < 0.01$ (significant). However, there was no significant improvement between sessions 1 and 2 ($\chi^2 = 4.41$; $p > 0.10$ (not significant)).

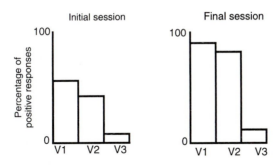

Mean scores at three velocities - linear displacement

Fig. 27.3 Game 2: mean scores at three velocities for linear displacement are shown. In the first session a significant difference was found between low and high velocities ($\chi^2 = 103$; $p < 0.01$ (significant)). In the second session no significant improvement was found between sessions 1 and 2 ($\chi^2 = 2.08$; $p > 0.10$ (not significant)).

Visual attention span was also a critical factor. Some children had a limited visual field, which required them to shift their gaze from the moving spot to the target back and forth. As a consequence, their performances were lowered. Some subjects attempted to follow the moving stimulus with their finger. Their score was improved when they were prevented from doing so. In this game, where the target was moving, size and contrast were not discriminating factors. Motion velocity was the major discriminating factor.

Game 3

The performances on this task were similar to the previous ones. The children had obviously gained experience from the previous task and quickly reached their individual limits. Fig. 27.4 shows scores obtained at three velocities of the sinusoidal displacement. A total of 300 responses were analysed for the three velocities used. A significant difference was found between Game 2 and Game 3. This means that a sinusoidal displacement yields poorer performance ($\chi^2 = 4, 8; 0.10 > p > 0.05$). The first two speeds are not discriminative of the performance.

Five out of the seven subjects made attempts to follow the spot with their finger, a behaviour that resulted in a deterioration of the performance, probably because it required mastery of the whole visual field in real time. It was decided to forbid the use of the finger, and the scores were improved as a consequence.

Game 4

The subject had to anticipate displacement and time. A total of 420 responses were anlaysed for the three velocities used. Most subjects (six out of seven) failed in this difficult task. The time allotted for a positive response, between

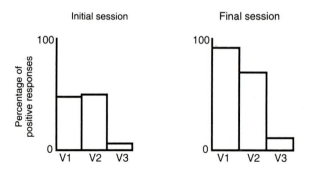

Fig. 27.4 Game 3: mean scores at three velocities for sinusoidal displacement are shown. In the first session a significant difference was found between low and high velocities ($\chi^2 = 4.08$; $p < 0.10$ (significant)). The first two velocities are not discriminative of the performance. In the second session there is a non-significant improvement for the first two velocities ($\chi^2 = 4.71$; $p > 0.10$ (significant)).

the emergence from the mask and the target, was too short. However, no subject had any difficulty guessing that the spot would reappear right in line with the initial segment of the path. This task could only be mastered by a subject older than 3 years. The scores were very low but may have improved for the lowest velocity used. The first two speeds were not discriminative of performance. However, these data from a single subject should be treated with caution.

Discussion

This clinical study of a rehabilitation procedure was designed to optimize the use of residual visual capacities in visually deficient children to obviate two limitations in the literature of visually deficient subjects. Very few studies have been performed before the age of 4–5 years, and most of them examine the promotion of vicarious sensory systems. It is generally considered that early training is largely beneficial (Hirst *et al.* 1993), although clear evidence has not been easily supported by well-controlled experiments (Tavernier 1993). Experiments with infants have to deal with motivational and attentional constraints, although it may appear that performance is better than expected when the atmosphere is made appropriate (Abramov *et al.* 1984). This limitation can only be exaggerated in handicapped and multi-handicapped subjects who often show a double difficulty in focusing and shifting their attention (Butter *et al.* 1989).

Our data do not allow us to isolate a specific effect of training from the benefit of the whole programme of special education and spontaneous development. However, some parameters, like detection of smaller stimulus sizes and velocity estimation, underwent more positive change than others, for example, chromatic contrast detection.

It is clear that infants with visual-field deficits developed more head and eye motility as they were more exposed to the Point Mobile program. A clear improvement of the global motility of the infants was observed in terms of walking smoothness and spatial performances, such as hand manipulation. Unfortunately, these clinical observations could not be measured properly in this study. However, the follow-up of these seven children, who are now aged 4–6 years, reveals that two of them will only use printed documents, two are trained in parallel in Braille and printed texts, one only Braille and two are still too young to determine their capabilities.

CONCLUSIONS

The series of four games proved to be efficient in developing spatial capacities in visually deficient infants. It can be used from 2.5 years of age. The difficulty in assessing specifically the final benefit of such a game, as opposed to spontaneous maturation and skill acquisition, requires a larger population of subjects with well-defined visual deficits.

ACKNOWLEDGEMENTS

This study was supported by Inserm and Cnamts-Inserm convention. We are thankful to the children of the Camsp, to the trainers devoted to alleviate their handicap, to N. Chounlamountri who made the figures, and to K. Knoblauch for his helpful comments on the manuscript.

REFERENCES

Abramov, I., Hainline, L., Turkel, J., Lemerise, E., Smith, H., Gordon, J., and Petry, S. (1984). Rocketship psychophysics. *Investigative Ophthalmology and Visual Science*, **25**, 1307–15.

Aitken, S. and Buultjens, M. (1991). Visual assessment of children with multiple impairments: a survey of ophthalmologists. *Journal of Visual Impairment and Blindness*, **85**, 170–3.

Arditi, A., Holtzamn, D., and Kosslyn, S. M. (1988). Mental imagery and sensory experience in congenital blindness. *Neuropsychologia*, **26**, 1–12.

Banks, M. S. and Salapatek, P. (1978). Acuity and contrast sensitivity in 1-, 2-, and 3-month-old human infants. *Investigative Ophthalmology and Visual Science*, **17**, 361–5.

Ben-Yishay, Y. and Diller, L. (1981). Rehabilitation of cognitive and perceptual defects in people with traumatic damage. *International Journal of Rehabilitation Research*, **4**, 208–10.

Birch, E. E. and Bane, M. C. (1991). Forced-choice preferential looking acuity of children with cortical visual impairment. *Development Medicine and Child Neurology*, **33**, 722–9.

Bower, T. G. R., Broughton, J. M., and Moore, M. K. (1970). Demonstration of intention in the reaching behavior of neonate humans. *Nature*, **5272**, 679–81.

Brossard, A. (1992). *La psychologie du regard: de la perception visuelle aux regards*. Delachaux et Nieslé, Paris.

Bullinger, A. (1984). *Instrumentation du système visuel déficient. Perspective psychobiologique*. Association de langue française des psychologues pour handicapés de la vue, Lausanne.

Bullinger, A. and Mellier, D. (1988). Influence de la cécité sur les conduites sensori-motrices chez l'enfant. *Cahiers de Psychologie Cognitive*, **8**, 191–203.

Butter, C. M., Buchtel, H. A., and Santucci, R. (1989). Spatial attentional shifts: further evidence for the role of polysensory mechanisms using visual and tactile stimuli. *Neuropsychologia*, **27**, 1231–40.

Cornell, E. H. and McDonnell, P. M. (1986). Infant's acuity at twenty feet. *Investigative Ophthalmology and Visual Science*, **27**, 1417–20.

Ducarne de Ribaucourt, B. and Barbeau, M. (1993). *Neuropsychologie visuelle*. DeBoeck Université, Bruxelles.

Favez, N., Gertsch-Bettens, C., Corboz-Warnery, A., and Fivaz-Depeursinge, E. (1992). Processus de l'interaction visuelle dans la triade précoce père–mère–bébé: une étude préliminaire. *Neuropsychiatrie de l'Enfance*, **40**, 521–30.

Fielder, A. R., Fulton, A. B., and Mayer, D. L. (1991). Visual development of infants with severe ocular disorders. *Ophthalmology*, **98**, 1306–9.

Gauthier, G. M. and Hofferer, J. M. (1983). Visual motor rehabilitation in children with cerebral palsy. *International Rehabilitation Medicine*, **5**, 118–27.

Hainline, L., Turkel, J., Abramov, I., Lemerise, E., and Harris, C. M. (1984). Character-istics of saccades in human infants. *Vision Research*, **24**, 1771–80.

Harris, C. M., Jacobs, M., Shawkat, F., and Taylor, D. (1993). The development of saccadic accuracy in the first seven months. *Clinical Vision Science*, **8**, 85–96.

Hirst, C., Poole, J. J., and Sian Snelling, G. (1993). Liverpool visual assessment team 1985–1989: 5 years on. *Child Care Health Development*, **19**, 185–95.

Kosslyn, S. M., Ball, T., and Riser, B. J. (1978). Visual images preserve metric spatial information: evidence from studies of image scanning. *Journal of Experimental Psychology: Human Perception and Performance*, **4**, 47–60.

Lacert, P. and Picard, A. (1987). Troubles optomoteurs de l'IMC ancien prématuré. Possibilités thérapeutiques. *Motricité Cérébrale*, **8**, 143–47.

MacKenzie, Ch. L. and Marteniuk, R. (1985). Motor skill: feedback, knowledge and structural issues. *Canadian Journal of Psychology*, **39**, 313–37.

Mohn, G. and van Hof-van Duin, J. (1983). Behavioural and electrophysiological measures of visual functions in children with neurological disorders. *Behavioural Brain Research*, **10**, 177–89.

Pommerenke, K. and Markowitsch, H. J. (1989). Rehabilitation training of homonymous visual field defects in patients with postgeniculate damage of the visual system. *Restorative Neurology and Neuroscience*, **1**, 47–63.

Ron, S. and Gur, S. (1986). Oculotherapy, or how eye movements can be made more effective. In *Sensorimotor plasticity; theoretical, experimental and clinical aspects*. Colloque Inserm Vol. 140, (ed. S. Ron, R. Schmid and M. Jeannerod), Les Editions Inserm, Paris.

Slater, A. (1996). The organisation of visual perception in early infancy. In *Infant vision*, (ed. F. Vital-Durand, J. Atkinson, and O. J. Braddick), pp. 309–26. Oxford University Press.

Sonksen, P. M., Petrie, A., and Drew, K. J. (1991). Promotion of visual development of severely visually impaired babies: evaluation of a developmentally based programme. *Developmental Medicine and Child Neurology*, **33**, 320–35.

Tavernier, G. G. F. (1993). The improvement of vision by vision stimulation and training: a review of the literature. *Journal of Visual Impairment and Blindness*, **87**, 143–8.

Tresidder, J., Fielder, A. R., and Nicholson, J. (1990). Delayed visual maturation: ophthalmic and neurodevelopmental aspects. *Developmental Medicine and Child Neurology*, **32**, 872–81.

Vital-Durand, F. (1992). Acuity card procedures and the linearity of grating resolution development during the first year of human infants. *Behavioural Brain Research*, **49**, 99–106.

Zihl, J. (1980). 'Blindsight' improvment of visually guided eye movements by systematic practice in patients with cerebral blindness. *Neuropsychologia*, **18**, 71–7.

Zihl, J. (1994). Rehabilitation of visual impairments in patients with brain damage. In *Low vision, research and new development in rehabilitation*, (ed. A. C. Kooijman, P. L. Looijestijn, J. A. A. Welling, and G. J. van der Wildt), pp. 287–95. IOS Press, Amsterdam.

Index